Healthcare Professionalism

Healthcare Professionalism
Improving Practice through Reflections on Workplace Dilemmas

Lynn V. Monrouxe
Chang Gung Memorial Hospital, Linkou, Taiwan

Charlotte E. Rees
Monash University, Melbourne, Australia

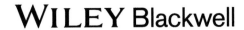

This edition first published [2017] © 2017 John Wiley & Sons Ltd

Registered Office
John Wiley & Sons Ltd, The Atrium, Southern Gate, Chichester, West Sussex, PO19 8SQ, UK

Editorial Offices
9600 Garsington Road, Oxford, OX4 2DQ, UK
1606 Golden Aspen Drive, Suites 103 and 104, Ames, Iowa 50010, USA

For details of our global editorial offices, for customer services and for information about how to apply for permission to reuse the copyright material in this book please see our website at www.wiley.com/wiley-blackwell

The right of Lynn V. Monrouxe and Charlotte E. Rees to be identified as the author of this work has been asserted in accordance with the UK Copyright, Designs and Patents Act 1988.

Library of Congress Cataloging-in-Publication data applied for

ISBN: 9781119044444

A catalogue record for this book is available from the British Library.

Wiley also publishes its books in a variety of electronic formats. Some content that appears in print may not be available in electronic books.

Cover design: Wiley
Cover image: Manfred Thumberger

Set in 10/12pt Warnock by SPi Global, Pondicherry, India

10 9 8 7 6 5 4 3 2 1

Dedication

We dedicate this book to the thousands of students who have shared their stories with us. We also dedicate this book to our late colleague, Professor Kieran Sweeney, who began this journey with us and who represented all that was great about humanity in healthcare.

Contents

Foreword

The ultimate goal of healthcare education is the delivery of optimal patient care by healthcare professionals. For this reason, *Healthcare Professionalism: Improving Practice through Reflections on Workplace Dilemmas* is an important book as it addresses issues that are fundamental to present and future models of healthcare delivery. Robert Merton, in the introduction to the first serious study of the sociology of medical education in the 1950s, wrote that the task of medical education is to give to the novice 'the best available knowledge and skills', and 'a professional identity' so that all graduates come 'to think, act, and feel like a physician'[1], a statement that applies equally to the education of all healthcare professionals. In their book, Lynn Monrouxe and Charlotte Rees do not directly address the transmission of the knowledge and skills necessary for practice as these issues pose fewer educational challenges. What concerns them and many other contemporary observers is how best to facilitate the development of physicians, dentists, nurses, pharmacists, physical therapists, and indeed any healthcare professional so that they come to 'think, act, and feel' like members of their professions. This requires that the learners accept and internalize the values and norms of their chosen profession.

The first words of their text are well chosen, reflecting the wide consensus that has appeared in educational circles during recent decades. They state that 'professionalism matters'. It matters to patients, to society and of course to professionals. The book seeks to help us understand how individuals actually become professionals. Monrouxe and Rees draw upon their truly unique experience of having examined over 2000 narratives of professional dilemmas from a programme of quantitative and qualitative research involving over 4000 healthcare students in four different countries. They do not restrict their analysis to the often negative impact of these dilemmas on students and faculty. Rather, the issues illuminated by the pervasive dilemmas faced by students in all healthcare disciplines serve as a base for an examination of the nature of professionalism and professional identity, how best to teach professionalism and to support professional identity formation, and how to assess professionalism.

They acknowledge the complexity of the issues, but the extraordinarily well-organized structure and organization of the book isolates the major issues without taking them out of context, encouraging readers to both reflect and learn. Each chapter is richly endowed with meaningful narratives, learning outcomes, key terms, take-home messages, and is well referenced. The many commonalities found in the education of the various healthcare professions are presented, along with differences. As an example, valuable contrasting information about codes of ethics in different professions and countries is included. An important chapter, co-authored by Ming-Jung Ho and Madawa Chandratilake, stresses the impact of culture and different national practices on the professionalism and professional identities of their healthcare students and professionals.

The authors have succeeded in their stated objective: 'to provide healthcare students, trainees and educators with a unique type of "core textbook" on healthcare professionalism', linking theory with practice. By basing their dialogue on the well-documented and well-recognized dilemmas faced in each healthcare profession, they highlight the tensions inherent in being a professional in contemporary society. It is not difficult to behave professionally when the choices are relatively easy. The true value of the professional becomes apparent in situations of complexity and uncertainty when both their knowledge and skills and their attitudes and values are called upon. The richness of the authors' experiences in documenting and analysing dilemmas contributes to the excellence of this book.

Lynn Monrouxe and Charlotte Rees reflect a quote from the education literature: 'Consciously, we teach what we know; unconsciously, we teach who we are.'[2] The book is a treasure trove of knowledge on a subject of great importance to society. The authors have consciously taught what they know. But, by their selection and organization of material and their attention to detail, they have also told us much about who they are. While clearly believing in the aspirational aspects of professionalism, many of the dilemmas record the failure of professionals in leadership roles in all healthcare disciplines to live up to the ideal. They also record the often corrosive impact of its internal power relationships and hierarchy. By highlighting areas with the potential to negatively impact the learning environment, the authors provide guidance for corrective action. Their intention is to support learners in developing their own professional identities, along with the educators who support them. They wish to ensure that healthcare students and professionals truly come to 'think, act, and feel' like a professional.

The Centre for Medical Education, McGill University

Sylvia R. Cruess, MD
Richard L. Cruess, MD

References

1 Merton RK. Some preliminaries to a sociology of medical education. In RK Merton, LG Reader, PL Kendall (Eds) *The Student Physician: Introductory Studies in the Sociology of Medical Education*. Cambridge MA: Harvard Univ Press, 1957: pp. 3–79.
2 Hamachek D. Effective teachers: what they do, how they do it, and the importance of self-knowledge. In RP Lipka, TM Brinthaupt (Eds) *The Role of Self in Teacher Development*. Albany NY: State Univ of NY Press, 1999: pp. 189–224.

About the Authors

Lynn V. Monrouxe is Professor and Director of the Chang Gung Medical Education Research Centre (CG-MERC) at Chang Gung Memorial Hospital, Linkou, Taiwan.

Charlotte E. Rees is Professor and Director of Health Professions Education & Education Research, and Director of Curriculum (Medicine), Faculty of Medicine, Nursing & Health Sciences, Monash University, Melbourne, Australia.

Acknowledgements

We have many people to thank for their contributions to this book and its underpinning research, without whom the book would never have materialized. While both of us were principal investigators for the underpinning research programme, the research was a team-based effort, so we thank all of our research collaborators for their enthusiasm, dedication, insight, intellect and creativity. In alphabetical order: Dr Rola Ajjawi, Dr Madawa Chandratilake, Dr Andrew Chen, Professor Ian Dennis, Professor Ruth Endacott, Ms Katherine Gosselin, Professor Ming-Jung Ho, Professor Wendy Hu, Dr Laura McDonald, Dr Laura Rees-Davies, Dr Sarah Sholl, Dr Edwina Ternan and Dr Stephanie Wells. We also thank the organizations who funded our underpinning research, including: the Association of the Study of Medical Education (ASME), the Association for Medical Education in Europe (AMEE), the British Academy, the Higher Education Academy (HEA) and NHS Education for Scotland (NES). Finally, in terms of our underpinning research, we thank those thousands of study participants who have so kindly and candidly shared their professionalism dilemma experiences with us. It has been a privilege to listen to your stories and we hope the book, as Arthur Frank might say, lets your stories breathe.[1]

In terms of the book-writing project itself, we also have many people to thank. Over the course of our research, preparations for the book, and book writing, we have been employed at various different universities and we would like to give our sincere thanks to our colleagues at those institutions for helping us to protect our time for writing. In chronological order: the then Institute of Clinical Education at Peninsula Medical School, Universities of Exeter and Plymouth, England; the then Office of Postgraduate Medical Education at Sydney Medical School, University of Sydney, Australia; the Institute of Medical Education at the School of Medicine, Cardiff University, Wales; the Centre for Medical Education at the School of Medicine, University of Dundee, Scotland; the Faculty of Medicine, Nursing and Health Sciences at Monash University, Australia; and the Chang Gung Medical Education Research Centre at Chang Gung Memorial Hospital, Taiwan. Lynn would also like to thank the Melbourne Medical School, Melbourne University, Australia for hosting her book-writing retreat in November–December 2015.

We would also like to thank the diverse range of people who have reviewed our book chapters, including academics, clinicians, students and trainees representing dental, medical, nursing, pharmacy and physiotherapy education and from lots of different countries across the globe. Thank you so much for your time and wise words: your comments have been hugely helpful in improving the content and presentation of our chapters but any failings that remain are completely our own. From Australia, we thank Dr Rola Ajjawi, Dr Reema Harrison, Dr Fiona Kent, Professor Jill Thistlethwaite and

Dr Sally Warmington. From Canada, we thank Professor Richard Cruess, Professor Sylvia Cruess and Dr Judi Fairholm. From England, we thank Professor Vikram Jha and Prof Hilary Neve. From New Zealand, we thank Dr Alan Merry. From Scotland, we thank Dr Sharon Coull, Dr David Felix, Dr Melanie Foy, Dr Lisi Gordon, Dr Stella Howden, Mr John Lee, Mr Paul McLean, Dr Susie Schofield, Dr Sarah Sholl and Mr Arun Verma. From Sri Lanka, we thank Dr Madawa Chandratilake. From Taiwan, we thank Professor Ming-Jung Ho. From the USA, we thank Associate Professor Jeff Cain, Associate Professor Katherine Chretien, Professor Fred Hafferty, Professor Nora Jacobson, Dr Ashley Palvic and Dr Sally Santen. From Wales, we thank Dr Lori Black, Dr Ben Hannigan, Professor Dai John, Dr Iona Johnson, Mr James Kilgour, Mr Rob Lundin, Ms Eleni Panagoulas, Dr Chantalle Rizan, Dr Ray Samuriwo and Dr Stephanie Wells. Additional thanks go to Sylvia and Richard Cruess for writing the foreword to this book, and special thanks go to our colleague Professor John McLachlan for his constructive feedback after proofreading our entire book once all chapters had been revised, and for his afterword for the book. John, we now owe you more than a prawn curry and bottle of red wine. We would also like to thank our colleagues from Wiley-Blackwell, particularly Fi Goodgame for commissioning our book and James Schultz for giving us feedback, helpful advice, kind words of reassurance and positive encouragement when we needed it.

Finally, we would like to thank our friends and family for their support and encouragement through this book-writing project, and for giving us some extra space to write. More specifically, we have some personal thanks to add.

Charlotte: I would like to thank you, Sid, for your support and encouragement and for the practicalities of life – doing the school run and keeping our family well fed. I would like to thank Kitty for putting up with Mummy on her computer surrounded by piles of papers on weekends and Jane and Emlyn for giving me my moral compass, work ethic and confidence to speak out when something is wrong. Thanks to Lynn for your ear, fun and for making me a better researcher. A final dedication from me goes to Murphy, my wonder dog, who stood his ground with dogs ten times his size to protect the pack. He was spirited and courageous to the end, put to sleep during the writing of this book by an amazing vet who demonstrated care, compassion and humanity. We miss you Murph.

Lynn: I would like to thank my mum and dad – Patricia and Malcolm Johnson – for the love I received as a child and for the loans as an adult. I am truly indebted; together these have facilitated my growth in many ways. I would like to thank my children – Jasmine and Delta – for enriching my life and for complaining extremely loudly when I'm too engrossed in my work: you're right, you *are* more important. I would also like to thank Charlotte, what a journey: between us, during the past ten years, we've been through the highs and lows of marriage, childbirth, divorce, deaths and multiple international relocations. Not only are we still talking, but also you're still the first person I go to whenever I come up against a personal or professional dilemma of my own.

Reference

1 Frank AW. *Letting Stories Breathe. A Socio-Narratology*. Chicago, Illinois: University of Chicago Press, 2010.

Author Contributions

This book has resulted from a tremendous partnership between us that has lasted over a decade. That partnership has been one characterized by equality of working practices and equality of effort. We decided a long time ago that Lynn would be first author and Charlotte second author for this book, based on Lynn collecting the bulk of the data for the first study on which this book is based (a qualitative interview study with 200 medical students) while Charlotte was on maternity leave. Other than that initial data collection period, the research underpinning the book and the writing of the book itself has been a joint effort.

At the start of our collaboration on the research underpinning this book, we worked together at the then Peninsula Medical School, Universities of Exeter and Plymouth, where we were both Lecturers in Human Sciences and Charlotte was the Academic Lead for Professionalism. As Academic Lead for Professionalism, Charlotte was caught up in all matters of professionalism education: curriculum, teaching and learning, assessment *and* professionalism dilemmas. The idea for this research came out of a project investigating patient involvement in medical education led by Charlotte. In this work our student participants began to talk to us about what we now term *professionalism dilemmas*. Our first research grant allowed us to qualitatively explore medical students' professionalism dilemmas at three schools in three different countries (two in the UK), and subsequent grants enabled us to explore professionalism dilemmas experienced by other healthcare students, both qualitatively and quantitatively and across many schools in various countries. This programme of research has continuously intersected with our career biographies, including our current and past educational, research and administrative roles and responsibilities.

We are both social scientists by background with psychology Bachelor degrees and PhDs in psychology: Lynn, cognitive psychology and Charlotte, health psychology. Lynn is currently Professor and Director of the national Chang Gung Medical Education Research Centre (CG-MERC) based at the Chang Gung Memorial Hospital, Taiwan. Charlotte is currently Professor and Director of Health Professions Education & Education Research and Director of Curriculum (Medicine) at the Faculty of Medicine, Nursing & Health Sciences, Monash University, Australia. Together we have developed a wider programme of research about patient-centred professionalism and workplace-based learning in health professions education and have numerous shared education research interests across the spectrum of undergraduate, postgraduate and continuing professional development, including professionalism, personal and professional identities, patient involvement, informal and hidden curriculum, educational transitions, student-teacher interactions, student-teacher-patient interactions and emotion.

We have led on the writing of different chapters for this book, often based on our different expertise and interests. Lynn has led on the writing and revision of the following chapters: Chapter 2 What is healthcare professionalism? Chapter 5 Identity-related professionalism dilemmas; Chapter 7 Patient safety-related professionalism dilemmas; Chapter 10 E-professionalism-related dilemmas; Chapter 11 Professionalism dilemmas across national cultures; and Chapter 13 Conclusions. Charlotte has led on the writing and revision of: Chapter 1 Introduction; Chapter 3: Teaching and learning healthcare professionalism; Chapter 4 Assessing healthcare professionalism; Chapter 6 Consent-related professionalism dilemmas; Chapter 8 Patient dignity-related professionalism dilemmas; Chapter 9 Abuse-related professionalism dilemmas; and Chapter 12 Professionalism dilemmas across professional cultures. While we have edited each other's writing and tried diligently to stick to jointly developed guidelines around formatting across the chapters to maintain consistency, you will note some flourishes of difference between the chapters based on variations in our writing styles. We hope that these differences are a breath of fresh air rather than a distraction.

1

Introduction

'The one that happened to me… that disturbed me greatly… I was watching a colonoscopy with the consultant and there was a reasonably young woman… and she was very anxious about having the colonoscopy… she was sedated but [the sedation] barely even touched the sides, it looked like she was still completely lucid… she started having the colonoscopy… and it was incredibly painful for her and they couldn't advance the colonoscope… he [consultant] was being… unnecessarily rough and she was screaming… she hadn't had the full amount of painkiller… he kept advancing it, he didn't kind of reassure her… she was just a body to him and it was so frightening… at one point the nurse came in and… really tentatively suggested, "Shall we give her more painkiller?" and he said, "No" and the woman was still screaming on the table completely conscious looking at her colon on the screen in front of her and he just kept pushing and pushing and pushing and then it got to the point where the nurse came in and… asked again about the painkiller and he said, "I said no!"… I was just standing there with my hand on the patient going, "Oh my God!"… He didn't back down, he continued with her colonoscopy and finished it and meanwhile the patient was screaming… the patient left to go to recovery and I kind of walked back out to… the nurses' station… I looked at the nurse and… just started bawling, it still makes me cry.'

Fiona, female, year 3, medical student, Australia

Professionalism matters: it is the cornerstone of safe and dignified healthcare practice. This book, intended chiefly for healthcare students, but with healthcare trainees and educators also in mind, aims to help raise professionalism standards in healthcare, to benefit learners, qualified practitioners and patients. Healthcare students and trainees learn professionalism and how to *become* professional through various learning activities. While they are taught professionalism through codes of practice mandated by regulatory bodies, they often witness and participate in events that breach those codes, including serious lapses of patient safety and dignity, as illustrated in Fiona's narrative. Events like these are relatively commonplace during healthcare education and comprise what we term in this book 'professionalism dilemmas', that is, day-to-day experiences in which individuals witness or participate in something that they believe to be unprofessional, unethical or immoral, which causes them some angst.[1] These can be seen as professionalism 'lapses' too, another term we use in our book, although

Healthcare Professionalism: Improving Practice through Reflections on Workplace Dilemmas, First Edition.
Lynn V. Monrouxe and Charlotte E. Rees.
© 2017 John Wiley & Sons Ltd. Published 2017 by John Wiley & Sons Ltd.

dilemmas and lapses are not always synonymous (students may, for example, witness or participate in professionalism lapses that are not apparently troublesome for them, such as e-professionalism lapses). Ultimately, professionalism dilemmas can cause individuals like Fiona to experience emotional distress, with learners often left feeling unable to act on their own professionalism ideals because of structural challenges like healthcare hierarchies.[2] Ultimately, healthcare students and trainees who feel unable to act professionally might eventually experience their own professionalism standards eroding as they develop a non-reflexive (un)professionalism,[1,3] resulting in less resistance to (and distress within) future professionalism dilemmas. Given the current drive towards increasing professionalism standards within healthcare worldwide, we need to develop stronger professionalism standards and practices within the healthcare workforce, including those among students and trainees.

This textbook is based on our decade-long programme of professionalism research in which we have collected over 2000 narratives (i.e. stories) of professionalism dilemmas from thousands of healthcare (dental, medical, nursing, pharmacy and physiotherapy) students from four different countries (Australia, Sri Lanka, Taiwan and the UK: including England, Northern Ireland, Scotland and Wales). These narratives are essentially stories of professionalism dilemma experiences with beginnings, middles and ends that have entered into the biographies of the students who narrate them.[4] Students shared their experiences with us as part of six interrelated funded research projects using either individual or group interviews (oral narratives) or online questionnaire surveys (written narratives). While we have published many of the results of these studies in journal articles,[2,5–18] this book still contains original findings and scores of narratives (all with pseudonyms) not previously published.

While we know that innumerable examples of good professional practice and exceptional role modelling exist in the healthcare workplace,[19] our programme of research did not employ appreciative inquiry. It has instead focused on 'dilemmas', which are inevitably negative, challenging and troublesome. We chose narrative inquiry for our research programme because the act of storytelling can help individuals make sense of their experiences, as well as their actions within those experiences, and their developing identities.[20] As a reader of this book, you will come to understand narratives as sense-making activities through reading the real-life narratives from healthcare students, starting with Fiona's, in this book. You will also come to understand that narratives have a social function in that narrators are motivated to portray themselves in a positive light.[21] One therefore needs to be continuously mindful that the stories in this book are representations of the structure of students' experiences rather than accounts of what happened *exactly*.[22]

This book comprises an evidence-based approach to educating healthcare students, trainees and educators about commonplace professionalism dilemmas encountered in the healthcare workplace, and how to respond appropriately when faced with such professionalism dilemmas. Using practical activities, and illustrated through authentic narratives providing real-life case studies, this textbook aims to facilitate a robust and reflective approach for addressing professionalism dilemmas, including learners having a better understanding of how dilemmas come about and how they can be prevented and managed for the good of the learner, the wider healthcare team and the patient. The book is organized into three parts, with Part I giving an overview of healthcare professionalism education, Part II illustrating common professionalism dilemmas recounted by healthcare students, and Part III synthesizing cross-cultural differences across professionalism dilemmas, namely by country and by healthcare professional group. While all three parts are pertinent to both healthcare learners and educators, Part I is especially germane to healthcare educators, and Parts II and III to healthcare learners.

Part I includes Chapters 2–4. Chapter 2 will help you understand healthcare professionalism codes of conduct common in the Western world, the diverse ways in which professionalism is defined across different professions and English-speaking countries, different discourses (ways of thinking and talking) in which professionalism is framed and finally, how *phronesis* (or practical wisdom) interacts with students' developing professional identities. Chapter 3 will discuss why teaching and learning professionalism is important, what constitutes professionalism curricula and the different teaching and learning methods, curriculum-related professionalism dilemmas and finally, how learners might act in the face of curriculum-related dilemmas. Chapter 4 will help you understand why and how professionalism is assessed, the key challenges facing professionalism assessment, assessment-related professionalism dilemmas, and how learners might act in the face of assessment-related dilemmas.

Part II includes Chapters 5–10. Chapter 5 will help you understand what identities are and why they are important, relationships between educational transitions and identity dilemmas, different identity-related professionalism dilemmas and their impact and finally, how learners can act in the face of identity dilemmas. Chapter 6 will discuss what consent is and why it matters, common myths about patient consent for student involvement in healthcare, consent-related professionalism dilemmas and their impact, and how learners might act in the face of consent dilemmas. Chapter 7 will outline what patient safety is and the factors affecting patient safety, patient safety-related professionalism dilemmas, the role of students in facilitating safe workplace cultures and finally, the prevention and management of patient safety lapses. Chapter 8 will help you understand what patient dignity is and why it matters, patient dignity-related professionalism dilemmas and how they arise, the impact of dignity dilemmas and how learners can act during dignity dilemmas. Chapter 9 will outline what workplace equality, diversity and dignity are and why they matter, relationships between power and workplace abuse, the causes and consequences of workplace abuse, abuse-related professionalism dilemmas and finally, how they can be prevented and managed. Chapter 10 will help you understand what comprises online social networks and how their use intersects with professionalism, policy-related e-professionalism guidelines, e-professionalism-related dilemmas and how they come about, and finally how e-professionalism lapses can be prevented and managed.

Part III includes Chapters 11–13. Chapter 11 will help you understand what culture is and how it influences professionalism, different dimensions of professionalism found across different countries, relationships between how professionalism dilemmas are interpreted according to different cultural frames of reference, strategies for engaging effectively in intercultural interactions and finally, the range of professionalism dilemmas occurring across different countries. Chapter 12 will discuss the key roles of different healthcare professionals, differences in professionalism dilemmas across different healthcare professions, interprofessional dilemmas and how they come about, students' reactions to interprofessional dilemmas and finally, how interprofessional conflict can be prevented and managed. Finally, we conclude our book with Chapter 13 by discussing key cross-cutting themes including power, hierarchy, conformity and resistance on the one hand, and negative emotions, empathy and moral distress on the other. We consider how we can move the current professionalism state of play forward through education and research, and we end the chapter and book with our own reflexivity around how we have simultaneously shaped this professionalism research and been shaped by it.

With the exception of this introduction and our conclusion chapter, all chapters are specifically designed to facilitate your learning. With specified learning outcomes for each chapter, numerous real-life narratives, 'stop and do' activities, summary points, discussion points, extra learning activities and recommended reading, we hope that you will engage with this text actively, reflecting critically on what you are reading and making links and connections between what you see on the page with your own experiences of being a healthcare learner or teaching healthcare students. While we have written this book to be read chronologically, each of the chapters can be read as stand-alone chapters, so you can dip in and out of the book (and at random) depending on what best suits your needs and at what time. Ultimately, we hope that this book will help you navigate your way through inevitable professionalism dilemmas occurring in the healthcare workplace learning environment, to better protect yourself, your colleagues and most importantly, your patients.

References

1 Feudtner C, Christakis D, Christakis N. Do clinical clerks suffer ethical erosion? Students' perceptions of their ethical environment and personal development. *Academic Medicine* 1994;69:670–679.

2 Monrouxe LV, Rees CE, Dennis A, Wells S. Professionalism dilemmas, moral distress and the healthcare student: insights from two online UK-wide questionnaire studies. *BMJ Open* 2015;5:e007518. doi:10.1136/bmjopen-2014-007518.

3 Coulehan J, Williams PC. Vanquishing virtue: the impact of medical education. *Academic Medicine* 2001;76:598–605.

4 Labov W. Some further steps in narrative analysis. *Journal of Narrative Life History* 1997;7:395–415.

5 Monrouxe LV, Rees CE, Hu W. Differences in medical students' explicit discourses of medical professionalism: acting, representing, becoming. *Medical Education* 2011;45:585–602.

6 Monrouxe LV, Rees CE. 'It's just a clash of cultures': emotional talk within medical students' narratives of professionalism dilemmas. *Advances in Health Sciences Education* 2012;17(5):671–701.

7 Monrouxe LV, Rees CE, Endacott R, Ternan E. 'Even now it makes me angry': healthcare students' professionalism dilemma narratives. *Medical Education* 2014;48:502–517.

8 Monrouxe LV, Rees CE. Hero, voyeur, judge: understanding medical students' moral identities through professionalism dilemma narratives. In K Mavor, M Platow and B Bizumic (Eds) *The Self, Social Identity and Education*. Oxford: Psychology Press, 2017: pp. 297–319.

9 Rees CE, Monrouxe LV. Medical students learning intimate examinations without valid consent: a multi-centre study. *Medical Education* 2011;45:261–272.

10 Rees CE, Monrouxe LV. 'A morning since eight of just pure grill': a multischool qualitative study of student abuse. *Academic Medicine* 2011;86(11):1374–1382.

11 Rees CE, Monrouxe LV, McDonald LA. Narrative, emotion, and action: analysing 'most memorable' professionalism dilemmas. *Medical Education* 2013;47(1):80–96.

12 Rees CE, Monrouxe LV. Laughter for coping: medical students narrating professionalism dilemmas. In CR Figley, P Huggard and CE Rees (Eds) *First do no Self-harm: Understanding and Promoting Physician Stress Resilience.* New York: Oxford University Press, 2013: pp. 67–87.

13 Rees CE, Monrouxe LV, Ajjawi R. Professionalism in workplace learning: Understanding interprofessional dilemmas through healthcare student narratives. In D Jindal-Snape and EFS Hannah (Eds) *Exploring the Dynamics of Personal, Professional and Interprofessional Ethics.* Bristol: Policy Press, 2014: pp. 295–310.

14 Rees CE, Monrouxe LV. Professionalism education as a jigsaw: Putting it together for nursing students. In T Brown and B Williams (Eds) *Evidence-based Education in the Health Professions: Promoting Best Practice in the Learning and Teaching of Students.* London: Radcliffe Publishing, 2015: pp. 96–110.

15 Rees CE, Monrouxe LV, McDonald LA. My mentor kicked a dying woman's bed: analysing UK nursing students' most memorable professionalism dilemmas. *Journal of Advanced Nursing* 2015;71(1):169–180.

16 Rees CE, Monrouxe LV, Ternan E, Endacott R. Workplace abuse narratives from dentistry, nursing, pharmacy and physiotherapy students: a multi-school qualitative study. *European Journal of Dental Education* 2015;19(2):95–106.

17 Ho M-J, Gosselin K, Chandratilake M, Monrouxe LV, Rees CE. Taiwanese medical students' narratives of intercultural professionalism dilemmas: exploring tensions between Western medicine and Taiwanese culture. *Advances in Health Sciences Education* 2016; doi:10.1007/s10459-016-9738-x.

18 Monrouxe LV, Chandratilake M, Gosselin K, Rees CE, Ho M. Taiwanese and Sri Lankan students' dimensions and discourses of professionalism. *Medical Education.* In press.

19 Karnieli-Miller O, Vu TR, Frankel RM, Holtman MC, Clyman SG, Hui SL, *et al.* Which experiences in the hidden curriculum teach students about professionalism. *Academic Medicine* 2011;86(3):369–377.

20 Smith B, Sparkes AC. Contrasting perspectives on narrative selves and identities: an invitation to dialogue. *Qualitative Research* 2008;8:5–35.

21 Riessman CK. *Narrative Methods for the Human Sciences.* Thousand Oaks, CA: Sage Publications, 2008.

22 Kleres J. Emotions and narrative analysis: a methodological approach. *Journal for the Theory of Social Behaviour* 2010;41(2):182–202.

2

What is Healthcare Professionalism?

'I know there's three Ps that's to promote dentistry... I don't know what the other two Ps are, but one is to maintain the profession through CPD [continuous professional development] and that kind of thing, and then acting yourself in a professional behaviour, so maintaining patient confidentiality and not getting drunk on whisky in front of your patients on nights out (laughs).'

Sarah, female, year 5, dentistry student, UK

LEARNING OUTCOMES

- To understand the role of healthcare regulatory bodies, alongside the legal and ethical underpinnings of professionalism codes of conduct
- To appreciate the diversity of ways in which professionalism is defined across different healthcare groups and countries
- To recognize the ways in which healthcare students understand professionalism and how this is similar and different across healthcare groups and national cultures
- To understand the different discourses (i.e. ways of thinking and talking) in which professionalism is framed
- To appreciate the concept of *phronesis* (i.e. practical wisdom) and how this interacts with students' developing professional identities

---

KEY TERMS

Ethical frameworks (e.g. virtues, principlism)
Professionalism dimensions
Professionalism discourses
Phronesis
Professional identities

Healthcare Professionalism: Improving Practice through Reflections on Workplace Dilemmas, First Edition.
Lynn V. Monrouxe and Charlotte E. Rees.
© 2017 John Wiley & Sons Ltd. Published 2017 by John Wiley & Sons Ltd.

Introduction

'Always say *please* and *thank you*', 'don't steal', 'tell the truth'. From the moment we are born, our lives are dominated by social rules (or norms); these become natural to us and part of who we are as we are socialized into them from birth. However, these rules do not come from nowhere: they are derived culturally, and comprise context-specific values, customs and traditions that are crucial for the smooth functioning of social groups. They tell us how we *should* act in certain contexts and even how to *think* in order to belong to a specific group. They also include messages about what will happen to us if we ignore the rules. Professional healthcare groups are much the same: each group has its own set of norms – or codes – which guide members of that profession in terms of how they should behave professionally. In other words, these norms enable us to understand the knowledge, skills and behaviours required of us to act with professionalism. But what is professionalism? We know that there is no one perspective or definition of what comprises healthcare professionalism, with professionalism understandings varying by person, culture and time.[1–9] This chapter aims to bring you a better understanding of healthcare professionalism from the perspective of regulatory bodies' codes of conduct through to how different healthcare professionals and students understand professionalism. We talk about different understandings as well as the different types of discourses (i.e. ways of thinking and talking) through which they operate. Knowing how different healthcare groups make sense of what it means to be a professional, along with the underpinning legal and ethical frameworks, will enable you to develop your own understanding about your professional identities – who you are and who you are becoming – and how you fit within the various multiprofessional teams in which you work and learn.

Who is Responsible for Setting Professionalism Codes of Conduct?

In around 400BC, the Hippocratic Oath required physicians to swear upon their healing gods that they would uphold the ethical standards of the day, including ensuring that patients suffered no harm as a result of their practice. Although versions of this oath are still used today, nowadays each professional group, often with lay representation, has its own code of conduct that invariably sets out what is expected of its members: codes that are in harmony with modern-day ethical and legal statutes. But who is responsible for setting these codes? And to whom do they apply?

Professional codes are designed and implemented by the profession's regulatory body, so differ according to different healthcare professions and countries. Furthermore, regulatory bodies can differ in terms of their scope and authority (see Table 2.1 for summary of key documents from healthcare regulatory bodies from different professions and different English-speaking countries). If we look at medicine, for example, the UK General Medical Council (GMC) sets the professional standards expected of all undergraduate students, trainees and doctors: they are responsible for ensuring that doctors continue to meet those standards through annual appraisals and revalidation;[10] and when problems arise, such as concerns about a doctor risking patient safety (see Chapter 7), it is the GMC's responsibility to investigate and act. The GMC can decide to restrict a doctor's

Table 2.1 Regulatory bodies for medicine, dentistry, nursing, physiotherapy and pharmacy practioners across the main four native English speaking countries in the world.

	Australia	Canada	United Kingdom	USA
Medicine	Australian Health Practitioner Regulation Agency[11]	Royal College of Physicians and Surgeons of Canada[12]	General Medical Council[10]	American Board of Internal Medicine Foundation-American College of Physicians-American Society of Internal Medicine-European Federation of Internal Medicine[13]
Dentistry	Australian Dental Council[14]	Royal College of Dental Surgeons of Ontario[15]	General Dental Council[16]	American Dental Association[17]
Nursing	Australian Nursing and Midwifery Council[18]	Canadian Nurses Association[19]	Nursing and Midwifery Council[20]	American Nurses Association[21]
Physiotherapy	Australian Physiotherapy Association[22]	National Physiotherapy Advisory Group[23]	Chartered Society of Physiotherapy[24]	American Physical Therapy Association[25]
Pharmacy	Pharmaceutical Society of Australia[26]	National Association of Pharmacy Regulatory Authorities[27]	General Pharmaceutical Council[28]	American Pharmacists Association[29]

Note: dates indicate the version of the document used in this chapter.

practice, ordering them to work under supervision, suspending their practice and (in serious cases) removing them entirely from the medical register. By contrast, the Australian Medical Council (AMC) only sets the standards for medical education and training in Australia, with the Medical Board of Australia (MBA) and the Australian Health Practitioner Regulation Agency (AHPRA) being responsible for registering doctors, developing standards, codes and guidelines for medical professionals and investigating complaints levelled against its members. Each one of the various professional regulatory bodies works within national legal frameworks. For example, the GMC is directly accountable to the Privy Council (a formal body of advisers to the United Kingdom sovereign), to which it makes its statutory reports for laying before Parliament under the single Act of Parliament that provides the legal framework for all 32 UK-regulated healthcare professions.

What is the Ethical Basis of Healthcare Professionalism?

It is important to remember that legal frameworks are interrelated with ethics. Although there are many approaches to understanding ethics, two key perspectives in healthcare education and practice are *principlism* and *virtue ethics*. Briefly, principlism refers to four interrelated principles originally developed by Beauchamp and Childress:[30] autonomy, beneficence, non-maleficence and justice (see Box 2.1). This perspective is often taught to healthcare students as a useful way of approaching ethical decision making (see Box 2.2 for Cassie's dilemma). However, due to the interrelatedness of the four principles, they can often be in conflict during professionalism dilemmas, as will be seen throughout this book. For example, the concept of patient autonomy can be at odds with a utilitarian perspective (see Chapter 6), which values the greatest good for the greatest number of people.[31] Virtue ethics, on the other hand, is essentially a person-based, rather than action-based, approach with its roots in Plato, Aristotle and Chinese philosophy.[32] Focusing on the three core concepts of *arête*, *phronesis* and *eudaimonia* (see Box 2.3), it considers the moral character of the individual's action. Within this approach to professionalism dilemmas, relations between different parties, alongside the broader needs of all those involved, plays a key role in understanding the most *appropriate* ways to act.[31]

Box 2.1 Information: Beauchamp and Childress[30] four principles

Autonomy: Respect for patients' rights to decide appropriate courses of action for themselves, so long as they have the capacity to consider and act on that plan. This links with informed consent (see Chapter 6).

Beneficence: Comprises *positive beneficence* (healthcare professionals providing benefit) and *utility* (healthcare professionals weighing the benefits and deficits for optimum outcomes). This can be challenged by respect of autonomy: one cannot act without the patient's consent.

Non-maleficence: Epitomized by the Latin phrase *primum non nocere*, first do no harm. This links with the deficit side when considering beneficence and the disclosure of risks associated with autonomy.

Justice: Addresses the conflict between the distribution of scarce healthcare resources, respect for people's rights and for morally acceptable laws.

Box 2.2 'Probably not adhering to best-practice'

'You know in terms of the bioethical principles they [educators] talk about it... beneficence and non-maleficence and autonomy... I've seen situations where a mistake has been made and the team hasn't told the family, which for me I think that's probably not adhering to best practice (said laughingly)... there was a patient who hadn't received medication... he started having seizures... they were absence seizures, it wasn't like an obvious fit, he was just lying in bed and the mum kept saying that he looked like he was sleeping with his eyes open... he did very much deteriorate... it was obviously lack of medication... and when they [doctors] found out they didn't tell the family... I came in when they were panicking when they'd just realized... so I saw the end bit where they were running round in panic... the patient and their family hadn't been told... [Interviewer: You didn't say anything about it?]... no, this is the dilemma (laughs)... cause it was you know my first day, I'm there asking them about a mistake they made and so I guess they were a little bit anti answering my questions.'

Cassie, female, year 4, medical student, UK

Box 2.3 Information: three main concepts within the virtue ethics approach

Arête: An embodied disposition as a morally desirable kind of person (virtuous), combined with a *conscious decision* to be that kind of person (e.g. honest, compassionate, courageous). But some virtues can also be faults when taken to their extremes.

Phronesis: Moral (or practical) wisdom. As virtues can lead to a person acting wrongly, the capacity to recognize that some features of a situation are more important than others is required. Phronesis is part of our rational choice as we decide how to act in particular situations.

Eudaimonia: Typically translated as happiness or flourishing. Living a virtuous life is necessary for happiness, so in pursuit of happiness one should be virtuous.

Box 2.4 Stop and do: get to know your regulatory body

- Which regulatory body oversees the professional activities for your healthcare group and in your country?
- What aspects of healthcare education and practice is that regulatory body responsible for overseeing?
- Go online to examine the goals and values for your regulatory body.
- What legal and ethical frameworks (if any) underpin the goals and values?
- How does your regulatory body deal with professional misconduct issues?

In this section we have begun to answer our 'What is professionalism?' question by exploring the relationships between professional regulatory bodies, law and ethics. Knowledge of the particular regulatory body that oversees professional activities for your healthcare practice, along with a familiarization of the underpinning legal and ethical basis, are an important first port of call for your understanding of professionalism. We suggest you now turn to Box 2.4 for our first 'stop and do' activity.

How is Professionalism Understood Across Regulatory Bodies' Codes of Conduct?

'Professionalism is a basket of qualities that enables us to trust our advisors.'

Dame Janet Smith[33 p.15]

We now explore how professionalism is understood in the regulatory bodies' various codes of conduct. Here we focus on the key documents produced for medical, dentistry, nursing, physiotherapy and pharmacy practitioners from the four main native English-speaking countries in the world (see Table 2.1). In doing this, we make comparisons between the documents by country and healthcare group, identifying the similarities and the differences.

Across all 20 documents in Table 2.1, we identified over one hundred different dimensions of professionalism. In terms of similarities, in Table 2.2 we list the various dimensions for which there is complete agreement across all countries; and healthcare groups (in bold). From this table, we can see that all healthcare practitioners are required to be respectful and competent. Prioritizing 'patient' care, they are also expected to protect patient confidentiality, and continuously maintain their skills and knowledge. In terms of differences, while the USA, UK, Canada and Australia are all Western countries, their codes are surprisingly different. For example, the concept of *altruism* is only explicitly cited in the North American medical, nursing and physiotherapy codes of conduct. Furthermore, only the UK codes specified *politeness* across all healthcare professions. What is important to recognize here is that concepts such as *altruism* and *politeness* are culturally defined: what is polite or altruistic in one situation or culture might not be in another (note we will touch on this aspect of language later when we consider the different discourses of professionalism).

Another interesting way to look at the dimensions identified in Table 2.2 is to consider the ways in which the professionalism codes contribute to the socialization of a particular kind of professional identity. Indeed, it has been argued that professionalism codes of practice are the outward, visible expressions of our identity: our professionalism.[34] In terms of the outward expression of professionalism, some professions stress certain aspects more than others, for example knowledge of the law (dental), wider societal responsibilities (medicine) and equality and diversity (nursing). This means that different professional groups are expected to embody different roles, values and behaviours for themselves: becoming certain kinds of people both personally and professionally, rather than merely behaving in ways aligned with their professional roles.

In this section we have explored the multitude of dimensions stipulated across various professionalism codes of practice and compared them by healthcare group and country. From this original analysis, we have begun to see that there is no single way of understanding professionalism even within the same healthcare group, although there are strong areas of agreement (e.g. competence, respect, honesty). While these codes are important for professions as a way of providing guidance, they are not necessarily black and white. For example, there may be occasions when two or more aspects of professionalism conflict (e.g. patient care priority vs. protects resources). It is therefore important that we understand professionalism dimensions as frameworks to be lived *through*, rather than as a set of rules to be lived *by*. In other words, it is through our

Table 2.2 Commonalities of personal and professional dimensions for the medical, dentistry, physiotherapy, nursing and pharmacy professions across the USA, UK, Canadian and Australian policy documents.

	Medicine	Dentistry	Nursing*	Physiotherapy*	Pharmacy*
Personal 'virtues'	Honest Integrity **Respectful** Trustworthy	Honest Integrity Ethical Kind **Respectful** Trustworthy	Integrity **Respectful** Trustworthy Embodies professional identity	Ethical **Respectful**	Integrity **Respectful** Trustworthy
Professional attributes (individual)	**Competent** Culturally aware Knowledgeable	**Competent** Legal knowledge	Accountability: personal **Competent** Culturally aware Effective teacher Knowledgeable	Accountability: personal **Competent** Knowledgeable	**Competent** Good communicator
Professional practice (interpersonal)	**Continues professional development** Evidence-based practitioner Obtaining informed consent Respects diversity **Patient care priority** Practises safely	**Continues professional development** Evidence-based practitioner Not over treating Obtaining informed consent **Patient care priority** Practises safely	**Continues professional development** Evidence-based practitioner Obtaining informed consent **Patient care priority** Practises safely **Protects confidentiality**	**Continues professional development** Obtaining informed consent **Patient care priority** **Protects confidentiality** Respects dignity Respects diversity	**Continues professional development** **Patient care priority** **Protects confidentiality** Shared decision making

(Continued)

Table 2.2 (Continued)

	Medicine	Dentistry	Nursing*	Physiotherapy*	Pharmacy*
	Protects confidentiality	**Protects confidentiality**	Respects dignity	Shared decision-making	
	Respects boundaries	Respects boundaries	Respects diversity	Team worker/collaborator	
	Shared decision-making	Respects dignity	Respects healthcare team		
	Team worker/collaborator		Self-care		
			Quality care		
Wider responsibilities (societal)	Declares conflicts of interest	**Raises concerns**	Accountability: professional	Accountability: social	
	Improves patient safety		**Raises concerns**	**Raises concerns**	
	Protects resources				
	Raises concerns				

Note: Bold dimensions refer to commonalities across all professions and countries; *We use the term patient as this was most commonly used, although the codes variously talked about *clients* and *consumers*.

Box 2.5 Stop and do: get to know your professionalism code of conduct

- Take a look at your own professional code of conduct.
- What does this document say in terms of expectations for your personal 'virtues', professional attributes and practices?
- How do these codes reflect what is expected of you as a student or trainee?
- Reflect on the extent to which these attributes are part of who you are both professionally and personally, and whether this has changed over time.
- To what extent does this code reflect the ethical perspectives of principlism or virtue ethics?
- Which of the professionalism dimensions do you think are most important and why?

---

understanding and appreciation of these codes of conduct that we come to develop more sophisticated ways of knowing the best course of action in any particular situation. Rather than knowing what is right or wrong, this entails going beyond the codes in order to understand what is right *here and now*. Also known as the development of *phronesis* (as defined earlier in Box 2.3), this is of utmost importance when faced with professionalism dilemmas that have no absolute *right* way of acting. We now ask you to undertake the 'stop and do' exercise in Box 2.5 before we broaden our understanding of professionalism by looking at professionalism discourses.

How is Professionalism Linguistically Framed Across Healthcare Professionalism Codes of Conduct?

We have so far discussed the dimensions of healthcare professionalism as specified within various policy documents. Here, we focus on the *discourses* of professionalism within them. Discourse is about language and the ways in which language shapes how we think about aspects of the world: so-called *discourse practice*. Within medical professionalism, for example, there are a number of practices and ideas of professionalism that run from and to the policy documents already discussed (note that we will see later how these discourses of professionalism eventually find their way into healthcare students' understandings of professionalism). It is important to consider the different ways in which healthcare professionalism is framed through the language we use, for this shapes the way that healthcare professionalism is taught and assessed (see Chapters 3 and 4), and ultimately how professionalism is practised.

Let us begin by considering the minutiae of language: words. So a word *signifies* (represents) a concept. The word *watch*, for example, signifies the physical object placed on your person that tells the time. Although watches come in different shapes and sizes, this signifier-signified relationship is reasonably simple. Now, let's think about a word signifying an abstract concept such as *professionalism, altruism* or *politeness* rather than a physical object like *watch*. When referring to such abstract concepts the signifier-signified relationship is complex, creating variations in understandings between different people and different contexts. For example, Wear and Nixon[35] demonstrate impressively the many ways that terms such as *altruism, duty*, and *excellence* outlined in *Project Professionalism*,[13] can be understood and enacted across a range of contexts.

Furthermore, different words can be used to describe the same object, concept or person, such as the words *patient*, *client* and *consumer* being used to refer to the person consulting the healthcare professional. Importantly, those different words can make us think very differently about, and act very differently towards, that person. Take a look at the word clouds in Figure 2.1 that we have created from the different professionalism codes for medicine, dentistry, nursing, physiotherapy and pharmacy identified in Table 2.1. Words that are largest appear more frequently in the documents than the smaller words. Read through the word clouds and complete the 'stop and do' activity in Box 2.6.

Not only can single words mean very different things to different people in different contexts, but they can also have different meanings depending upon how they are used within wider discourses. By way of an example, think about a word commonly used across the various policy documents: *accountability*. Accountability is a word with different meanings depending on how it is used. In the nursing literature alone, accountability has been embedded, described and associated with: professional socialization, professional values, virtue ethics, professional identity, ethical behaviours, moral agency and character development.[36]

Sometimes accountability is constructed separately from responsibility, at other times the two concepts are intertwined.[37] In Table 2.2 we can see how *accountability* is constructed differently across different policy documents through different discourses. Sometimes it is constructed through an individualistic discourse: as a healthcare student or practitioner you are *personally* accountable for your actions. At other times it is constructed through a collectivist discourse: as a healthcare student or practitioner you have a duty to uphold the *collective* body of the profession in which society places trust. Accountability has also been constructed through an interpersonal discourse highlighting the social interaction *between* individuals: 'accountability means being prepared to explain and justify one's… actions and omissions to those involved or influenced by one's actions'.[38] [p. 301] Finally, accountability can be constructed through a *complexity* discourse seen as a 'dynamic construct of actors and structures shifting across time'.[9] [p. 587] Within this frame, healthcare practitioners are required to have sensitivity to the various accountability mechanisms that might create tensions for them and an understanding of how and when one might act on issues of accountability, and when a lack of action is justifiable. This complexity understanding of accountability resonates with the notion of *phronesis* discussed earlier (see Box 2.3).

What are Stakeholders' Understandings of Professionalism Across Different Country Cultures?

Having considered how professionalism is understood by examining dimensions and discourses within various professionalism codes of conduct, we now explore some of the national cultural differences in how professionalism is construed by different stakeholders. For reasons of brevity, we use medical professionalism case studies as this links well with our further exploration of cross-cultural professionalism dilemmas in Chapter 11. However, we encourage you to explore such differences in the literature for your professional group.[39-42]

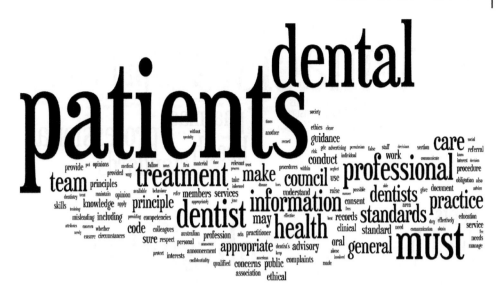

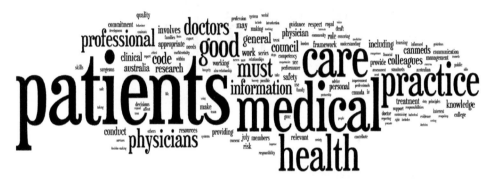

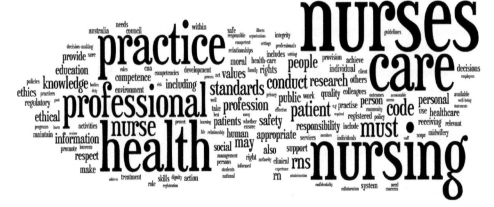

Figure 2.1 Word clouds of the professionalism codes for dentistry, medicine, nursing, pharmacy and physiotherapy respectively (in Table 2.2).

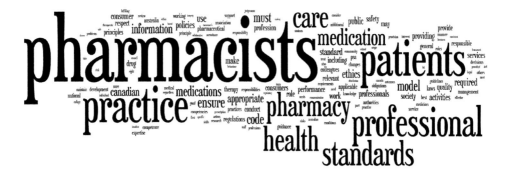

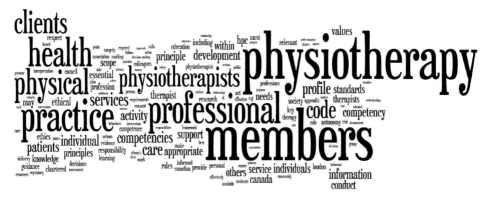

Figure 2.1 (*Continued*)

Box 2.6 Stop and do: it's all in a word

Take a look at the word clouds in Figure 2.1 that we created from the different professionalism codes for medical, dentistry, nursing, physiotherapy and pharmacy documents in Table 2.2. Words that are largest appear more frequently in the documents than smaller words.

- What do you notice about the most and least prominent words in each document?
- What are the similarities and differences across healthcare professional groups?
- The cluster of words for each healthcare professional group can be thought of as discourses for that profession. Try to summarize each profession according to the prominent words in terms of who that professional is, their relationship to significant others and their governing bodies.

In Box 2.4 we asked you to go online to look at your own regulatory body's professionalism guide. Take a moment to create your own word cloud using this document: http://www.wordle.net/create

Focusing on the word cloud that you have created: to what extent do you feel comfortable with the words and why? Do these words represent how you talk and think about your chosen profession? Do these words represent how you behave?

Medical Professionalism Case Study

Here, we summarize two recent papers that have explored cultural differences in understandings of medical professionalism.[5,7] First, Chandratilake *et al.*[5] explored perceptions of essential attributes of medical professionalism across the UK, Europe, North America and Asia. Using a questionnaire, they asked medical professionals to rate 55 different dimensions of professionalism using a five-point scale. They found a high degree of agreement across all regional groups (29 dimensions), many of which can be seen in Table 2.2. However, the emphasis given to 11 dimensions differed by region, for example: being accessible to patients (emphasized by European, Asian and North American doctors), being culturally sensitive (North American doctors only), being punctual and adaptable to changes in the workplace (Asian doctors only) and having the skills to train colleagues (European doctors only).

Using the nominal group interviewing technique, Ho *et al.*[7] found differences in understandings of medical professionalism between Chinese and Taiwanese stakeholders (including doctors, nurses, patients, public health experts and school administrators). For example, economic considerations (not profiting from prescribing certain drugs), health promotion and teamwork (including mutual professional support) were exclusively emphasized as specific professionalism dimensions by Chinese participants, whereas teamwork was considered to be part of the *accountability* dimension for the Taiwanese participants. So we can see from these two cross-cultural medical professionalism studies how we can glean a wider perspective on what it means to be a particular type of healthcare professional in terms of national culture. While we have so far considered the viewpoints of regulators through policy documents and key stakeholders who have been mainly qualified healthcare professionals, we next turn to consider students' viewpoints of what comprises healthcare professionalism.

What are Students' Understandings of Professionalism Across Country Cultures?

For this section we draw on our own programme of research, where we asked over 400 medical, dental, nursing, physiotherapy and pharmacy students in the UK, Australia, Taiwan and Sri Lanka the seemingly simple question: 'What does professionalism mean to you?'[9,43] Before reading further, complete the 'stop and do' exercise in Box 2.7.

What was noticeable in our studies, across students from all countries and healthcare groups, was that they often struggled to define professionalism, as evidenced by their

---

Box 2.7 Stop and do: what does professionalism mean to you?

- Given what you have read so far, alongside your own thinking about professionalism for your healthcare profession, write down your own definition of professionalism.
- Once you have your own definition, reflect on the difficulty of defining professionalism.
- Later, come back to your definition and compare this with what students from our professionalism dilemma study thought. Which of the dimensions coming up are reflected in your definition?

Table 2.3 Students' understandings of professionalism: 19 dimensions.

Individual attributes*	Such as punctuality, manners, integrity, honesty, leadership, etc.	**Integration**	Suggests that one cannot completely segregate personal and professional lives.
Development	Developing attitudes, skills, knowledge and behaviours for future practice.	**Contextual**	Environmental influences on professionalism (e.g. time, hierarchy).
Stasis	Having a full set of responsibilities from the beginning.	**Rules***	Being governed by, and abiding to, rules: from policymakers, clinical and educational settings, society, etc.
Internalized self	Relates to the embodied development of professional identity.	**Patient-centredness***	Patient care priority, affording dignity, sharing decision making.
Presentation*	Professionalism is enacted through clothes and talk (not embodied).	**Role models**	Includes qualified professionals and student peers as role models to students.
Special*	Belonging to a privileged self-regulated group, having a compact with society.	**Hierarchy**	Knowing your place in the hierarchy (within your profession, and across others).
Knowledge	Knowledge-based (including keeping up to date with knowledge).	**Team-playing**	Part of a dynamic process requiring good communication and carrying a responsibility for team development.
Competence*	Being competent at the appropriate level and knowing limits.	**Service provider**	Providing services to patients, often called *clients*, *consumers* or *customers*.
Phronesis	Practical wisdom – as defined in Box 2.3.	**Self-care**	Protecting yourself emotionally and legally.
Segregation	Segregates professional and personal life, setting boundaries between the two.		

Note: Dimensions with an asterisk are the five most commonly mentioned and the only ones mentioned by all healthcare groups and across all countries.

frequent silences, hesitations and laughter. However, once they got going, they collectively identified 19 different dimensions of professionalism (see Table 2.3), some of which concur with the dimensions found in the policy documents discussed previously. For example, professionalism as competence and understanding one's limits, professionalism as knowledge and the requirement to keep up to date, prioritizing patients (professionalism as patient-centredness) along with professionalism as individual attributes (virtues), are just some of the overlapping dimensions. Competence, individual attributes and patient-centredness, along with rules and presentation constituted the 'top-five' most cited dimensions and we discuss these in more depth next as these were the only dimensions discussed by students across all healthcare groups and countries.

Professionalism as Rules

By far the most common dimension of professionalism identified by all student groups was that of rule following (recall the opening quote by Sarah who talks about the 'three Ps'). These rules constituted both the explicit rules laid down by professional regulators as in the formal curriculum (see Charles' definition in Box 2.8) and the often-implicit ethical and moral rules learnt by students from the clinical environment (as in the informal and hidden curriculum, discussed in Chapter 3), from patients and society more generally. Students sometimes talked about needing to strictly adhere to rules, and at other times they talked about rules as guiding frameworks for 'ideal-type' behaviours that could be bent so long as such bending was acceptable by the profession.

Professionalism as Patient Centredness

As the second most commonly talked about dimension, patient centredness comprised many different but related aspects: placing the patient as the first priority, treating them respectfully, in a non-judgemental manner (Susan in Box 2.8), treating the whole patient, developing trust with the patient, communicating with patients appropriately (and, for the Taiwanese students in particular, with family members), and affording patients dignity, autonomy and confidentiality. As such, this dimension of professionalism draws heavily on the principlism approach to ethics. What is interesting here is where students' notions of patient-centred professionalism came from, including formal lectures on ethics, informal learning through role models and from formal assessments (we will discuss teaching, learning and assessment in Chapters 3 and 4).

Professionalism as Presentation

One of the most important dimensions of professionalism, according to students, was the requirement to act and dress like a professional. This presentational aspect included the manner in which students spoke, their attitude, eye contact, body language, the clothes they wore, along with other aspects such as punctuality and hygiene (see the group discussion, Box 2.8). For many students this represents quite an artificial side of them, something that did not come naturally and was not necessarily part of who they were. In particular, students felt they had to act more 'grown up' than they felt, which included having to stop saying 'cool' and swearing when talking with patients. They talked about 'pretending to be' a professional and putting on 'the hat and cloak' of professionalism and even 'stepping into another body'. Furthermore, students often expressed frustration around this aspect of professionalism, in that it was 'in the eye of the beholder' and as such what one person felt was important presentationally, another did not (Box 2.8).

Professionalism as Attributes of the Individual

Professionalism was frequently defined according to specific personal attributes or values of individual people including: being respectful, punctual, honest, polite and truthful, along with having the appropriate manners and possessing integrity and empathy (Karen's definition, Box 2.8). Definitions highlighting this dimension of professionalism drew heavily on the individualist discourse discussed above, along with virtue ethics, with members of the professions being expected to be morally desirable kind of people with strong ethical values.

Box 2.8 Information box: top five most cited professionalism dimensions with illustrative quotes

Professionalism as rules

'Being a professional you have certain standards to achieve… like for us, pharmacists, we have our own code of ethics to start with, and that is like the basis of professionalism, that's where our professionalism lies in the code of ethics and then it goes from there.'

Charles, male, year 2, pharmacy student, UK

Professionalism as patient-centredness

'Well [we're] certainly graded… one of them is like discrimination… do you treat all your patients the same, whether they're not, sort of a difficult patient or a particularly nice patient, you have to treat them all the same.'

Susan, female, year 3, nursing student, UK

Professionalism as presentation

BEN: We have a lecture on professionalism… how you even wear your hair and what you dress like, not to wear trainers…

JAMES: Stuff like having long hair and you should tie it back, looking smart and not wearing creased clothes.

BEN: Yeah a lot of it was on appearance and visibility things.

NICK: Yeah, something about not having facial hair but it is okay to have a beard (laughter) you can't be in between, so you, at no stage can you grow a beard. You have to have one or not.

JACK: A consultant placement for the fourth years… told them in advance before his clinic that they would all have to be very smart… that would include clean wet shaven facial hair, or the lack of, top buttons and ties and everything else… and one of the students wasn't quite clean shaven enough, apparently he used an electric razor… (laughs) it didn't provide quite the necessary look he was after, so he refused him for his clinic.

LESLEY: Blimey that's very extreme.

JANET: I heard of a consultant who said to all his female students that he expected them all to be dressed in skirts… that trousers wasn't professional for female medical students.

JACK: That just sounds really sexist doesn't it?

JAMES: Yeah I think the point here is, it is a bit subjective isn't it, sometimes, professionalism?

Mixed gender group discussion, year 3, medical students, UK

Professionalism as attributes of the individual

'I think also acting with integrity… you always should be doing what you think is the best thing.'

Karen, female, year 2, dentistry student, UK

Professionalism as competence

'At university you're taught manual techniques for example, and when you're on placement you may be taught additional ones, but it's knowing the certain techniques you might not be able to do until you've gone on postgraduate courses or whatever… so it's knowing sort of what level you can practice.'

Georgia, female, year 3, physiotherapy student, UK

Professionalism as Competence

Healthcare students talked liberally about the importance of being clinically and ethically competent, alongside knowing the limits of their competence (Georgia's definition, Box 2.8). This meant students refusing to act in situations where their limits were exceeded, unless there was adequate supervision. Other aspects of this definition included the requirement to continue to keep skills up to date, linking with the universally agreed aspect of professionalism around engaging with continuing professional development (Table 2.2).

Final Thoughts

Although we have presented the five most common dimensions here, one of the most interesting aspects within our research was the way that professionalism was hotly debated as healthcare students grappled with trying to understand this complex issue: what exactly professionalism is, who is entitled to be called a professional and what it means to work professionally. To illustrate this complex debate with no black and white answers, read Box 2.9, which presents a discussion between six final-year UK medical students as they grapple with the question: 'What is professionalism?' Interestingly, this discussion resonates with Friedson's definition presented later in Box 3.1.

Professionalism: Embodied Identities?

Having considered the many ways in which healthcare professionalism is understood through regulators' professionalism documents and by different stakeholders, we now consider the concept of professional identity. We have already seen that competency is considered to be a key component of healthcare professionalism and this is perhaps unsurprising given the international backdrop of competency-based education over the past decade.[44-48] While we have this strong competency discourse in healthcare professionalism currently, other discourses are beginning to come to the fore that emphasize the importance of not just *doing* but also *being*: this is the identity discourse.[49,50]

Becoming a healthcare professional is more than just learning the competencies (i.e. skills, knowledge and behaviours) set out by healthcare regulators. It also entails a process of *becoming* a healthcare practitioner, identifying with other practitioners and embodying professionalism as part of *who you are*, not just *what you do*.[51,52] In this sense, learning to become a healthcare professional is a process of developing an evolving identity that often begins with following the rules and acting like a professional (as in rules and presentation above). However, as students develop their professional identities, they will develop more sophisticated understandings of professionalism, moving from black and white thinking (e.g. rules are to be followed always), towards an understanding that the rules are simply guidance, and sometimes the 'right' thing to do is to step outside the rules (Box 2.10). This requires a strong identity developed over time as a particular kind of healthcare practitioner with practical wisdom (*phronesis*). This moves students from having competence alone to developing broader capabilities (i.e. knowing their competence in any given situation and developing their ability to exercise this wisely, making moral judgements in response to complex situations).

Box 2.9 'But that's the whole point of being professional'	
JIM:	Whenever an institution has regulations… they've got to follow the regulations… I regard that as professionalism…
EDWARD:	I think the thing that for me makes that, doesn't allow bricklaying to fall into the category of professional, or profession, is that you aren't dealing with privileged confidential information that affects other people and people's lives… in a profession… you are entrusted and empowered with information and privileged to make decisions and perform actions that actually have a bearing on people's ability to survive.
CASSIE:	But then that could actually be taken into a civil servant working in social security, to people looking after your IT information, and to banking et cetera because they have huge impact on lives…
EDWARD:	I agree but… in IT, then what you're doing is you are following a series of steps and rules aren't you?
CASSIE:	…I was just about to say is, is a leadership element to professionalism?
EDWARD:	You're doing a job involving data. You're not actually making decisions based on that data that will affect the people who the data's been generated from…
CASSIE:	And that leadership element, I mean are politicians professionals too?
MARTHA:	I bracket politicians sort of under lawyers and things like that… so yes I probably would. And then you've got, as with any other profession, you've got your ranks in professionals…
CASSIE:	But then they [politicians] sort make up their code of practice as they go along don't they? (laughs)
MARTHA:	But doctors have the ability to do that as well…
DARREN:	So there's degrees of professionalism… so could you still classify say bricklayers as a professional, but not as kind of with the same complexity…
CASSIE:	I think, if a bricklayer could lay his bricks anyway he chose and still come up with a result that built the wall, then I would say that. But he has to lay his bricks in a particular way, there's no other way for him to lay those bricks, correct me if I'm wrong…
MARTHA:	A bricklayer does have the ability to step outside of those.
DARREN:	So you're saying it's a creative element?
MARTHA:	Yes it is a creative element. It's a control element. It's the leadership element. That's why it's so difficult to define… coming back to bricklaying (group laughs)… you could certainly act in a professional way which I would say, for example, if you were asked to build a gas chamber at Belsen [Nazi concentration camp] and you knew what you were doing, and you refused to do so, then that would be a professional decision.
DARREN:	Would it not just be an ethical decision?
DAVID:	I think ethics and professionalism are… intimately intertwined aren't they? I mean dealing with ethics is what professionals do isn't it?
MARTHA:	But it's ethics defined by a point of view. If you were a Nazi German bricklayer (laughter) then you wouldn't have any problems building your gas chamber at Belsen.
DAVID:	Then the professional thing to do would be to build it wouldn't it?
MARTHA:	Yes. So it's the ethics defining your point of view…
DAVID:	And then justify your standpoint to your peers.
CASSIE:	Of course, it might be very unwise to refuse to do it. (laughs)
DAVID:	Ah, but that's the whole point of being professional. You have that fortitude to put society and others above personal gain.

Mixed gender group discussion, year 5, medical students, UK

Box 2.10 'A certain amount of professional judgement'

'Apart from being like clinically competent just being ethically competent... understanding and being able to extrapolate appropriate behaviours from the limited guidelines that we are given in terms of like ethics.'

Vicky, female, year 2, medical student, Australia

'They set out these rules and they set out these guidelines and say, *"you must not do this, you must do this"*, but... as a pharmacist you're given a certain amount of professional judgement to act within and outside of these guidelines, so you're sort of given a responsibility as well, so professionalism comes with responsibility I'd say definitely.'

Sonia, female, year 4, pharmacy student, UK

Finally, the embodiment of a professional identity links strongly with the notion of becoming a fully responsible and accountable professional (see Sonia's comment, Box 2.10). Embodying this aspect of accountability in its fullest sense, links strongly with students' active resistance to complying with negative aspects of the hidden curriculum (discussed later in Chapter 3) and refusing to go along with situations that students and trainees believe to be unprofessional. You will see, as you work though this book, examples of how students' strong professional identities lead them to speak out or act in a way to uphold what they believe is right.

Chapter Summary

This chapter has provided an overview of what comprises professionalism, based on an analysis of professionalism documents from regulatory bodies and stakeholders' talk. We have explored the similarities and differences in understandings (dimensions and discourses) of professionalism across different healthcare groups and countries. And we have talked about the importance of healthcare students developing their professionalism through embodied professional identities, moving beyond competence to develop phronesis. We present the chapter summary in Box 2.11. In Box 2.12 you will find our suggestions for small group discussions, with learning activities in Box 2.13, and recommended reading in Box 2.14.

Box 2.11 Chapter summary points

- Professionalism is a complex concept with many different understandings across different healthcare groups and countries.
- Even when there is agreement on specific dimensions of professionalism (e.g. accountability), the meanings can differ according to the different underpinning discourses (e.g. individual accountability versus collective accountability).
- Becoming a professional requires going beyond the development of competency; it is about developing a professional identity and how this identity intertwines with how students and trainees act in the face of professionalism dilemmas.

Box 2.12 Chapter discussion points

- What does professionalism mean to you? In what way do you agree and disagree with your regulatory body's professionalism code? What would you add to this code?
- Do you think it is possible and desirable to develop a truly embodied professional identity, and if so, at what point in your journey do you think this will happen?
- What, if any, prior experiences might facilitate your development of a professional identity along with phronesis?

Box 2.13 Chapter learning activities

- Thinking about who you were when you began your healthcare education, do you feel that you have changed as a person? If so, in what way?
- How might your reading from this chapter help you in your development of professionalism across your upcoming healthcare education?
- How do you think your undergraduate or postgraduate experiences have helped, or could help, you in developing your identity as a healthcare professional?

Box 2.14 Chapter recommended reading

Health and Care Professions Council *Professionalism in Healthcare Professionals.* 2014. http://www.hpc-uk.org/assets/documents/10003771Professionalismin healthcareprofessionals.pdf (Accessed Jan 20th 2017).

Hodges B. The professional identity of the future. In R Cruess, S Cruess, Y Steinert (Eds) *Teaching Medical Professionalism,* 2nd Edition. *Supporting the Development of a Professional Identity.* Cambridge: Cambridge University Press. 2016 pp. 277–287.

Monrouxe LV, Rees, C, Hu, W. Differences in medical students' explicit discourses of professionalism: acting, representing, becoming. *Medical Education* 2011;45(6):585–602.

Schryer CF, Spoel P. Genre theory, health-care discourse, and professional identity formation. *Journal of Business and Technical Communication* 2005;19(3):249–278.

Wear D, Nixon LL. Literary inquiry and professional development in medicine: against abstractions. *Perspectives in Biology and Medicine* 2002;45(1), 104–124.

References

1 Swick H. Toward a normative definition of medical professionalism. *Academic Medicine* 2000;75:612–616.

2 Hafferty F, W, Castellani B. A sociological framing of medicine's modern-day professionalism movement. *Medical Education* 2009;43:826–828.

3 Hafferty FW, Levinson D. Moving beyond nostalgia and motives: towards a complexity science view of medical professionalism. *Perspectives in Biology and Medicine* 2008;51:599–615.

4 Anijar K. Discourse as rock formation – fruitcake as professionalism. *American Journal of Bioethics* 2004;4:8–w10.

5 Chandratilake M, McAleer S, Gibson J. Cultural similarities and differences in medical professionalism: a multi-region study. *Medical Education* 2012;46:257–266.

6 Cruess SR. Professionalism and medicine's social contract with society. *Clinical Orthopaedics and Related Research* 2006;449:170–176.

7 Ho MJ, Yu KH, Pan H, Norris JL, Liang YS, Li JN, *et al.* A tale of two cities: understanding the differences in medical professionalism between two Chinese cultural contexts. *Academic Medicine* 2014;89:944–950.

8 Martimianakis MA, Maniate J, M, Hodges BD. Sociological interpretations of professionalism. *Medical Education* 2009;43:829–837.

9 Monrouxe LV, Rees CE, Hu W. Differences in medical students' explicit discourses of professionalism: acting, representing, becoming. *Medical Education* 2011;45:585–602.

10 General Medical Council. Good medical practice 2013. General Medical Council, hthttp://www.medicalboard.gov.au/Codes-Guidelines-Policies/Code-of-conduct.aspx (Accessed 2 March 2016).

11 Australian Medical Council. Good medical practice: a code of conduct for doctors in Australia. http://www.medicalboard.gov.au/Codes-Guidelines-Policies/Code-of-conduct.aspx (Accessed 2 December 2016).

12 Royal College of Physicians and Surgeons of Canada. The draft CanMEDS 2015 physician competency framework. http://www.royalcollege.ca/portal/page/portal/rc/common/docu ments/canmeds/framework/framework_series_1_e.pdf, 2015 (Accessed 2 December 2016).

13 American Board of Internal Medicine Foundation-American College of Physicians-American Society of Internal Medicine-European Federation of Internal Medicine. Medical professionalism in the new millennium: a physician charter. *Annals of Internal Medicine* 2002;136:243–246.

14 Australian Dental Council. Professional attributes and competencies of the newly qualified dentist. Australian Dental Council: Melbourne, 2013.

15 Royal College of Dental Surgeons of Ontario. Code of ethics. http://www.rcdso.org/Assets/DOCUMENTS/Professional_Practice/Code_of_Ethics/RCDSO_Code_of_Ethics.PDF, 2004 (Accessed 2 December 2016).

16 General Dental Council. Standards for dental practice. http://www.gdc-uk.org/Dentalprofessionals/Standards/Documents/Standards%20for%20Dental%20Professionals.pdf (Accessed 2 December 2016.)

17 American Dental Association. ADA principles of ethics and code of professional conduct (ADA code). http://www.ada.org/~/media/ADA/Publications/Files/ADA_Code_of_Ethics_2016.pdf?la=en (Accessed 2 December 2016).

18 Australian Nursing and Midwifery Council. Code of professional conduct for nurses in Australia. http://www.nursingmidwiferyboard.gov.au/Codes-Guidelines-Statements/Professional-standards.aspx (Accessed 2 December 2016).

19 Canadian Nurses Association. Framework for the practice of registered nurses in Canada. (2008 Rebranded). http://www.nursingmidwiferyboard.gov.au/Codes-Guidelines-Statements/Professional-standards.aspx (Accessed 2 December 2016).

20 Nursing and Midwifery Council. The code: standards of conduct, performance and ethics for nurses and midwives. https://www.nmc.org.uk/globalassets/sitedocuments/nmc-publications/nmc-code.pdf (Accessed 2 December 2016).

21 American Nurses Association. Code of ethics for nurses. http://www.nursingworld.org/codeofethics (Accessed 2 December 2016).

22 Australian Physiotherapy Association. APA code of conduct. https://www.physiotherapy.asn.au/DocumentsFolder/APAWCM/The%20APA/Governance/Code_of_Conduct_V2013.pdf (Accessed 2 December 2016).

23 National Physiotherapy Advisory Group. Essential competency profile for physiotherapists in Canada. http://npag.ca/PDFs/Joint%20Initiatives/PT%20profile%202009%20English.pdf (Accessed 2 December 2016).

24 Chartered Society of Physiotherapy. Code of professional values and behaviour. http://www.csp.org.uk/publications/code-members-professional-values-behaviour (Accessed 2 December 2016).

25 American Physical Therapy Association. APTA guide for professional conduct. http://www.apta.org/uploadedFiles/APTAorg/Practice_and_Patient_Care/Ethics/GuideforProfessionalConduct.pdf (Accessed 2 December 2016).

26 Pharmaceutical Society of Australia. Code of ethics for pharmacists. https://www.psa.org.au/download/codes/code-of-ethics-2011.pdf (Accessed 2 December 2016).

27 National Association of Pharmacy Regulatory Authorities. Model standards of practice for Canadian pharmacists. http://napra.ca/Content_Files/Files/Model_Standards_of_Prac_for_Cdn_Pharm_March09_Final_b.pdf (Accessed 2 December 2016).

28 General Pharmaceutical Council. Standards of conduct, ethics and performance. https://www.pharmacyregulation.org/sites/default/files/standards_of_conduct_ethics_and_performance_july_2014.pdf (Accessed 2 December 2016).

29 American Pharmacists Association. Code of ethics for pharmacists. http://www.pharmacist.com/code-ethics (Accessed 2 December 2016).

30 Beauchamp TL, Childress JF. *Principles of Biomedical Ethics*, 6th Edition. Oxford: Oxford University Press, 2008.

31 Arries E. Virtue ethics: an approach to moral dilemmas in nursing. *Curationis.* 2005;28:64–72.

32 Oakley J, Cocking D. *Virtue Ethics and Professional Roles.* Cambridge: Cambridge University Press, 2006.

33 Royal College of Physicians. Doctors in society: medical professionalism in a changing world. Royal College of Physicians Working Party, 2005. https://cdn.shopify.com/s/files/1/0924/4392/files/doctors_in_society_reportweb.pdf?15745311214883953343 (Accessed 2 December 2016).

34 Irvine D. Patients want to be sure that they have a good doctor: relating public expectations to professional regulation, professional identity and professionalism.
In R Cruess, S Cruess, Y Steinert (Eds) *Teaching Medical Professionalism: Supporting the Development of a Professional Identity*, 2nd Edition. Cambridge: Cambridge University Press, 2016.

35 Wear D, Nixon LL. Literary inquiry and professional development in medicine: against abstractions. *Perspectives in Biology and Medicine.* 2002;45:104–124.

36 Krautscheid LC. Defining professional nursing accountability: a literature review. *Journal of Professional Nursing* 2014;30:43–47.

37 Dohmann E. *Accountability in Nursing. Six Strategies To Build and Maintain a Culture of Commitment.* Marblehead, MA: HCPro, Inc, 2009.

38 Milton C. Accountability in nursing: reflecting on ethical codes and professional standards of nursing practice from a global perspective. *Nursing Science Quarterly* 2008;21:300–303.

39 Williams KF. Re-examining 'professionalism' in pharmacy: a South African perspective. *Social Science & Medicine* 2007;64:1285–1296.

40 Ghadirian F, Salsali M, Cheraghi MA. Nursing professionalism: an evolutionary concept analysis. *The Journal of Nursing iranian and Midwifery Research* 2014;19:1–10.

41 Lerkiatbundit S. Professionalism in Thai pharmacy students. *Journal of Social and Administrative Pharmacy* 2000;17:51–58.

42 Hutchings HA, Rapport FL, Wright S, Doel MA, Wainwright P. Obtaining consensus regarding patient-centred professionalism in community pharmacy: nominal group work activity with professionals, stakeholders and members of the public. *International Journal of Pharmacy Practice* 2010;18:149–158.

43 Monrouxe LV, Chandratilake M, Gosselin K, Rees CE, Ho M. Taiwanese and Sri Lankan students' dimensions and discourses of professionalism. *Medical Education*. In press.

44 DePaola DP, Slavkin HC. Reforming dental health professions education: a white paper. *Journal of Dental Education* 2004;68:1139–1150.

45 Fan J-Y, Wang YH, Chao LF, Jane S-W, Hsu L-L. Performance evaluation of nursing students following competency-based education. *Nurse Education Today* 2015;35:97–103.

46 Fastré GJ, van der Klink M, Amsing-Smit P, van Merriënboer JG. Assessment criteria for competency-based education: a study in nursing education. *Instructional Science* 2014;42:971–994.

47 McCormick G, Marshall E. Mandatory continuing professional education. A review. *Australian Journal of Physiotherapy* 1994;40:17–22.

48 Smith E. A review of twenty years of competency-based training in the Australian vocational education and training system. *International Journal of Training and Development* 2010;14:54–64.

49 Crigger N, Godfrey N. From the inside out: a new approach to teaching professional identity formation and professional ethics. *Journal of Professional Nursing* 2014;30:376–382.

50 Jarvis-Selinger S, Pratt DD, Regehr G. Competency is not enough: integrating identity formation into the medical education discourse. *Academic Medicine* 2012;87:1185–1190.

51 Monrouxe LV. Theoretical insights into the nature and nurture of professional identities. In R Cruess, S Cruess, Y Steinert (Eds) *Teaching Medical Professionalism: Supporting the Development of a Professional Identity*, 2nd Edition. Cambridge: Cambridge University Press, 2016: pp 37–56.

52 Monrouxe LV, Rees CE. Theoretical perspectives on identity: researching identities in healthcare education. In JA Cleland, SJ Durning (Eds) *Researching Medical Education*. Oxford: Wiley, 2015: pp.129–140.

3

Teaching and Learning Healthcare Professionalism

'The [GP in clinical setting] actually said to us, "You know in real life you wouldn't actually spend so long washing your hands". I mean when we have competencies in clinical skills they... watch you do each step and they mark you down if you miss anything out, so then going to a GP [placement] and for them [to] say, "Oh don't spend so long washing your hands it makes the patient feel uncomfortable while waiting", and you're kind of under pressure then... I mean I just tend to do all the steps but ultra-quickly so that I'm making sure I'm doing it (laughs) but I'm not making the patient wait for ages... it makes you feel uncomfortable that the GP is kind of scoffing really... at the fact that you're spending so long washing your hands.' (laughs)

Kate, female, year 2, medical student, UK

LEARNING OUTCOMES

- To understand why teaching and learning professionalism is important
- To understand what constitutes the different elements of healthcare professionalism curricula
- To explore how healthcare professionalism is taught and learnt through different methods
- To discover the range of curricula-related professionalism dilemmas occurring across different healthcare professions
- To reflect on the various ways one could act in the face of curricula-related professionalism dilemmas

---

KEY TERMS

Formal, informal and hidden curricula
Professionalism teaching and learning
Role modelling
Professionalism curricula-related dilemmas
Moral distress
Socialization and resistance

Healthcare Professionalism: Improving Practice through Reflections on Workplace Dilemmas, First Edition.
Lynn V. Monrouxe and Charlotte E. Rees.
© 2017 John Wiley & Sons Ltd. Published 2017 by John Wiley & Sons Ltd.

Introduction

Professionalism is nowadays an explicit part of healthcare curricula across the world. In this chapter, we provide an overview of how professionalism is taught as part of formal, informal and hidden curricula. We know that healthcare students and trainees commonly engage in professionalism teaching and learning across their healthcare education, and that university- and hospital-based academics and clinicians teach professionalism to students and trainees, even when they are primarily teaching something else (e.g. anatomy dissection). While powerful learning can occur when aspects of the formal, informal and hidden curricula reinforce one another,[1] teaching and learning professionalism is not easy, particularly as students and trainees sometimes receive mixed messages from different elements of curricula about how they should embody professionalism. This is illustrated starkly in Kate's hand-washing dilemma above where she is taught a thorough hand-washing method in the simulated clinical skills environment, but which is subsequently dismissed in the real life of general practice. These mixed messages then leave her flummoxed about how she should best wash her hands professionally. In this chapter, we cover various contradictions between formal, informal and hidden professionalism curricula and how such disconnects can create professionalism dilemmas for students and trainees. We will cover numerous examples of curricula-related professionalism dilemmas across the healthcare professions and consider how students and trainees can be supported to best negotiate the conflicting messages found within healthcare curricula.

Why Teach and Learn Professionalism?

> '*Clinical excellence and unprofessional behavior rarely coexist despite the commonly held beliefs to the contrary.*'[2, p. 1043]

At a most basic level, professionalism enables members of an occupation such as medicine, nursing and allied health to earn an income while controlling their own work (see Box 3.1 for the interdependent elements of professionalism).[3] Various regulatory bodies worldwide now include professionalism among their core health professions curricula, as discussed in Chapter 2. There are three fundamental reasons for this. First, in recent decades, healthcare professions as collectives have been perceived to possess weak standards and poor self-regulation. This has resulted in a loss of patient and public trust, alongside questions being raised about the privileged positions professions hold in society.[4] Second, research shows that healthcare professionals' professionalism lapses contribute to poor patient care (leading to adverse patient events and outcomes, patient dissatisfaction, complaints and litigation). Furthermore, lapses may result in poor staff morale and reduced team collaboration.[2,5] Finally, there is growing recognition that professionalism is not something that can be developed through passive absorption: it is far too important to be left to chance.[2] Indeed, research shows that professionalism curricula can improve learners' and teachers' perceptions of students' and trainees' professionalism.[6] Ultimately, the explicit teaching of professionalism is thought to be a necessary antidote to suboptimal professionalism at the levels of the profession, the professional and the curriculum.[4,7]

> **Box 3.1 Information: interdependent elements of professionalism (Freidson)**[3, p. 127]
>
> - Specialized work based on a body of knowledge and skill and thus accorded special status
> - Authority in a particular division of labour established and monitored by occupational cooperation
> - A protected position in the labour market based on qualifications invented by the occupation
> - Formal education involving higher education producing the occupation-controlled qualifications
> - Occupational ideology of doing good quality work rather than economic efficiency

What is a Curriculum?

Although there are many different types of curricula talked about in the educational literature, we talk about three commonly discussed aspects of health professions education curricula here: formal, informal and hidden curricula. We will explain what each are in general terms in this section and how they interrelate.

Formal curricula can be described as those which are: 'stated, intended and formally offered and endorsed.'[8, p. 404] These include the planned content and methods of teaching and assessment, course handbooks, syllabi and learning objectives, and professional standards and codes of conduct stipulated by regulatory bodies (such as those already outlined in Chapter 2). The focus within formal curricula is firmly on explicit teaching (which we cover in this chapter) and assessment (covered in Chapter 4). Formal teaching and assessment can take place anywhere in health professions education, including in the clinical workplace through methods such as bedside teaching encounters. However, when we think of formal curricula, we typically think of education that happens in the structured and planned environment of the classroom: in lectures, small groups, workshops and simulation exercises.

Informal curricula have been defined as: 'opportunistic, idiosyncratic, pop-up, and often unplanned instruction that takes place between anyone who is teaching... and trainees.'[9, p. 452] This includes any serendipitous or opportunistic learning that takes place through teacher-learner interactions that are essentially unplanned. Such serendipitous teaching can often result in unanticipated learning outcomes. The educational focus within informal curricula is on what is learnt rather than what is taught (bearing in mind that teaching and learning are not necessarily the same thing). Although informal learning can take place anywhere in health professions education (including in formal classroom settings such as impromptu student questions in lectures), when we think of informal curricula we typically think of education that happens in the seemingly complex and messy environment of the clinical workplace.

Finally, hidden curricula have been described as enormous networks of: 'unwritten social and cultural values, rules, assumptions and expectations.'[9, p. 452] Learners are thought to assimilate these as they become socialized into particular communities of practice such as medicine, nursing, pharmacy, dentistry and physiotherapy. Such norms,

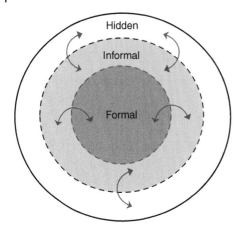

Figure 3.1 Interrelated aspects of curriculum.

values and belief systems are embedded within both curricula and the daily practices of healthcare schools and workplaces. These are: 'imparted to students through daily routines, curricular content and social relationships'.[10, p. 6] As with informal curricula, hidden curricula focuses on learning. This is concerned with what students learn through often-implicit messages transmitted to learners through the structures and cultures of the learning environment. For example, through hidden curricula students may learn that professionalism is unimportant for their future healthcare practice if it is not taught or assessed within their healthcare school (equally, students might learn through hidden curricula that professionalism *is* important if it is taught and assessed; the hidden curriculum is not always bad).[1] Given that hidden curricula are about the structures and cultures of institutions, and what these communicate to students about what is and what is not valued, it truly is anywhere and everywhere.

In Figure 3.1, we provide a visual representation of how we see the interrelations between formal, informal and hidden curricula. We choose three concentric circles instead of the Venn diagrams used by others for two reasons.[11,12] First, we think it reflects the differing amounts of professionalism learning that occurs for students as part of each curricular element, with most occurring as part of hidden curricula, and least as part of formal curricula. Second, we think formal curricula always include aspects of informal and hidden curricula, and that informal curricula in turn includes aspects of hidden curricula, but the reverse of this is not necessarily true. Hidden curricula, for example, can be manifest in the physical built environment (such as the fabric of a building), which might have little to do with formal curricula or interpersonal relationships. While some scholars seem to (erroneously) use the words 'informal' and 'hidden' curricula interchangeably, we see them as very different despite their similar educational focus on learning. Key differences between the two include their different foci, with informal curricula related to micro-level interpersonal relationships and hidden curricula concerned with macro-level organizational structures and cultures. We see hidden curricula, therefore, as omnipresent and 'bigger' than informal curricula.[13] Finally, we employ dotted rather than hard lines between these three concentric circles to illustrate the fuzzy boundaries between curricula and how they flow in and out of each other.

How is Professionalism Taught and Learnt?

Professionalism and its constituent elements are things that medical educators may think can be taught, learnt and assessed, rather like clinical communication skills.[11] In this section, we discuss the different ways in which professionalism is taught and learnt as part of formal, informal and hidden curricula. We do not talk here about *what* it is that students and trainees learn by way of professionalism (knowledge, skills, attitudes, behaviours and practices) as these are discussed in Chapter 2. Before reading the next section, stop and think about professionalism teaching and learning in your own institutional context and work through Box 3.2.

How is Professionalism Taught Through Formal Curricula?

Professionalism is thought to be one of the hardest subjects to integrate into formal healthcare curricula,[11] partly because it 'crosses departmental lines'.[4, p. 262] Considerable variation exists in formal professionalism curricula from school to school and stage to stage (e.g. pre-clinical versus clinical; undergraduate versus postgraduate). This often reflects different philosophies and resource limitations.[2] Such variation in formal professionalism curricula typically arises from differences in the levels of integration between professionalism and broader healthcare curricula, along with differences in teaching and learning methods (see Box 3.3 for further details about integration). Some scholars, for example, argue that professionalism learning should take place in the most 'authentic' context, specific to the stage of study. For example, small group learning may be more appropriate in the early years, through to less standardized clinical environments in later years.[4,11] While most educators accept such institutional variation, they

---

Box 3.2 Stop and do: reflect on professionalism teaching and learning in your own institution

- How has professionalism been taught and learnt in your school, or during your training programme?
- From your perspective as a learner, what are the strengths and weaknesses of these teaching and learning methods?
- How do these strengths and weaknesses relate to those discussed in the literature?

Box 3.3 Information: professionalism and curricular integration

Horizontal integration: The extent to which professionalism is integrated with other courses taught in the same year. Sometimes professionalism is integrated with other courses such as clinical and communication skills or ethics. At other times professionalism is provided as a stand-alone course so is not integrated.[14]

Vertical integration: The extent to which professionalism is integrated across different years of study. At some institutions, professionalism is a longitudinal thread running through all years of healthcare curricula. In other places courses are timetabled in particular years only.[11]

still expect some consistency in terms of professionalism learning outcomes,[1] as set down by regulatory bodies outlined in Chapter 2.

The literature outlines various teaching and learning methods for professionalism as part of formal curricula (see Chapter 4 for an in-depth discussion about professionalism assessment methods). Teaching and learning methods include school-based activities (such as workshops, debates, interactive lectures, small group discussions, undergraduate ethics teaching, simulation-based education, role-play exercises, videotaped consultation analyses including interactive virtual patients, and significant event analyses, arts and humanities), workplace-based activities (such as experiential and reflective learning, patient encounters with tutor feedback, case presentations, bedside teaching, mentorship and educational portfolios), and finally independent learning such as self-directed reading.[5,7,12,15–22] Interestingly, Passi *et al.*[16] identified three themes across the forty professionalism teaching and learning papers included in their systematic review: the importance of learning patient-centred approaches; reflective practice; and ethical approaches to practice.

It is not unusual for students and trainees to feel dissatisfied with formal professionalism curricula.[17] Indeed, we have repeatedly heard professionalism being referred to derogatorily as 'pink and fluffy'. Furthermore, students also notice when professionalism is not well integrated into other aspects of curricula, such as during anatomy dissection (see Box 3.4). In Box 3.4, we see a group of first-year medical students talking about a professionalism lapse of one of their colleagues during formal anatomy dissection. Despite being encouraged to write a poem about donating bodies as part of their formal curricula, they imply that their anatomy demonstrators make this student's professionalism lapse possible because of their lack of formal instruction (or supervision) during dissection classes. Interestingly, research has shown that learner satisfaction with formal professionalism curricula can increase with increased amounts of time spent engaging with formal courses on professionalism.[17]

Box 3.4 'That just leads to unprofessionalism'
JANE: I think I felt uncomfortable when… we were dissecting a vagina and… our lady [the cadaver] was quite large and he [fellow male student] cut the fat around from outside of her vagina and… he sort split the legs… then he started making it [labia] talk and I felt really uncomfortable… I was like, 'Can you just stop that… that's not treating the body with respect'.
PETER: Disrespectful.
JANE: Yeah it's disrespectful and luckily he just sort of went, 'Oh yeah', and just kind of carried on doing something else.
MEL: We had to write a poem about it [donating bodies] as part of our course and most people had actually said they'd never donate their bodies because of the way… they saw like medical students, including ourselves, treating their bodies.
DAMIAN: They [anatomy demonstrators] don't really give you much in the way of like tutorials and things… You sort of have one person wandering round like six tables so you do feel a bit lost with it and that just leads to unprofessionalism.
Jane, Peter, Mel and Damian, year 1, medical students, UK

There is no consensus about how best to teach professionalism,[15] and few studies have explored the effectiveness of different teaching and learning methods for professionalism. Indeed, Passi *et al.*[16] labelled the forty papers included in their review as typically descriptive, with each paper illustrating a single method with little comparison against other methods or evaluation of different methods. In their recent systematic review of 43 'best evidence' papers on how to teach professionalism, Birden *et al.*[15] explained that personal reflections facilitated by faculty, mentoring and role modelling were widely held to be the most effective methods for developing professionalism. Consistent with this, one recent online survey with medical students and faculty found that one third of students and faculty thought that role modelling was the most effective teaching method for professionalism. However, faculty were more likely than students to report that all methods were equally important (e.g. rules, mentoring, clinical skills simulation, reflective essays, and self-evaluation).[23] Although these findings need to be interpreted with caution given the small sample size (102 students and 14 faculties) at a single USA site and reliance on subjective opinion, much professionalism literature talks about the importance of role modelling.[2]

How is Professionalism Learnt through Informal Curricula?

As mentioned earlier, informal curricula involve the serendipitous and unplanned learning that occurs through learner-educator interactions. In the context of professionalism learning, students and trainees are thought to learn professionalism from their educators (their role models). This may be through consciously and unconsciously modelling their attitudes, skills, behaviours and practices.[24] Indeed, many scholars argue that role modelling is the principal means by which healthcare students learn professionalism,[2,5,25,26] and should be harnessed as an effective teaching tool.[16] Role models can be found across all learning environments, including university and healthcare workplace settings. They are typically defined positively, such as, 'people we can identify with, who have the qualities we would like to have, and are in positions we would like to reach'.[27, p. 707] Role models are thought to possess clinical competence (e.g. clinical knowledge, skills and reasoning), teaching skills (e.g. student-centred, communication skills) and personal qualities (e.g. compassion, honesty, integrity enthusiasm).[24,27–29] Such characteristics can be seen in the following narrative from a medical student from the USA, published by Karnieli-Miller *et al.*[30] (see narrative 1, Box 3.5).

In another narrative, this time from an Iranian nursing student, published by Karimi *et al.*,[31] we see how the doctor role models professionalism to the nursing student and her friend by emptying a patient's urine bag, a task normally done by healthcare assistants (see narrative 2, Box 3.5). Interesting, we see this doctor role model constructed as 'ideal' and thus more influential than the 'usual' nurse. Alternatively, we know that students and trainees can be disappointed by their supposed role models when those role models demonstrate behaviours antithetical to those the learners want to emulate, as illustrated in narrative 3, Box 3.5. Here, Deborah, a UK nursing student from our study, expresses her shock and sadness at the derogatory comments made by a nurse she was working with about two professional carers. She recognizes that this nurse was meant to be her role model and as such finds her comments all the more inappropriate to say in her presence.

Box 3.5 Professionalism narratives and the informal curriculum

Narrative 1: 'I saw my resident absolutely shine'

'The night my resident was supposed to be on call, I witnessed how the team concept of medicine functions… As the "bell was about to ring" for no new admissions, our team suddenly got three new admissions. The intern that was scheduled to leave was suddenly devastated as it was his first anniversary and he had been looking forward to getting home and spending it with his wife… though my resident was on call and had a very long night in front of him, he told the intern to go home and that he would handle the new admissions… I saw my resident absolutely shine as he juggled his patients, other doctors' patients, and new patients in stride without wasting a moment.'

Year 3, medical student, USA [30, p. 375]

Narrative 2: 'a physician came and emptied the bag'

'The patient's urine bag was full. One of my friends wanted to empty that because it was harassing for the patient, and we knew what complications it might bring about. But a nurse said: "No, don't do that; it's a nurse assistant's duty." Then we saw that a physician came and emptied the bag. It was really instructive for us. Well, physicians are very ideal in our minds, and ideals are always more influential than those usual individuals.'

Nursing student, Iran [31, p. 5]

Narrative 3: 'they are supposed to be a role model'

'Remarks made by a nurse I was working with directed at two other healthcare professionals were derogatory. I was sitting in a car with the qualified nurse I was working with, we had just pulled up outside our patient's house. Two carers got out of a car in front of us and walking into the same house we were going into. The nurse I was working with said, "Look at… those two, it makes you wonder where they get these people from"… I was shocked at what she had said… [I feel] sad that people have these sorts of attitudes towards other people and feel it is inappropriate to say something like this to someone they are supposed to be a role model to.'

Deborah, female, year 3, nursing student, UK

Narrative 4: 'we try to learn the new way'

'They want you to… take history in efficient way, yeah, and we often see that in the OPD [outpatient department], because the outpatient department we got, the professors were very famous, and they will kind of like [have] 120 patients and they have to finish it in the morning and that's mission impossible, but they have to do it as fast as they can… Even there's one teacher in the paediatrics department we are now in, he taught us about how can we be efficient and ask questions to make, to finish the patient as soon as possible… it's quite counteracting our previous learning in the medical school. But he said… "it's… our reality and you're in Taiwan so you have to do this"… so I think it's… the most major challenge, one of the most major challenges when we came into the clinical situation in Taiwan… it's like they [medical school] telling you to ask open questions, and in the clinical situation "closed ended questions are best" (soft laughter)… so whenever we get to a new department (soft laughter) we try to learn… the new way.'

Yang, male, year 4, medical student, Taiwan

Bandura's[32] classic social learning theory illustrates that learners' responsiveness to role modelling is dependent on: the attributes of the role models; the characteristics of the learners; and the perceived response consequences of the learner matching the model's behaviours. Role models with high status and power are more influential in evoking matched behaviour in learners than role models with low status/power.[32] This is illustrated neatly in narrative 2, Box 3.5 above. More recently, Cruess *et al.*[24] have postulated that learning from role models occurs by active observation of role models and either: (1) unconscious incorporation of the observed behaviours into students' and trainees' practices; or (2) conscious reflection and attunement to emotion and values. The latter are then translated into principles and action, meaning that learners may consciously decide to adopt or resist the observed behaviours of their role models. The impact of such conscious reflection and attunement to emotion and values on the subsequent behaviour of students is apparent in narrative 4 from Yang, a Taiwanese medical student (see Box 3.5). In this narrative, he shares the dilemma of observing celebrated professors (those with high status and power) in his hospital interviewing patients very quickly with closed questions in order to get through large numbers of consultations in a short time frame. He consciously reflects that this behaviour contradicts the patient-centred approach he has been taught in medical school. He tunes into his emotion by stating twice that this is a 'most major challenge', also using laughter to potentially cope with the discomfort that this dilemma causes him and his fellow students. However, despite this conscious reflection and attunement to emotion and values, Yang still adopts the observed practices of his celebrated professors.

What is important for healthcare students and trainees is that they should reflect on such negative role modelling, understand why such lapses may occur, and use that reflection to guide their own professionalism.[16] From educators' perspectives, role modelling could be improved by increasing educators' awareness of being professionalism role models (known as role modelling consciousness).[28] It could also be improved through being explicit to students and trainees about what they are modelling to them and why, alongside being reflexive about which professionalism behaviours they are modelling (or not) and participating in faculty development for professionalism.[4,24] Cruess *et al.*[24] also talk about how institutional cultures for role modelling can be improved through identifying and addressing barriers to effective role modelling (e.g. increased time to teach).

How is Professionalism Learnt through Hidden Curricula?

As discussed above, hidden curricula are manifest in institutional structures and cultures, which communicate to learners often unspoken and implicit survival rules.[8,33] Several authors, therefore, argue that learners' grasp of hidden curricula is just as important as their grasp of formal curricula.[9] While hidden curricula can function as positive and negative forces,[1] many researchers have focused on the negative aspects of hidden curricula. For example, over a decade ago, Lempp and Seale[33] outlined the (often negative) 'content' of hidden curricula in medical education, including: loss of idealism; adoption of ritualized professional identities; emotional silence; decreased ethical integrity; acceptance of hierarchy; and learning informally aspects of being a good doctor. In their interviews with 36 medical students across all years in one school, they found the medical school to be hierarchical and competitive with haphazard and belittling teaching.[33] Sadly our own multi-site research across healthcare professions and involving thousands of students shows a similar picture a decade on.[34-37]

Students and trainees can learn professionalism through hidden curricula by paying attention to various things including: (1) the role of the physical environment; (2) the importance of the body; and (3) intentional socialization practices plus resistance to those same socialization practices.[38] Futhermore, Hafferty[8] talks about the importance of language such as institutional slang for communicating important messages to students and trainees about what is and is not valued and the way things are 'done around here'. Regarding the physical environment, students and trainees learn in a multiplicity of settings, including university, hospital and community-based facilities. Within the university, students can learn what subjects are most and least valued by their schools through, for example, the stature, prominence and layout of different classrooms used for different subjects, and by the timetabling of subject teaching within the curriculum.[38,39] For example, healthcare students can quickly learn that biomedical sciences are highly valued if they are taught in the most well-maintained classrooms, have the greatest prominence in the timetable in terms of teaching hours, and are taught during the most popular times of the day. Likewise, healthcare students can swiftly learn that professionalism is unimportant if it is taught in neglected classrooms, has little timetabled contact hours, and is repeatedly taught in unpopular slots such as late Friday afternoon.

Within the clinical setting, students can also learn important (yet implicit) messages about professionalism from the physical environment. For example, several pharmacy students told us how patients attending the pharmacy for methadone needed to come to the back door to get their prescriptions rather than entering the front of the shop like other patients. This sent powerful messages to students that patients requiring methadone were second-class citizens – untouchables – who should not mix with other patients. Furthermore, many healthcare students across our data narrated professionalism lapses involving patient dignity that related to the physical layout of hospital wards with their multiple beds separated by flimsy curtains (see Chapter 8). In the following narrative from Olivia, a UK medical student, she makes it clear how the physical layout of the ward, combined with the thoughtless treatment of the patient by the doctor, all serve to breach the privacy and dignity of an elderly dying woman (see narrative 1, Box 3.6). What is clear from this narrative is that healthcare students can learn from the physical ward environment alone that patient privacy and dignity is not as important as formal curricula suggest.

In terms of the body, according to Gair and Mullins[38, p. 31] hidden curricula are manifest in the: 'gendered, racialized, class-based bodies of students and faculty'. Healthcare students across our study spoke severally about physical manifestations of professionalism by way of appearance, including personal grooming and clothing (see 'professionalism as presentation', discussed in Chapter 2). While some students talked about receiving lectures as part of their formal curricula about how they should dress, students typically learnt what constitutes a professional appearance through hidden curricula by observing how healthcare professionals dressed (e.g. wearing smart and clean conservative clothes or profession-specific uniforms, being well-groomed with good hygiene, etc.). Furthermore, some students explained how they learnt about dressing professionally by receiving feedback from their clinical teachers on their own appearance. As illustrated by narrative 2 (Box 3.6) such feedback was often received as unwelcome. Here, Tessa, a UK nursing student explains her upset when she is told her attire is 'too

---

Box 3.6 Professionalism dilemmas and the hidden curriculum

Narrative 1: 'I asked whether we could move the lady to a side room'

'[the dilemma took place on a] Care of the Elderly [COTE] placement. Patient dying with death rattle from aspiration pneumonia. Doctor called three students to come and see. Family had not arrived. [It was in a] cubicle on four-bed bay. Curtains drawn… doctor decided to teach us about death in a bay where other patients could hear rather than moving patient to another room. I asked whether we could move the lady to a side room so the other patients wouldn't hear what was going on to respect the dying lady and her confidentiality. [I feel] sad that I stayed to see the woman and watch her die. It seemed callous… and three of us looked like a parade, it wasn't respectful.'

Olivia, female, year 5, medical student, UK

Narrative 2: 'I was not projecting the health visitors' professional image'

'I was told that they [health visitors] all had been conferring and concluded I was not projecting the health visitors' professional image, I was wear[ing] a black shift dress, black cardigan and black tights and it was too "sexually" focused. The health visitor had pulled me into a room on my own but she was referring to the three health visitors and health visitor student. She walked out, I started crying, and she sent me home. [I] contacted my learning team facilitator at the university who then asked for a meeting. [I did that because] I felt alone and had four women completely knock my confidence. I needed help and the university was the only place I could go. [I feel] sick, bullied, angry. These women made my placement impossible for me… [In the end], the university asked me to apologize to the health visitors which I refused as they were ganging up on me [and] when one of them is wearing a denim mini skirt! I've lost all my confidence and I'm not sure I want to be associated with people who think that behaviour is acceptable.'

Tessa, female, year 3, nursing student, UK

Narrative 3: 'I knew my treatment technique was correct'

'[The] physio challenged me as to why I used particular treatment technique, asking why I was doing this technique over more commonly used techniques. This made patient ask tricky questions, and question me about treatment. I told physio why exactly I was doing this particular treatment, explaining my reasons for this. I then turned to patient and explained what I would be doing and asked again whether he consented to treatment. [I did that because our] university training taught us specific situations and how to deal with it, therefore I knew my treatment technique was correct and answered questions accordingly.'

Dee, female, year 3, physiotherapy student, UK

---

sexually focused', particularly given that one of the health visitors was wearing a denim mini-skirt, which Tessa implies was more unprofessional than what she was wearing.

With respect to intentional socialization practices, Hafferty[8] talks about policies contained within recruitment brochures and student and faculty handbooks that convey implicit messages about what is and what is not valued by institutions. Michaelec and

Hafferty[39, p. 394] argue, for example, that medical schools suggest both directly and tacitly to medical students through hidden curricula that they are the crème de la crème: 'superior, smarter and of more social worth than those outside of medicine'. This reinforces traditional interprofessional hierarchies, divisions of labour and conflicts (see Chapter 12).[40,41] Intentional socialization practices are what healthcare schools do in order to reproduce the 'right' social roles, habits of mind and interests in their students and faculty, reinforced further through rewards such as awards and promotions.[8,38] For example, a medical school within a research-intensive university will most probably want to produce research-orientated medical graduates. Meanwhile, a nursing school committed to social accountability will most likely want to produce nursing graduates committed to patient and public involvement. One could argue that formal healthcare professionalism curricula are intentional socialization practices in their own right. They aim to produce professional healthcare graduates with the 'right' social roles (e.g. nurse as patient advocate) and habits of mind (e.g. honesty, integrity, patient-centredness, etc.). Although such intentional socialization practices can and do produce graduates of the 'right' ilk, we know that such practices can also yield strategic compliance (i.e. bending to institutional constraints but choosing to retain opposing beliefs) and resistance (i.e. challenging the prevailing cultures).[38] Such resistance to intentional socialization practices can be seen in narrative 3, Box 3.6, where Dee, a physiotherapy student explains how her physiotherapy teacher challenged a certain treatment technique she was using in front of the patient. Despite this challenge being uncomfortable for Dee, she resists her teacher's advice, instead explaining to her teacher (and the patient) why she was using her preferred treatment technique.

What Curricula-related Professionalism Dilemmas do Healthcare Students Experience?

We know from our own and others' research that learners are commonly bombarded with mixed messages from different aspects of curricula about how they should embody professionalism. Indeed, the narratives presented so far illustrate a range of mixed messages experienced by healthcare students including: 'wash your hands thoroughly' versus 'wash your hands quickly'; 'maintain the cadaver's dignity' versus 'it's okay to make jokes about the cadaver to help you cope'; 'treat your healthcare colleagues with respect' versus 'it's okay to disrespect other healthcare colleagues'; 'use patient-centred communication skills' versus 'use doctor-centred communication in order to see patients quickly'; 'maintain the dignity and privacy of dying patients' versus 'it's okay to treat dying patients as a spectacle to help students learn'; 'students deserve respect from their teachers' versus 'it's okay for teachers to disrespect students as part of the learning process'; and finally 'use the most appropriate treatment technique' versus 'use the most common/expected treatment technique'. What we see from all of the narratives presented so far is that there is a central disconnect between what healthcare students are explicitly taught (the way things *should* be done) versus the way things *are* done. At this point, stop and think about curricula-related professionalism dilemmas you have experienced and work through Box 3.7.

Although students are not always concerned by such mixed messages (see Box 3.8 by way of illustration), they typically do experience frustration when they are taught one

---

Box 3.7 Stop and do: reflect on curricula-related professionalism dilemmas you have experienced

- Have you experienced any curricula-related professionalism dilemmas?
- If so, write down your experience(s) thinking about where you were and who was present, what happened, what you did and why and how you felt? Try to articulate what your dilemma was at the time.
- What might you do differently if faced with a similar curricula-related professionalism dilemma in the future?

Box 3.8 'I noticed that was wrong and against what I'd been taught'

Senior dentist was checking patient without gloves on. [I was] in hospital (on the dental clinics), nursing for dental student X who had a patient who was being checked by Professor Y (who is a dentist). [The] senior dentist was checking patient without gloves on. [I did] nothing [because I] did not want to call him up in front of the patient, especially as he was one of my main tutors. [I] don't care [about it now], he didn't really do anything invasive. This wasn't a huge dilemma but it was something I noticed that was wrong and against what I'd been taught.'

Stan, male, year 2, dental student, UK

---

thing and see another.[42] Moreover, such mixed messages can go beyond mere frustration for healthcare students with them sometimes experiencing severe moral distress as a result of professionalism dilemmas. This may arise when they know the ethically correct behaviour but feel thwarted to act in such a manner.[43] We will see such examples of dilemmas and moral distress throughout Sections 2 and 3, where we provide numerous illustrations, including those involving identity (Chapter 5), consent (Chapter 6), safety (Chapter 7), dignity (Chapter 8), student abuse (Chapter 9), e-professionalism (Chapter 10), cross-cultural (Chapter 11) and interprofessional dilemmas (Chapter 12).

We provide just one example here from Tania, an Australian medical student, who shares her experience of various dignity lapses involving patients undergoing pelvic examinations by a particular gynaecologist in a rural practice (see Box 3.9). Tania has been taught to maintain patient dignity during pelvic examinations in various ways, ways that her gynaecologist teacher flouts, leaving her feeling: 'really, really uncomfortable'. Her own discomfort, coupled with her friends' horror, gives Tania the impetus to challenge the gynaecologist, first indirectly (through asking him where she should get a sheet from, to which he tells her not to worry) and then more directly (through telling him she thinks the women would be more comfortable with the sheet, a concern which he also dismisses). Thus the gynaecologist thwarts Tania's attempts to act professionally, resulting in severe moral distress for Tania (e.g. 'absolutely horrendous', 'so uncomfortable', coupled with laughter for coping). This leads her peer, Christine, to comment explicitly on the gap between 'what you get taught and what you see', and to explain that such gaps become more acceptable as students progress through their course as they understand better why such gaps exist and start to justify those gaps.

So, given these mixed messages and the distress they can cause healthcare students, how should students and educators deal with such curricular gaps? While some authors

---

Box 3.9 'There's always a gap between what you get taught and what you see'

TANIA: When I was out at country [rural practice] I was with a gynaecologist… usually in a gynaecology room you know there's a sheet for women to put over themselves when they're lying down half naked and I soon realized that there was no sheet… a lot of these women were undressing without a curtain, getting up onto the table, being examined and then still lying on the table half undressed. He would chat to them about what was going on and what he wanted to do about it and I found it really, really uncomfortable… then I talked about [it] with some girls that I lived with and they were just horrified and so the next time… I went in and helped set up the room and said, 'Oh, there's a sheet missing, where would I get a sheet from', and he was like, 'Oh we don't worry about that out here', and I said, 'Really? 'cause I mean I'm sure that they would feel more comfortable if there was…', 'Oh don't worry about it, it's fine,' and… that was the end of that… it was horrendous *it was absolutely horrendous* (said laughingly). I felt so uncomfortable for these women and you could tell they were so uncomfortable…

CHRISTINE: There's always… a gap between what you get taught and what you see.

TANIA: Huge.

CHRISTINE: And the further you get into the programme I think the more acceptable that gap sometimes gets… you start realizing why that gap exists and in a way you start justifying it… time constraints, this, this and that, because we start seeing that then we start justifying it, you know?

TANIA: Absolutely, I mean he's a gynaecologist for twenty odd years, he's seen a hundred million thousand vaginas, he doesn't care but he's forgotten that to that woman it's different… I don't want to be treated as though I'm another hundred thousandth vagina… I'm a person and I have my modesty… it doesn't get much more (said laughingly)… undignified than being half naked with your legs wide open… you know like 'jeez'. (laughs)

(Tania and Christine, female, year 4, medical students, Australia)

---

argue that we should all be striving to eliminate gaps, for example by ensuring that all educators behave according to institutional values and agreed definitions,[11] we think this is improbable given the complexities of the healthcare workplace, which is often described as challenging and stressful.[2] Instead of removing contradictions for students and trainees entirely, we think they need help to navigate their way through the mixed messages and for them to reconnect the disconnects between formal, informal and hidden curricula themselves. Many authors have suggested that students and trainees need to have a place within formal curricula to discuss their professionalism dilemmas and we would agree with this approach. For example, numerous healthcare educators have employed small group discussion including professionalism narratives as a professionalism teaching tool, and one that can help students integrate the disconnects between formal, informal and hidden curricula.[30,44,45] This book is one such attempt to help students reflect on their professionalism dilemmas and understand that they are not alone in their experiences. In turn, this book aims to help learners work out how best to tackle such dilemmas in the future to protect themselves, their colleagues and importantly, patients.

Chapter Summary

This chapter has provided an overview of why we teach and learn professionalism, what the interrelated elements of professionalism curricula are and how professionalism is taught and learnt. While we know that powerful learning can occur when aspects of the formal, informal and hidden curricula reinforce one another and that learning from the hidden curriculum is not always bad;[1] this chapter has illustrated how disconnects between formal, informal and hidden curricula for professionalism can create professionalism dilemmas for students and trainees and moral distress when learners' desires to act in ethically appropriate ways are thwarted. We have learnt about various common curricula-related dilemmas in this chapter, and how students and trainees can be helped to connect the disconnects between the mixed messages they receive. We outline how this can be done by reflecting critically on their own professionalism dilemma narratives, sharing and discussing them with others, and recommitting to their professionalism ideals.[46] Stop and think about learners' and educators' curricula-related professionalism dilemmas and work through Box 3.10.

The key take-home messages for healthcare students, trainees and educators from this chapter are summarized in Box 3.11. Suggestions for small group discussions around the topic of curricula-related dilemmas can be found in Box 3.12. Finally, Boxes 3.13 and 3.14 outline some reflective exercises and recommended reading.

Box 3.10 Stop and do: reflect on curricula-related professionalism dilemmas presented in this chapter

- Re-read all the curricula-related professionalism dilemmas in this chapter, being mindful of the complexities of learning professionalism through formal, informal and hidden curricula.
- Thinking about learners' dilemmas, how might learners cope better with the mixed messages they receive about professionalism? How might learners manage the moral distress they may feel when their desires to act professionally/ethically are thwarted?
- Thinking about teachers' dilemmas, how might teachers develop strategies to model professionalism wherever possible? How might teachers explain their professionalism lapses to students? How might teachers help students to manage the mixed messages they receive about professionalism?

Box 3.11 Chapter summary points

- It is important to teach and learn professionalism for optimal patient care and because professionalism cannot be learnt by chance.
- Learners and teachers need to appreciate the different methods of teaching and learning professionalism as part of formal, informal and hidden curricula.
- Key challenges facing professionalism curricula, teaching and learning exist, including mixed messages from different aspects of curricula.
- Learners and teachers should consider how best to navigate their way through common curricula-related professionalism dilemmas.

Box 3.12 Chapter discussion points

- What do you think is the most powerful aspect of curricula in terms of learning professionalism, and why?
- What do you think are the most effective teaching and learning methods for professionalism, and why?
- How might students and trainees be better empowered to resist the professionalism lapses of their role models?

Box 3.13 Chapter learning activities

- Think about a recent or most-memorable curricula-related professionalism dilemma of your own (different to Box 3.7.)
- Write down the details of the dilemma: what was the gist of your dilemma, where and when did it take place, who was there, what happened, what did you do and why, how did you feel?
- How can you understand your experience better by applying what you now know about professionalism curricula, teaching and learning from this chapter?
- Using what you now know, how could you cope better with this dilemma if it happened again? What could you do differently next time?
- What advice would you give to one of your peers if they had this same experience?

Box 3.14 Chapter recommended reading

Bahaziq W, Crosby E. Physician professional behavior affects outcomes: a framework for teaching professionalism during anesthesia residency. *Canadian Journal of Anesthesia* 2011;58:1039–1050.

Cruess SR, Cruess RL, Steinert Y. Role modelling – making the most of a powerful teaching strategy. *British Medical Journal* 2008;336:718–721.

Felstead I. Role modelling and students' professional development. *British Journal of Nursing* 2013;22(4):223–227.

Hafferty FW. Beyond curriculum reform: confronting medicine's hidden curriculum. *Academic Medicine* 1998;73(4):403–407.

Passi V, Doug M, Peile E, Thistlethwaite J, Johnson N. Developing medical professionalism in future doctors: a systematic review. *International Journal of Medical Education* 2010;1:19–29.

References

1 Hafferty FE, O'Donnell JF. The next generation of work on the hidden curriculum. In FW Hafferty, JF O'Donnell (Eds) *The Hidden Curriculum in Health Professional Education.* New Hampshire: Dartmouth College Press, 2014: pp. 233–263.

2 Bahaziq W, Crosby E. Physician professional behavior affects outcomes: a framework for teaching professionalism during anesthesia residency. *Canadian Journal of Anesthesia* 2011;58:1039–1050.

3 Freidson E. *Professionalism. The Third Logic.* Oxford: Polity Press, 2001.

4 Cruess SR, Cruess RL. Teaching professionalism – why, what and how. *Facts, Views & Visions in OBGYN* 2012;4(4):259–265.

5 Deptula P, Chun MBJ. A literature review of professionalism in surgical education: suggested components for development of a curriculum. *Journal of Surgical Education* 2013;70(3):408–422.

6 Hochberg MS, Berman RS, Kalet AL, Zabar SR, Gillespie C, Pachter HL, *et al.* The professionalism curriculum as a cultural change agent in surgical residency education. *The American Journal of Surgery* 2012;203:14–20.

7 Steinert Y, Cruess S, Cruess R, Snell L. Faculty development for teaching and evaluating professionalism: from program design to curriculum change. *Medical Education* 2005;39:127–136.

8 Hafferty FW. Beyond curriculum reform: confronting medicine's hidden curriculum. *Academic Medicine* 1998;73(4):403–407.

9 Wear D, Skillicorn J. Hidden in plain sight: the formal, informal and hidden curricula of a psychiatry clerkship. *Academic Medicine* 2009;84(4):451–458.

10 Margolis E. Peekaboo. Hiding and outing the curriculum. In E Margolis (Ed.) *The Hidden Curriculum in Higher Education.* New York: Routledge, 2001: pp.1–19.

11 O'Sullivan H, van Mook W, Fewtrell R, Wass V. Integrating professionalism into the curriculum: AMEE Guide No. 61. *Medical Teacher* 2012;34:e64–e77.

12 Schafheutle EI, Hassell K, Ashcroft DM, Harrison S. Organizational philosophy as a new perspective on understanding the learning of professionalism. *American Journal of Pharmaceutical Education* 2013;77(10):214. doi: 10.5688/ajpe7710214.

13 O'Donnell JF. The hidden curriculum – a focus on learning and closing the gap. In FW Hafferty, JF O'Donnell (Eds) *The Hidden Curriculum in Health Professional Education.* New Hampshire: Dartmouth College Press, 2014: pp. 1–20.

14 Walsh Lang C, Smith PJ, Friedman Ross L. Ethics and professionalism in the pediatric curriculum: a survey of pediatric program directors. *Pediatrics* 2009;124(4):1143–1151.

15 Birden H, Glass N, Wilson A, Harrison M, Usherwood T, Nass D. Teaching professionalism in medical education: a best evidence medical education (BEME) systematic review. BEME guide no. 25. *Medical Teacher* 2013;35:e1252–e1266.

16 Passi V, Doug M, Peile E, Thistlethwaite J, Johnson N. Developing medical professionalism in future doctors: a systematic review. *International Journal of Medical Education* 2010;1:19–29.

17 Van Mook WNKA, de Grave WS, van Luik SJ, O'Sullivan H, Wass V, Schuwirth LW, *et al.* Training and learning professionalism in the medical school curriculum: current considerations. *European Journal of Internal Medicine* 2009;20:e96–e100.

18 Rutter PM, Duncan G. Can professionalism be measured? Evidence from the pharmacy literature. *Pharmacy Practice* 2012;8(1):18–28.

19 Strawbridge JD, Barrett AM, Barlow JW. Interprofessional ethics and professionalism debates: findings from a study involving physiotherapy and pharmacy students. *Journal of Interprofessional Care* 2014;28(1):64–65.

20 Schwartz B, Bohay R. Can patients help teach professionalism and empathy to dental students? Adding patient videos to a lecture course. *Journal of Dental Education* 2012;76(2):174–184.

21 Numminen O, Leino-Kilpi H, van der Arend A, Katajisto J. Comparison of nurse educators' and nursing students' descriptions of teaching codes of ethics. *Nursing Ethics* 2011;18(5):710–724.

22 Ernstzen DV, Statham SB, Hanekom SD. Learning experiences of physiotherapy students during primary healthcare clinical placements. *African Journal of Health Professions Education* 2014;6(2)S1:211–216.

23 Morihara SK, Jackson DS, Chun MBJ. Making the professionalism curriculum for undergraduate medical education more relevant. *Medical Teacher* 2013;35:908–914.

24 Cruess SR, Cruess RL, Steinert Y. Role modelling – making the most of a powerful teaching strategy. *British Medical Journal* 2008;336:718–721.

25 Brown J, Stevens J, Kermode S. Supporting student nurse professionalization: the role of the clinical teacher. *Nurse Education Today* 2012;32:606–610.

26 Felstead I. Role modeling and students' professional development. *British Journal of Nursing* 2013;22(4):223–227.

27 Paice E, Heard S, Moss F. How important are role models in making good doctors? *British Medical Journal* 2002;325(7366):707–710.

28 Wright SM, Carrese JA. Excellence in role modeling: insight and perspectives from the pros. *Canadian Medical Association Journal* 2002;167(6):638–643.

29 Burgess A, Goulston K, Oates K. Role modeling of clinical tutors: a focus group study among medical students. *BioMed Central Medical Education* 2015;15:17. doi: 10.1186/s12909-015-0303-8.

30 Karnieli-Miller O, Vu R, Frankel RM, Holtman MC, Clyman SG, Hui SL, *et al.* Which experiences in the hidden curriculum teach students about professionalism? *Academic Medicine* 2011;86(3):369–377.

31 Karimi Z, Ashktorab T, Mohammadi E, Ali Abedi H. Using the hidden curriculum to teach professionalism in nursing students. *Iranian Red Crescent Medical Journal* 2014; 16(3):e15532.

32 Bandura A. *Social Learning Theory*. New York: General Learning Press, 1971.

33 Lempp H, Seale C. The hidden curriculum in undergraduate medical education: qualitative study of medical students' perceptions of teaching. *British Medical Journal* 2004;329:770–773.

34 Monrouxe LV, Rees CE. 'It's just a clash of cultures': emotional talk within medical students' narratives of professionalism dilemmas. *Advances in Health Sciences Education* 2012;17(5):671–701.

35 Monrouxe LV, Rees CE, Endacott R, Ternan E. 'Even now it makes me angry': healthcare students' professionalism dilemma narratives. *Medical Education* 2014;48:502–517.

36 Rees CE, Monrouxe LV, McDonald LA. My mentor kicked a dying woman's bed: analysing UK nursing students' most memorable professionalism dilemmas. *Journal of Advanced Nursing* 2015;71(1):169–180.

37 Rees CE, Monrouxe LV, McDonald LA. Narrative, emotion, and action: analysing 'most memorable' professionalism dilemmas. *Medical Education* 2013; 47(1):80–96.

38 Gair M, Mullins G. Hiding in plain sight. In E Margolis (Ed.) *The Hidden Curriculum in Higher Education*. New York: Routledge, 2001: pp. 21–41.

39 Michaelec B, Hafferty FW. Stunting professionalism: the potency and durability of the hidden curriculum within medical education. *Social Theory & Health* 2013;11(4): 388–406.

40 Rees CE, Monrouxe LV. Professionalism education as a jigsaw. Putting it together for nursing students. In T Brown, B Williams (Eds) *Evidence-Based Education in the Health*

Professions. Promoting Best Practice in the Learning and Teaching of Students. London: Radcliffe, 2015: pp. 96–110.

41 Rees CE, Monrouxe LV, Ajjawi R. Professionalism in workplace learning: understanding interprofessional dilemmas through healthcare student narratives. In D Jindal-Snape, EFS Hannah (Eds) *Exploring the Dynamics of Personal, Professional and Interprofessional Ethics*. Bristol: Policy Press, 2014: pp. 295–310.

42 Leo T, Eagen K. Professionalism education: the medical student response. *Perspectives in Biology & Medicine* 2008;51(4):508–516.

43 Monrouxe LV, Rees CE, Dennis A, Wells S. Professionalism dilemmas, moral distress and the healthcare student: insights from two online UK-wide questionnaire studies. *British Medical Journal Open* 5:e007518. doi:10.1136/bmjopen-2014-007518.

44 Kittmer T, Hoogenes J, Pemberton J, Cameron BH. Exploring the hidden curriculum: a qualitative analysis of clerks' reflections on professionalism in surgical clerkship. *The American Journal of Surgery* 2013;205:426–433.

45 Rogers DA, Boehler ML, Roberts NK, Johnson V. Using the hidden curriculum to teach professionalism during the surgery clerkship. *Journal of Surgical Education* 2012;69(3): 423–427.

46 Christakis DA, Feudtner MA. Ethics in a short white coat: the ethical dilemmas that medical students confront. *Academic Medicine* 1993;68:249–54.

4

Assessing Healthcare Professionalism

'I got so worried [about doing the dental impressions] I got him [clinical supervisor] to check every stage and... so I waited and he did it [checked the X-ray] a bit slow so it took about 15 minutes on the appointment waiting for him, he knew I was waiting there and he said... knowing that 15 minutes has gone by... "Yeah just wanted to know if you were trying to check the patient because... you've wasted 15 minutes of the patient's time", and so he got me in trouble for wasting time... he actually gave me [professionalism] penalty points for that... you only get six penalty points [per year] and he gave me two... I said to [person in charge of professionalism assessment system] "If we're governed by clinicians in the point system what's governing clinicians?... there should be a system for clinicians as well"'

Christopher, male, year 5, dental student, UK

LEARNING OUTCOMES

- To understand why healthcare professionalism is assessed
- To explore how healthcare professionalism is assessed through different methods
- To understand key challenges facing professionalism assessment
- To discover the range of assessment-related professionalism dilemmas occurring across different healthcare professions
- To reflect on the various ways one could act in the face of assessment-related professionalism dilemmas

---

KEY TERMS

Professionalism assessment
Workplace-based assessment
Feedback
Professionalism assessment-related dilemmas

Healthcare Professionalism: Improving Practice through Reflections on Workplace Dilemmas, First Edition.
Lynn V. Monrouxe and Charlotte E. Rees.
© 2017 John Wiley & Sons Ltd. Published 2017 by John Wiley & Sons Ltd.

Introduction

We live within organizational cultures of measurement and accountability. Within such cultures, healthcare students and trainees typically have their professionalism assessed at multiple times and in numerous different ways. Similarly, healthcare educators, particularly clinical teachers, will inevitably face the requirement to assess students' and trainees' professionalism, as well as give them feedback to facilitate their professionalism development. However, professionalism assessment is a tricky business: how can we really measure something that may be hidden away deep inside individuals? How can we assess something that might in large part be a feature of the surrounding context rather than a characteristic possessed by an individual learner? Given such difficulties, it should be no surprise that healthcare learners and teachers often experience a range of assessment-related professionalism dilemmas. These include students receiving purportedly unjust professionalism assessments, like Christopher above, learners failing to challenge the professionalism lapses of their teachers for fear of being failed, students receiving abusive feedback and assessment from their teachers and teachers being reluctant to fail learners for their underperformance in professionalism. In this chapter, we cover all of these interrelated issues to help you navigate your way through the minefield of healthcare professionalism assessment.

Why Assess Professionalism?

Before we tackle why professionalism is assessed, we first need to think about why we assess anything in health professions education. Assessment may be formative (where the focus is on facilitating students' and trainees' learning through constructive feedback) or summative (where pass/fail decisions are made about student and trainees' progress). In terms of formative assessment, professionalism assessment is important as it helps students develop their professional attitudes, behaviours and practices in a way that is consistent with the expectations set out by regulatory bodies as illustrated in Chapter 2,[1-4] and ultimately society (particularly in the face of high-profile examples of professionalism lapses).[5] As for summative assessment, professionalism assessment is important for two very different reasons. First, the protection of patients and colleagues is paramount and professionalism assessment can prevent professionalism lapses.[6] We know from the research literature, for example, that qualified doctors who face disciplinary action from regulatory bodies had higher incidences of professionalism lapses when they were students.[7] This suggests that the professionalism lapses of healthcare students might be a predictor for their later lapses as qualified healthcare practitioners. Second, we know that students and trainees value and learn what is assessed. Conversely, they devalue and do not learn what is not assessed, a hidden curriculum issue (as discussed in Chapter 3). By assessing professionalism summatively, healthcare schools and postgraduate training programmes send implicit yet powerful messages to students and trainees that professionalism is vital to healthcare practice; that it is valued by the school/programme, its teachers and regulatory bodies; and that it is crucial for their successful progression within their chosen profession.[8] Indeed, if learners demonstrate unsatisfactory performance in professionalism assessment (and if remediation attempts prove unsuccessful) they will be required to exit their studies. Ultimately, there is no message more powerful than this in communicating the importance of professionalism to future and current healthcare practitioners.

How is Professionalism Assessed?

Given the complexity of what professionalism might be (see Chapter 2), it is understandable that various medical educators argue for a longitudinal and multi-method approach to assessing professionalism: multiple methods that go beyond simply observing the professional behaviours of students and trainees.[8–10] The selection of assessment methods should, of course, depend on the purpose of the assessment (formative or summative) and the characteristics of the assessment methods, such as reliability (i.e. reproducibility of assessment scores) and validity (i.e. the test measures what it is supposed to measure).[6] Obviously, medical educators are more concerned about the reliability and validity of summative (rather than formative) professionalism assessments to ensure that any pass/fail decisions are defensible.[11] Although some authors argue for the assessment of professionalism at individual, interpersonal and institutional levels,[10,12] we will focus on the individual level in this chapter, as this is the primary concern of healthcare students.

At this point, it is perhaps helpful to consider an often-cited framework in the assessment literature: Miller's framework for clinical assessment – *knows, knows how, shows how* and *does* – which has previously been linked to professionalism assessment.[8,10,11,13] Miller's 'pyramid' has at its foundation students' and trainees' knowledge (*knows*), on which their competence (*knows how*) is based. Grounded on such knowledge and competence is students' and trainees' performance (*shows how*), and their ultimate action (*does*). Adequate achievement at the foundational levels (*knows* and *knows how*) are thought to be essential for attainment of higher levels but are not sufficient in themselves to predict performance at the *shows how* and *does* levels.[11,14] In Figure 4.1, inspired by the PhD of one of our colleagues (Dr Madawa Chandratilake), we have inverted Miller's classic pyramid to illustrate how we see professionalism assessment as typically

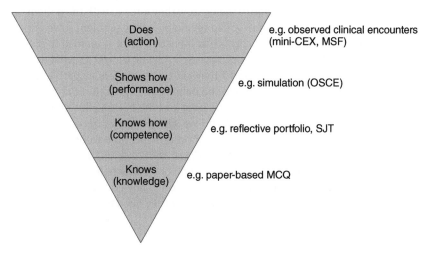

Figure 4.1 Framework for professionalism assessment based on Miller[13].

at the *shows how* and *does* levels.[13] Note that we would describe the boundaries between these four levels as fuzzy.

Professionalism Action: *does*

Many professionalism measures nowadays rely on assessors making judgements about learners' observable professionalism behaviours.[10,15] Students' and trainees' professionalism behaviours and practices within the clinical workplace are typically assessed using observed clinical encounters such as the mini-Clinical Evaluation Exercise (mini-CEX), the Professionalism Mini-Evaluation Exercise (P-MEX) based on the mini-CEX format,[16] or multi-source feedback (MSF).[17] It is outside the scope of this chapter to discuss all of these, so instead we consider the mini-CEX as this is probably the most widely used tool internationally, at both undergraduate and postgraduate levels of education (see Wilkinson *et al.*[17] for an overview of other methods of assessing observable behaviours).

The mini-CEX is used by clinical teachers on the basis of their 15–30 minute observations of learners' interactions with real patients in the clinical workplace. Clinical teachers are required to rate, via graded 'tick-boxes', the extent to which they think students and trainees meet their expectations at their particular stage of training in various domains such as medical interviewing, physical examination skills, communication skills, clinical judgement, organization skills and professionalism. In addition to the rating scales, the mini-CEX also encourages qualitative comments from the clinical teacher about the learners' behaviours. While reliability and validity findings for the mini-CEX have been variable, studies have found it to be reliable with ten encounters, with acceptable construct and criterion validity, plus it is thought to be 'authentic'.[18,19]

By way of illustration, let us consider Box 4.1, from our Academy of Medical Royal Colleges-funded study exploring supervised learning events (SLEs) and workplace-

---

Box 4.1 'It's real life'

'We have a trainee who's currently in difficulty and we had an extra assessment for her a couple of months ago… in the mini-CEX when you're in a clerk situation, the patient is there, you're seeing the whole package, you're seeing how they interact with the patient, you're seeing how [their] knowledge base is, you're seeing how they problem solve and it… was the most valuable tool for us in this particular trainee because it seemed to pick out where the gaps were… I think it's a good tool because… it's real life and it's what their job is, what they'll be doing day-in day-out and if they can't do that there's a problem… she didn't take a good history, she didn't listen to the patient who was a nurse and gave a very good history… and her knowledge base was poor and she became flustered and out-of-depth and it became obvious doing that and we sat in with her because it was a problem… we're never trained in these things and no one has time to do it with a person… beforehand a lot of the boxes were just ticked, just tick boxes and no text, so the comments are where you get the valid information and no one either had time to put in comments or didn't feel comfortable putting comments on… any consultant doing it either won't have time to do it properly or aren't aware that they need to pinpoint either good or poor practice.'

Jane, female, postgraduate trainer, UK[20]

based assessments (WPBAs) in the UK Foundation Programme.[20] Here, Jane, a clinical teacher, explains how she prefers the mini-CEX to other methods of WPBA because they are more authentic assessments. She shares this view by narrating a specific experience with a trainee in difficulty, in which she purposely used the mini-CEX to observe the trainee's actions thereby opening the door to remediation opportunities. Interestingly, Jane finishes her narrative by explaining that while the most valuable part of the mini-CEX is the opportunity to provide free-text comments, busy doctors are more likely to just tick the boxes, which is a common criticism of such rating scales.[9] The reasons she cites for this lack of engagement are trainers' lack of time, their lack of knowledge around good assessment practice and the social aspects of assessment. We will return to these issues later when we discuss educators' assessment-related dilemmas around *failure to fail* practices.

Professionalism Performance: *shows how*

Medical educators commonly assess students' professionalism by observing their performance while interacting with simulated patients within Objective Structured Clinical Examinations (OSCEs). While OSCEs vary from one institution to the next, they typically involve multiple 'stations'. For example, the United States Medical Licensing Examination (USMLE) Step 2 Clinical Skills OSCE is a 12-station examination where each candidate is allowed 15 minutes for each patient encounter, along with 10 minutes to record each patient note. The trained simulated patients assess the patient encounters and trained physician raters assess the student's written patient notes. Students are scored in terms of three sub-components in the USMLE: (1) integrated clinical encounter (e.g. data gathering, data interpretation); (2) communication and interpersonal skills (e.g. patient-centredness); and (3) spoken English proficiency (e.g. pronunciation, word choice).[21] Although OSCEs are standardized and reliable with sufficient station numbers of reasonable durations, and have reasonable face and content validity, they can be resource intensive and lack the authenticity of workplace-based assessments.[6,22]

Professionalism Competence: *knows how*

Students and trainees sometimes have their professionalism assessed in terms of their ability to apply their knowledge of professionalism principles in order to reason through real professionalism dilemmas they have experienced themselves. Such assessments can be in the form of critical incident reports (often as part of reflective portfolios) or through paper- or video-based tests that present professionalism dilemmas to learners and ask them how best they should act within those situations. This latter type of assessment includes the situational judgement test (SJT), which has gained in popularity over the last few years and is now part of selections assessments for healthcare schools and postgraduate healthcare education in some countries.[23,24] While SJTs vary from one programme to the next, the SJT for the UK Foundation Programme is a 140-minute examination consisting of 70 questions, each including a vignette and one of two response formats: ranking five responses in order of appropriateness or choosing three from eight possible responses as appropriate (see Box 4.2). While such tests can have acceptable reliability with sufficient numbers of items and construct validity, test scores

---

Box 4.2 Information: example of SJT 'professionalism dilemma test'

At your morning briefing you are informed by Infection Control that all hospital staff must roll their sleeves up when they have any clinical interaction with patients. During your shift you notice that your FY1 colleague always has her sleeves down.

Rank in order the appropriateness of the following actions in response to this situation (1 = Most appropriate; 5 = Least appropriate).

A Tell Infection Control that your colleague is not complying with their policy (5)
B Speak directly to your FY1 colleague about your observation (1)
C Raise your observation with the nurse in charge of the ward (3)
D Do not say anything immediately but monitor the situation over the course of the next few days (4)
E Discuss the situation with your registrar/specialty trainee (2)

Example of item on the SJT Practice Paper for UK Foundation Programme and SJT Answers (see: http://www.foundationprogramme.nhs.uk/pages/medical-students/SJT-EPM)

---

do not necessarily predict professionalism performance or action in simulated or real settings.[6,17,23] However, there is some emerging evidence that SJTs may better predict the in-role performance of trainees with lower SJT scores at the postgraduate level.[25,26]

Professionalism Knowledge: *knows*

Professionalism assessment methods that measure knowledge (*knows*) without its application (*knows how*) are extremely rare in the literature. Blue *et al.*,[27] for example, assessed the knowledge and attitudes of three cohorts of students at two institutions during their orientation. They employed two professionalism knowledge instruments, a vignette-based instrument like the SJT discussed above (measuring *knows how*) and an instrument asking students to select the best answer for 17 multiple choice and true/false questions reflecting one of the professionalism attributes such as humanistic values, ethics and moral values, self-reflection, accountability and subordinating self-interest (measuring *knows*). Combining together these *knows how* and *knows* items, Blue *et al.*[27] found that the five scales of the instrument lacked reliability and did not correlate with their professionalism attitudes scales. However, others argue that multiple choice tests generally can have excellent face and content validity and can test students' underlying knowledge about principles of professionalism, such as those espoused by regulatory bodies.[6,17] They cannot, however, assess how students might apply that knowledge to real-life practice.[6,17]

What are the Key Challenges Facing Professionalism Assessment?

So far, we have explored why we assess professionalism and the common types of assessment at Miller's *does, shows how, knows how and knows* levels.[13] We have already begun to talk about the challenges facing professionalism assessment methods, in terms

---

Box 4.3 Stop and do: reflect on how your professionalism has been assessed within your institution

- How has your professionalism been assessed in your school, or during your training programme, according to Miller's four levels?
- From your perspective as a learner, what are the strengths and weaknesses of these assessment methods?
- How do these strengths and weaknesses relate to those found in the literature (see recommended reading later)?

---

of their psychometric properties (e.g. reliability, validity), especially when they are used for summative assessment purposes.[28] At this point, stop and think about your own experiences of professionalism assessment methods and work through Box 4.3.

In this section, rather than continue our discussion about the psychometric challenges of different assessment methods, we instead talk about some other key concerns that map onto our own research and lived experiences of teaching and assessing professionalism. First, it is hard to measure something that is difficult to define.[11] As we have seen from Chapter 2, there is no universal agreement about what professionalism is: instead, it is something that is constructed differently by different people, within different cultures and within different time periods.[29]

Second, there are challenges around assessment methods that focus purely on observational behaviours rather than knowledge, attitudes, perceptions and reasoning.[27] We have previously discussed such challenges and similarly argued for professionalism assessment methods that extend beyond observational methods.[30] For example, we have discussed how attitudes are poor predictors of behaviours when contextual constraints such as social pressure to act in an unprofessional manner are strong.[30] While students are perfectly capable of 'faking' professionalism for the purposes of professionalism assessments based on observation, students might similarly exhibit professionalism lapses because of contextual pressures such as role-modelling (as discussed in Chapter 3) rather than because their behaviour is indicative of any underpinning unprofessional attitudes.[30]

Third, assessment methods often collect quantitative (or tick-box) data with a simultaneous dearth of qualitative comments, thereby denying learners meaningful developmental feedback to help them improve their future professionalism.[9,20] Such tick-boxes also have the added problem of eliciting *halo* and *horn* effects.[9] For example, interviews with 19 internal medicine attendees at two Canadian universities revealed that they tended to overlook or excuse deficiencies of residents thought to be excellent (*halo* effect), and similarly ignored the competence and excellence exhibited by residents labelled as problematic (*horn* effect).[15] We also know that professionalism assessors are often reluctant to fail students or provide them with negative feedback about their professionalism behaviours, also known as the 'leniency error'.[11,31]

Finally, as mentioned above, professionalism is dependent on broader contextual factors, including students' and trainees' relationships with their senior colleagues and those seniors role-modelling appropriate behaviours and practices to students and trainees.[10,12] Linked with this, there are thought to be inequities in professionalism assessment across organizational hierarchies, with assessments typically directed at

> **Box 4.4 Stop and do: reflect on any assessment-related professionalism dilemmas you have experienced**
>
> - Have you experienced any assessment-related professionalism dilemmas?
> - If so, write down your experience(s) thinking about where you were and who was present, what happened, what you did and why and how you felt. Try to articulate exactly what your dilemma was at the time.
> - What might you do differently if faced with a similar assessment-related professionalism dilemma in the future?

those occupying the lowest rather than the highest rungs of the hierarchy.[10,32] It is perhaps unsurprising that with these professionalism challenges come innumerable assessment-related professionalism dilemmas, which we turn to next. Before reading the following section, stop and think about your own experiences of assessment-related professionalism dilemmas and work through Box 4.4.

What Assessment-related Professionalism Dilemmas are Learners Experiencing?

We have elicited many assessment-related professionalism dilemmas within our research programme across a variety of healthcare student groups, including students receiving purportedly unjust professionalism assessments (recall Christopher's narrative earlier), healthcare students not challenging clinical teachers' professionalism lapses within the workplace for fear of being failed by them, healthcare students receiving abusive feedback and clinical teachers being reluctant to fail underperformance in students. We consider these issues in turn next.

Receiving Unjust Professionalism Assessments

We elicited various narratives in our study where students reported receiving what they thought to be unjust professionalism assessments. These include students being criticized for elements of professionalism based on the personal opinions of clinical teachers that went beyond professionalism guidelines set down by regulatory bodies (see Chapter 2). Other dilemmas concerned differences of opinion between students and clinical teachers about students' behaviour and students getting blamed for things that they did not think were their fault.

Narrative 1 of Box 4.5 illustrates an example of purportedly unjust professionalism assessment from a UK dental student. Michael complains about receiving a professionalism lapse card from his clinical teacher for sporting a beard, despite Michael believing his appearance to be professional. He challenges his professionalism lapse card because he cannot find any evidence in the National Health Service (NHS) dress code to say that he should not wear a beard and he explains that he continues to wear his beard as a 'sign of resistance'.

In narrative 2, Box 4.5, we see Derek, a physiotherapy student, being accused of sexism by his female physiotherapy teacher for things that he has said, which according

---

Box 4.5 Dilemma narratives about students receiving unjust professionalism assessments

---

Narrative 1: 'he then issues me with a lapse of professionalism card'

'Professor challenged my personal appearance in front of a patient… [The] professor decided that my beard was not a professional appearance (which was trimmed and shaped everyday, about 2–3 mm in length) and began to tell me off in front of patient and other student. He rhymed off NHS dress code in front of patient. He then issued me with a lapse of professionalism card… I then challenged the lapse of professionalism through the proper channels. [I did this because] I felt that I was perfectly professional in appearance and that the professor was forcing his perception of what is professional on me. There was nothing within the NHS dress code document that backed up his argument… I still have my beard which I will keep until I graduate as a sign of resistance to that prof.'

Michael, male, year 2, dental student, UK

Narrative 2: 'felt that I had been wrongly accused'

'Felt I was being treated unfairly and things I said were always taken in the worst possible way or in a way that it wasn't meant to be taken and false accusations of being sexist… [The] final assessment [was] to be filled out [but I was] taken into an office behind a closed door. [I was] accused of several ridiculous things and things that I had said [were] blown out of proportion and interpreted in a sinister way. [I] genuinely felt that it was a sexist driven attack (female towards male). [I] put my points forward and asked her to explain why she felt that what she was saying was correct. [I did this because I] felt that I had been wrongly accused and wanted to know why she felt the way she did… [I] thought it was a huge joke, totally blown out of proportion.'

Derek, male, year 2, physiotherapy student, UK

---

to Derek had been misconstrued. He explains how his physiotherapy teacher takes him into an office at the end of his placement to give him feedback, which he describes as 'ridiculous' and which he constructs as a 'sexist driven attack' towards him. He describes the experience as a 'joke' because he believes his behaviour was 'totally blown out of proportion.'

Finally, to return to the narrative at the start of this chapter, Christopher, a UK dental student shares his experience with us where he received two professionalism penalty points (a third of his allowance for the whole year) from his clinical teacher for keeping a patient waiting while he got an X-ray checked by that same teacher. Christopher also constructs himself as professional in his narrative in that he seeks feedback from his clinical teacher about the quality of his work before proceeding with dental impressions. His narrative suggests that he thinks that these penalty points are unjust because it is his clinical teacher who keeps him waiting for the X-ray thus delaying the patient. Christopher bemoans the hypocrisy of a professionalism assessment system that penalizes *his* professionalism lapses, but not those of his clinical teacher who kept him (and the patient) waiting. Such critique is found elsewhere in the literature where students complain of professionalism assessment systems having a disproportionate focus on professionalism lapses rather than promoting and rewarding professionalism, and systems with double standards, which focus almost exclusively on students' professionalism rather than that of their clinical teachers and indeed, turns a blind eye to the professionalism lapses of their clinical teachers.[32] Although professionalism assessments for clinical teachers are beginning to be developed, such as the Professionalism Assessment of Clinical Teachers (PACT) tool developed in Canada, the research literature has yet to establish fully the psychometrics of such tools.[33]

The Student's Dilemma: Fear of being Failed

Across our data we have numerous examples from all healthcare student groups of students 'going along with' their clinical teachers' professionalism lapses due to fear of being failed. This is illustrated in narrative 1, Box 4.6, where Margaret, a medical student, explains how she failed to make a direct challenge towards her clinical teacher for insulting a patient about her weight because she thought he might fail her. Although she explains how she did not challenging him directly, she does report him to the medical school on her feedback form and expresses her 'hope' that the medical school acts on her feedback.

However, some students do respond in the face of professionalism lapses (see narrative 2, Box 4.6). Sarah, a nursing student, explains how she challenged professionalism lapses on her placement in a private nursing home. She describes how she repeatedly complained to the management of the nursing home and that her complaints eventually led to the manager threatening to fail her and get her thrown off her nursing course. She describes how she reported the situation to the university (who asked her to turn a blind eye) and to the Care Quality Commission (who conducted an inspection after the manager had rectified the perceived problems). Sarah constructs herself as saddened by this experience and now anxious about returning to her placements.

In the final narrative in this section, we see how James, a medical student, also challenges what he perceives to be professionalism lapses on his clinical psychology placement (see narrative 3, Box 4.6). He explains how he challenges the clinical team's interviewing of a teenage girl, which he thinks contributes to the girl's reluctance to talk. He describes how his placement partner warns him to expect a bad mark for his professionalism assessment (an MSF form) after his challenge, and his peer Fiona explains that students worry too much about their professionalism marks. What is interesting about all of the examples in this section is that while students fear being failed for challenging, when they do challenge professionalism lapses (as shown in narratives 2 and 3, Box 4.6) their fears are not realized.

The Student's Dilemma: Receiving Abusive Feedback in the Workplace

In Chapter 9, we discuss in great detail the abuse experienced by healthcare students as part of their workplace learning experiences. Here, we talk specifically about the abuse experienced as part of students' assessment and feedback experiences, plus the abuse that students actively take without complaint in order to secure positive assessments of their performance (so similar to the above section). This is illustrated in a narrative by Sally, a medical student, who explains that she and her colleagues were verbally abused by a clinical teacher because they could not answer questions on topics beyond their level of competence (see narrative 1, Box 4.7). She describes how she regrets not challenging him but felt that if she had complained it would not have been taken seriously, an issue commonly mentioned across the narratives.[34,35]

Box 4.6 Professionalism dilemma narratives around students' fear of failure

Narrative 1: 'he was my assessor and could have failed me'

'A doctor insulting a patient about her weight in front of her because she didn't speak English. [I was on a] GP placement, one other student [was present]. He was comparing her to him and how much she had "let herself go". [I] told the med school on the feedback form and acted cold towards the doctor. [I did that because] he was my assessor and could have failed me if I challenged him directly. I hope the med school have read and acted on the feedback.'

Margaret, female, year 5, medical student, UK

Narrative 2: 'threatened to fail me and have me thrown off the course'

'I was on placement at a nursing home where they didn't use PPE [personal protective equipment] or correct manual handling procedure. I reported it to the deputy manager... It carried on so I brought it up again and then reported it to the manager who on a num- ber of occasions was very aggressive and threatened to fail me on everything and to have me thrown off the course... I then spoke to the university who said I need[ed] to turn a blind eye. I then contacted CQC [Care Quality Commission], as I felt patients were at risk, who came in and did an inspection at which point the manager made sure all the appro- priate staff had the knowledge of what to do in certain situations and put PPE out around the home on show... I feel very sad about it all still as because of this experience I am now very nervous to return to practice...'

Sarah, female, year 1, nursing student, UK

Narrative 3: 'you're going to get a really bad PPD mark now'

JAMES: We had like clinical psychologist placement... there's... a young 15-year-old girl with her mum and it [interview room] had blacked out windows on one side of the room... and then two cameras on either side of the room and then three micro- phones built in sort of strategically round the room... there was a registrar in the room with her, a specialist nurse and a clinical psychologist, a trainee clinical psy- chologist and two medical students sat behind the various screens and they were trying to get her to talk about her deepest feelings... it was an entire hour of... questioning her and she said about three words during the entire [interview]... after the meeting they were all sat around (laughs) speculating about what could be wrong with this girl and I said... "What's the harm in just interviewing her in a normal room in a normal situation with just one or two people present... what's the harm in having a couple of women interviewing her"... my placement partner (laughs) came out laughing, she says, "You know you're going to get a really bad PPD [personal professional development] mark now because they're going to go back and moan about you to the medical school"...

FIONA: A lot of people do worry too much about whether they are going to get a good PPD.

James and Fiona, male and female, medical students, UK

Box 4.7 Professionalism dilemmas around students receiving abusive feedback

Narrative 1: 'too scared to report, was being assessed'

'[I was] verbally abused by clinician who threatened to fail us. [This happened during a] feedback session with two other students. He grilled us on topics we had not yet covered as this was our first week of first year. We were competent in the particular speciality we had been placed with but this was ignored… [I was] too scared to report, [because I] was being assessed. [I am] still upset and wish [I] had challenged. [I] feel a complaint would not be taken seriously'

Sally, female, year 3, medical student, UK

Narrative 2: 'I wanted to make sure they gave me a really good reference'

'I had a horrible placement in the summer… because the staff weren't very nice to me and they… spoke down to me quite a lot in front of… the patients… the pharmacist was there, he didn't stop it and sort of laughed along with it… they sort of said a few things to me like, "Don't worry about that the child will do it… the little kid, you can come and do it"… and then I would go off to do whatever menial task they'd like left me to do… they were like deliberately picking horrible jobs for me to do… I didn't say anything 'cause I didn't want them to say, "Oh she can't stick out four weeks in a shop… she can't hack it"… I wanted to make sure they gave me a really good reference so I could get my pre-reg 'cause I wanted it with this company, I was like, "I'll just keep quiet and I'll just get through it"'

Iris, female, year 4, pharmacy student, UK

Narrative 3: 'I was too scared that anything I do or say might result in an actual FAIL'

'My consultant did not acknowledge me at all even though I turned up to most of the teaching sessions and seemed to treat my male colleague with utmost respect and seemed to be eager to aid his learning… The same question asked by me and my colleague got two different responses from him – he snapped at me, but he was okay with my colleague. When it came to coursework… not surprisingly, my colleague got really good marks and I got a "safe" mark… [I did] nothing [because] I was too scared that anything I do or say might result in an actual FAIL in the exam or should I end up working under my consultant, there might be repercussions. I feel alright about it now, as I know I did not do anything to make my consultant dislike me, so I put it down to differences in race and sex'

Hayley, female, year 4, medical student, UK

In narrative 2, Box 4.7, Iris, a pharmacy student narrates her 'horrible' summer placement experience because she was the recipient of abuse from the community pharmacy staff. She explains that the pharmacist went along with the jokes from the pharmacy staff and did nothing to challenge them. As can be seen from Iris' narrative, she takes this abuse without complaint because she does not want the pharmacy staff to think she cannot handle their taunts, and she also wants to receive a good reference from the pharmacist because she wants to do her pre-registration training with the same company. Although this reference is not a university-based professionalism assessment as such, it is still an assessment to be used for her to secure her pre-registration place and so essential for her career progression.

We see a similar story from Hayley, a medical student, who explains receiving abuse from her clinical teacher (see narrative 3, Box 4.7). She contrasts her treatment with that of her male colleague, who was treated much better, Hayley putting this down to her different race and gender. However, she does nothing to challenge this consultant for fear of receiving an 'actual fail' or to prevent any repercussions should she work with this consultant again.

The Assessor's Dilemma: Fear of Failing

At the end of Jane's mini-CEX narrative in Box 4.1 earlier, she explains that clinical teachers sometimes lack the time, comfort or awareness in terms of providing qualitative comments on assessment forms, thereby denying learners opportunities for constructive feedback. Such reluctance to provide any feedback, let alone feedback that could be construed as negative, can be really problematic for both formative and summative professionalism assessment and has been illustrated in the literature.[31]

For example, we conducted a qualitative interview study with 70 medical educators from two different UK schools in order to explore their reluctance to fail underperforming students and give them constructive feedback about their underperformance (including professionalism assessment).[31] In that study, we identified numerous different reasons for clinical teachers' failure to fail including: they like the student (tutors' attitudes towards the students), they expect negative outcomes from failing the student such as additional work (tutors' attitudes towards failing students), other colleagues think the student's professionalism is acceptable (tutors' normative beliefs and motivation to comply), the tutor doubts their own professional judgement (tutors' self-efficacy), the tutor is unclear what the expected standards of professionalism are by level of training (tutors' skills and knowledge), or the tutor has insufficient time to fail the student and/or give them negative feedback (environmental constraints).

In narrative 1, Box 4.8, Emma, a clinical tutor explains how she gave one of her medical students an overall 'satisfactory' for an MSF professionalism assessment form, despite ticking some elements on the form as 'unsatisfactory'. She explains that she decided on assessing the student as 'satisfactory' overall because the student had health issues and second, because she did not like the student. Her reluctance to fail the student can therefore be seen as the tutor trying to take into account her illness and compensating for her dislike of the student.

However, not all assessors *fail to fail* students' underperformance or fail to give them constructive feedback, as illustrated in narrative 2, Box 4.8, from Tess, a UK nurse postgraduate trainer who participated in our supervised learning event (SLE) study.[20,36] She shares her experience of giving feedback to a struggling trainee, which she describes as 'challenging' and 'difficult' for several reasons: the trainee had spent limited time within that placement in order to understand fully nurse-doctor relationships (environmental constraints); the trainee was upset by the feedback and did not like being criticized (tutor's attitudes towards the student); and the trainee did not accept the constructive feedback as readily as perhaps another student would (tutor's attitudes towards the student).

Box 4.8 Professionalism dilemmas around teachers' fear of failure

---

Narrative 1: 'I can't mark her down just because I don't like her'

'I was thinking of one student I had, a third-year student I had last year… I gave her some unsatisfactory ticks and there were two issues that made me err on the side of going for an overall satisfactory. One of which, she had some health issues which meant that her attendance was appalling and you know there was lots of illness… she alluded to the fact she was going to have surgery and various other things going on. And so I thought … "I've sort of got to take that into account", and I was also aware of the fact that there was something about her that I didn't warm to, you know, I was aware of a negative reaction and I sort of was again compensating for that, thinking, "I can't mark her down just because I don't like her."'

Emma, female, GP and small group tutor, UK[31, p. 803]

Narrative 2: 'it's never nice is it, giving constructive criticism?'

'I've had a recent example with an F1 and a consultant actually asking me to assess this person taking a mental state from a patient and it being quite … challenging (laughs)… [the mental state] wasn't taken in the way I would've taken it… but it was quite difficult as well to give the feedback… after the interview with the patient I actually spent quite a bit of time with the F1 and told them how I would've done it differently and what it was about their interaction that I felt wasn't as helpful as it could've been… I think initially the person concerned was a bit upset but it's never nice is it, giving constructive criticism? (laughs)… but we have [to]… I think it's different with different people, some people accept it a lot easier than others and this particular person didn't much like being… criticized although I didn't feel like I was criticizing.'

Tess, female, nurse postgraduate trainer, UK[20,36]

Narrative 3: 'I wouldn't want my family to be treated by them'

'I think it's quite difficult to fail… and I see that in the school system, and the university system as well, where people never actually get taken to task if they're not good enough. It's always about more and more support… they [assessors] are becoming a little bit more assertive in identifying people that are not good enough to complete the course. I think SLE [supervised learning events], you don't necessarily have to fail a person, but I think you should still have the opportunity to be quite exact and honest in your feedback, and there you can still say, "This is not good enough…" I also feel that sometimes the feedback that is given to students is not always entirely open, I feel there's a lot of veiling going on and euphemisms, because they [assessors] don't want to upset students… which I find very irritating. Sometimes people just need to hear, "You're not good enough", you know, "Pull up your socks, or there's a consequence"… and I think if students have passed and they're not good enough, I wouldn't want my family to be treated by them.'

Martin, male, postgraduate trainer, UK[20]

We give the last word to Martin in this section (see narrative 3, Box 4.8), another UK postgraduate trainer from our SLE study.[20] Martin complains about the issue of *failure to fail*, suggesting that the issue arises from an overly positive and nurturing educational culture, starting at school and continuing at university, where students are given more and more support rather than critical feedback. Although Martin suggests that the situation may be improving in medical school with the better identification of students who are under-performing, he expresses how assessors in the postgraduate realm are still anxious about giving 'honest' feedback to trainees for fear of upsetting them, as has been suggested by other authors.[37] He brings the issue of *failure to fail* back round to the main reason for assessing students' and trainees' professionalism summatively: the importance of patient safety (discussed at the start of this chapter). As he very powerfully points out, he would not want his family to be treated by doctors who had passed their professionalism assessment but were 'not good enough'. This highlights a common professionalism assessment conundrum faced by healthcare educators: the need to balance a duty of care to students in the here and now with a duty of care to patients in the future.

Chapter Summary

This chapter has provided an overview of why we assess professionalism in healthcare education, how professionalism is assessed at Miller's four levels, the key challenges facing professionalism assessment and various assessment-related professionalism dilemmas. We must not forget that professionalism assessment, and in particular, constructive feedback on performance is crucial in helping learners develop their professionalism, as illustrated by Helen, a foundation year 2 doctor participating in our SLE study: 'We took it up a notch and really focused on... how I could really improve and to be honest I'm actually realizing this now as I spoke to you that Mini-CEX it's probably one of the reasons why I've improved for FY2.'[20] However, from our professionalism dilemmas study, we know that learners experience numerous assessment-related dilemmas, including: receiving unjust professionalism assessments, not challenging teachers' professionalism lapses for fear of being failed and receiving abusive feedback by clinical teachers. While some students do nothing in the face of these dilemmas, others resist through direct challenges of clinical teachers or reporting lapses to their healthcare schools, and even to external agencies. What is interesting about these learners' dilemmas is that their fears of being failed should they challenge were often unfounded. Linked to this, assessors' dilemmas are often around *failing to fail* underperforming learners for a multiplicity of individual, interpersonal and contextual reasons. Stop and think about both learners' and assessors' professionalism-assessment related dilemmas and work through Box 4.9.

The key take-home messages for healthcare students, trainees and educators from this chapter are summarized in Box 4.10. Suggestions for small group discussions around the topic of assessment-related professionalism dilemmas can be found in Box 4.11. Finally, Boxes 4.12 and 4.13 outline some learning activities and recommended reading.

Box 4.9 Stop and do: reflect on the assessment-related professionalism dilemmas in this chapter

- Re-read all the professionalism assessment-related dilemmas in this chapter, being mindful that assessment and feedback is a two-way process.
- Thinking about learners' dilemmas, how might learners reduce their fears of being failed? How might learners increase their receptivity to negative/constructive feedback? How might they reduce any defensiveness and resistance to such feedback?
- Thinking about assessors' dilemmas, how might assessors address their fears of failing students and giving them negative/constructive feedback? How might assessors develop their abilities to give negative/constructive feedback? How might assessors cope with learners' defensiveness and resistance to feedback?

Box 4.10 Chapter summary points

- It is important to assess professionalism so that students receive developmental feedback and patients are protected
- Learners and teachers should appreciate the strengths and weaknesses of key approaches to professionalism assessment
- Multiple challenges exist with respect to assessing professionalism
- Learners and teachers should consider how best to navigate their way through common assessment-related professionalism dilemmas

---

Box 4.11 Chapter discussion points

- Leo and Eagan[32] talk about an 'aura of negativity [from students] whenever the word professionalism is mentioned'. Why might this be? What can be done to reduce such negativity?
- How could professionalism be rewarded through formative and summative assessment?
- How might learners and assessors understand each other's dilemmas better?

Box 4.12 Chapter learning activities

- Think about a recent or most-memorable assessment-related professionalism dilemma of your own (different to Box 4.4.)
- Write down the details of the dilemma: what was the gist of your dilemma, where and when did it take place, who was there, what happened, what did you do and why and how did you feel?
- How can you understand your experience better by applying what you now know about professionalism assessment from this chapter?
- Using what you now know, how could you cope better with this dilemma if it happened again? What could you do differently next time?
- What advice would you give a peer if they had this same experience?

Box 4.13 Chapter recommended reading

Leo T, Eagen K. Professionalism education: the medical student response. *Perspectives in Biology & Medicine* 2008;51(4):508–516.

Wilkinson TJ, Wade WB, Knock LD. A blueprint to assess professionalism: results from a systematic review. *Academic Medicine* 2009;84:551–558.

Zijlstra-Shaw S, Robinson PG, Roberts T. Assessing professionalism within dental education; the need for a definition. *European Journal of Dental Education* 2011;16:e128–e136.

References

1 General Medical Council. Good Medical Practice. Manchester: General Medical Council, 2013, http://www.gmc-uk.org/static/documents/content/GMP_.pdf (Accessed 2 December 2016).

2 General Dental Council. Standards for the Dental Team. London: General Dental Council, 2013, http://www.gdc-uk.org/Dentalprofessionals/Standards/Documents/Standards%20for%20the%20Dental%20Team.pdf (Accessed 2 December 2016).

3 Health & Care Professions Council. Council Standards of Conduct, Performance and Ethics. London: HCPC, 2012, http://www.hcpc-uk.org/assets/documents/10004EDF Standardsofconduct,performanceandethics.pdf (Accessed 2 December 2016).

4 Nursing & Midwifery Council. The Code: Standards of Conduct, Performance and Ethics for Nurses and Midwives. London: NMC, 2015, https://www.nmc.org.uk/globalassets/sitedocuments/nmc-publications/nmc-code.pdf (Accessed 2 December 2016).

5 Francis R. *Report of the Mid Staffordshire NHS Foundation Trust Public Inquiry. Executive Summary*. London: The Stationery Office, 2013.

6 Sullivan C, Arnold A. Assessment and remediation in programs of teaching professionalism. In RL Cruess, SR Cruess and Y Steinert (Eds) *Teaching Medical Professionalism*. New York: Cambridge University Press, 2009: pp. 124–149.

7 Papadakis M, Arnold GK, Blank LL, Holmboe ES, Lipner RS. Performance during internal medicine residency training and subsequent disciplinary action by State Licensing Boards. *Annals of Internal Medicine* 2008;148:869–876.

8 Zijlstra-Shaw S, Robinson PG, Roberts T. Assessing professionalism within dental education; the need for a definition. *European Journal of Dental Education* 2011;16:e128–e136.

9 Van Mook WNKA, Gorter SL, O'Sullivan H, Wass V, Schuwirth LW, van der Vleuten CPM. Approaches to professional behavior assessment: tools in the professionalism toolbox. *European Journal of Internal Medicine* 2009;20:e153–e157.

10 Goldie J. Assessment of professionalism: a consolidation of current thinking. *Medical Teacher* 2013;35:e952–956.

11 Hawkins RE, Katsufrakis PJ, Holtman MC, Clauser BE. Assessment of medical professionalism: who, what, when, where, how and why? *Medical Teacher* 2009;31:348–361.

12 Hodges BD, Ginsburg S, Cruess R, Cruess S, Delport R, Hafferty F, *et al.* Assessment of professionalism: recommendations from the Ottawa 2010 Conference. *Medical Teacher* 2011;33:354–363.

13 Miller GE. The assessment of clinical skills/competence/performance. *Academic Medicine* 1990;65(9):S63–67.

14 Clauser BE, Margolis MJ, Holtman MC, Katsufrakis PJ, Hawkins RE. Validity considerations in the assessment of professionalism. *Advances in Health Sciences Education* 2012;17:165–181.

15 Ginsburg S, McIlroy J, Oulanova O, Eva K, Regehr G. Toward authentic clinical evaluation: pitfalls in the pursuit of competency. *Academic Medicine* 2010;85(5):780–786.

16 Cruess R, McIlroy JH, Cruess S, Ginsburg S, Steinert Y. The professionalism mini-evaluation exercise: a preliminary investigation. *Academic Medicine* 2006;81(1):S74–S78.

17 Wilkinson TJ, Wade WB, Knock LD. A blueprint to assess professionalism: results from a systematic review. *Academic Medicine* 2009;84:551–558.

18 Al Ansari A, Ali SK, Donnan T. The construct and criterion validity of the mini-CEX: a meta-analysis of the published research. *Academic Medicine* 2013;88(3):413–20.

19 Pelgrim EAM, Kramer AWM, Mokkink HGA, van den Elsen L, Grol RPTM, van der Vleuten CPM. In-training assessment using direct observation of single-patient encounters: a literature review. *Advances in Health Sciences Education* 2011;16:131–142.

20 Rees CE, Cleland JA, Dennis A, Kelly N, Mattick K, Monrouxe LV. Supervised learning events in the UK Foundation Programme: a nationwide narrative interview study. *British Medical Journal Open* 2014;16:4(10) e005980. doi:10.1136/bmjopen-2014-005980.

21 United States Medical Licensing Examination. Step 2 Clinical Skills (CS). Content description and general information. National Board of Medical Examiners and the Educational Commission for Foreign Medical Graduates, 2014, http://www.usmle.org/pdfs/step-2-cs/cs-info-manual.pdf (Accessed 2 December 2016).

22 Smith V, Muldoon K, Biesty L. The objective structured clinical examination (OSCE) as a strategy for assessing clinical competence in midwifery education in Ireland: a critical review. *Nurse Education in Practice* 2012;12:242–247.

23 Patterson F, Ashworth V, Zibarras L, Coan P, Kerrin M, O'Neill P. Evaluations of situational judgement tests to assess non-academic attributes in selection. *Medical Education* 2012;46:850–868.

24 Patterson F, Ashworth V, Mehra S, Falcon H. Could situational judgement tests be used for selection into dental foundation training? *British Dental Journal* 2012;213(1):23–26.

25 Cousans F, Patterson F, Edwards H, Walker K, McLachlan JC, Good D. Evaluating the complementary roles of an SJT and academic assessment for entry into clinical practice. *Advances in Health Sciences Education* 2016. https://doi.org/10.17863/CAM.4578.

26 Patterson F, Zibarras L, Ashworth V. Situational judgement tests in medical education and training: research, theory and practice: AMEE Guide No. 100. *Medical Teacher* 2016;38:3–17.

27 Blue AV, Crandall S, Nowacek G, Luecht R, Cauvin S, Wick H. Assessment of matriculating medical students' knowledge and attitudes towards professionalism. *Medical Teacher* 2009;31:928–932.

28 Veloski JJ, Fields SK, Boex JR, Blank LL. Measuring professionalism: a review of studies with instruments reported in the literature between 1982 and 2002. *Academic Medicine* 2005;80:366–370.

29 Hafferty FW. Definitions of professionalism. A search for meaning and identity. *Clinical Orthopaedics and Related Research* 2006;449:193–204.

30 Rees CE, Knight LV. The trouble with assessing students' professionalism: theoretical insights from sociocognitive psychology. *Academic Medicine* 2007;82(1):46–50.

31 Cleland JA, Knight LV, Rees CE, Tracey S, Bond CM. Is it me or is it them? Factors that influence the passing of underperforming students. *Medical Education* 2008;42:800–809.

32 Leo T, Eagan K. Professionalism education: the medical student response. *Perspectives in Biology & Medicine* 2008;51(4):508–5.

33 Young ME, Cruess SR, Cruess RL, Steinert Y. The Professionalism Assessment of Clinical Teachers (PACT): the reliability and validity of a novel tool to evaluate professional and clinical teaching behaviours. *Advances in Health Sciences Education* 2014;19:99–113.

34 Rees CE, Monrouxe LV, Ternan E, Endacott R. Workplace abuse narratives from dentistry, nursing, pharmacy and physiotherapy students: a multi-school qualitative study. *European Journal of Dental Education* 2015;19(2):95–106.

35 Rees CE, Monrouxe LV. A morning since eight of just pure grill: a multischool qualitative study of student abuse. *Academic Medicine* 2011;86(11):1374–1382.

36 Dennis AA, Foy MJ, Monrouxe LV, Rees CE. Exploring trainer and trainee emotional talk in workplace-based feedback narratives. *Advances in Health Sciences Education*. Under review.

37 Molloy E, Borrell-Carrio F, Epstein, R. The impact of emotions in feedback. In D Boud, E Molloy (Eds). *Feedback in Higher and Professional Education*. London and New York: Routledge, 2013: pp. 50–71.

5

Identity-related Professionalism Dilemmas

'I played in a football match last year and one of the guys broke his leg and everyone just kind of looked at me (laughs) as if I would know what to do... I just didn't do anything, I just left it to the referee because the referee would know more first aid... I don't have any clue (laughs)... like loads of people were like, "Oh, you know what to do" and I was like, "I really don't" (everybody laughs)... but people kind of expect you to know and be able to help with any medical thing.'

Gus, male, year 2, medical student, UK

LEARNING OUTCOMES

- To understand what identities are and why they matter for healthcare professionalism
- To appreciate key transitions in healthcare education and their relationships with identity-related professionalism dilemmas
- To discuss different types of identity-related professionalism dilemmas occurring across different healthcare professions
- To discuss the impact of identity-related dilemmas on healthcare learners
- To reflect on the various ways healthcare learners act in the face of identity-related professionalism dilemmas

---

KEY TERMS

Personal identities
Professional identities
In-groups and out-groups
Transitions
Identity-related professionalism dilemmas

Introduction

Who are you? This seemingly simple question has a multitude of answers. You might be a brother or sister, daughter, son or parent. You could be an accomplished musician, sportsperson or artist. You also have your own specific ethnic or racial identity. If you

Healthcare Professionalism: Improving Practice through Reflections on Workplace Dilemmas, First Edition.
Lynn V. Monrouxe and Charlotte E. Rees.
© 2017 John Wiley & Sons Ltd. Published 2017 by John Wiley & Sons Ltd.

are reading this book, you will either be a healthcare student, junior clinician, trainee or educator. All these are part of what makes you unique, they are all aspects of your own individual identity. While some of your identities are prescribed at birth (e.g. child or sibling), others come later and require a process of *becoming.* As students become healthcare practitioners, there will be times when they feel they are *role-playing*, that the people they are trying to become is not quite *them*, particularly in the early years (see professionalism as *presentation*, Chapter 2). At some point, however, learners may stop playing a role and really become that person, acquiring a new identity as a healthcare professional. Therefore, the development of healthcare students and practitioners comprises numerous *transitions*: from school to university or training environment as they begin to commit to their future vocation, their first patient encounters as they go through training, their transitions into practice upon graduation, and later, as they move into more senior positions. All of these transitions bring greater levels of responsibility and new professional challenges. Furthermore, other people look on learners differently as they go through these transitions of becoming. Sometimes the way others perceive learners is very different to who they feel they are: as illustrated by Gus at the start of this chapter. Therefore, a person's identity is not just an individual and personal aspect of them, but is also a *social* aspect. This chapter is about this process of becoming, why it is important for students, trainees and educators to understand how people develop their group-based identities, why it is important that professionals develop their own professional identities and about the different types of identity-related professionalism dilemmas that can be encountered through various transition periods. While this is a broad area for discussion, we specifically address these issues by drawing on a body of psychological research on professional identities and our own research about professional identities and graduates' feelings of preparedness for clinical practice.

How do Professional Identities Relate to Learning?

Healthcare education is not just about learning the knowledge, skills and behaviours required to be a doctor, dentist, nurse, physiotherapist or pharmacist. It is also about learners developing identities as healthcare professionals: internalizing professional ways and practices and taking them on as part of *who they are*, rather than just *what they do* (see Chapter 2).[1–3] Learners develop these identities over time as they learn and work within and across various *communities of practice*.[4] It is within these environments that the process of becoming healthcare practitioners emerges from a mutual interplay between the learner, educators and learning contexts.[5] These contexts include patient or client interactions. Essentially, this process includes aspects such as how learners experience their student or trainee roles, how they interpret their positions within the healthcare environment (including their sense of *fit*), their understanding of their roles as they learn and work within that environment, what they know and do not know and what they learn and choose not to learn. These aspects are negotiated as learners interact with their educators and patients within the healthcare community of practice.[4] This becoming results in a sense of belonging and identification with their own particular community of practice and is an essential aspect of their developing identities.[6]

Such belonging and identification enables healthcare students and trainees to imagine their future selves as particular kinds of healthcare practitioners, with particular sets of

---

Box 5.1 Stop and do: who are you?

- Take a moment to consider the question: 'Who are you?' Write down your immediate responses in terms of your personal and professional identities.
- Has your self-identity changed over the past year or two, and if so, how? Do others see you differently, and if so, how?
- Thinking about your professional identities, what facilitators and barriers have you experienced in terms of developing them?
- How might having a strong professional identity be beneficial or problematic in terms of professionalism?

---

moral and ethical ways of being.[7,8] It also brings learners to view the world differently, including how they view other groups (e.g. patients, other healthcare students and professional groups). Furthermore, as learners engage with particular teams and departments, their relationships with them are often reflected in the ways they talk about them, commonly referring to team members as *we* or *us* and non-members or those belonging to other professions, and even patients, as *they* or *them*.[9–12] Such positioning of others has the potential to impact on the delivery of patient care. Before moving on, take a moment to do the exercise in Box 5.1.

The processes of professional identity formation will be different for everyone, partly because students, for example, will enter university with various personal identities (as explored in Box 5.1). But what happens as students begin to assimilate newly developing professional identities alongside their personal identities? The very process of such development includes students having images of what healthcare practitioners look, act, think and even feel like. These images might be similar (consonant with) or different to how students themselves look, act, think and feel. We turn to this identity consonance and dissonance in the next section.

Are Professional Identities Easily Developed?

Research examining the impact of learners' personal identities (e.g. race, gender and socio-economic class) within professional (e.g. law and social work) schools suggests that, despite entering with the same qualifications, the very process of learning within these schools, intertwined with individuals' different personal identities, leads to feelings of identity consonance or dissonance, ultimately affecting their grades.[5] This suggests that for some people, subtle aspects of the learning environment, such as the buildings and bodies within, can seem familiar and comfortable (see our earlier discussion about the hidden curriculum, Chapter 3). For these learners, their developing professional identity can feel natural, or *consonant*. For others (e.g. women, non-white, people with disabilities or from lower socio-economic classes), the physical and interactional learning environments can feel unfamiliar, potentially leading to a sense of *dissonance*. This can result in professional identity formation being problematic: feelings around not fitting in leading to a loss of self-esteem and suboptimal academic performance.[5] Such a situation can lead students to attempt 'making it by faking it';[5, p. 183] consciously playing their professional role to avoid alienation, while never feeling a sense of belonging (note, this *faking it* is quite different to the *acting-like* in Chapter 2).

In addition to more subtle messages of fit operationalized through the hidden curriculum, healthcare students can sometimes experience more direct messages about their personal identities through various forms of abuse; mistreatment that also serves to impact on their developing professional identities. We discuss students' abuse-related professionalism dilemmas later in Chapter 9.

Finally, we all, at some point, experience ourselves as identifying with a range of different identities (me as a student, as female, as a sibling, as a future nurse). For example, when the social context emphasises our professional identity we are likely to perceive our colleagues as similar to us, irrespective of gender. However, when gender is contextually salient (e.g. during cervical screening) we might feel very different about that same colleague dependent upon their gender. In the face of such complexity it has been suggested that different people manage identities in different ways.[13]

What are the Consequences of Professional Identities?

Research has shown that developing professional identities can have positive and negative consequences at both individual and team-based levels. In terms of positive consequences, having a strong sense of professional identity has been shown to be beneficial for individuals' decision-making in areas such as work performance and career development.[14] It is also related to positive mental health, including feelings of personal well-being and life satisfaction,[15] and lower levels of depression and anxiety.[16] Furthermore, a strong professional identity can lead to ethical behaviour with, for example, nurses' professional identities being related to their ethical decision-making styles.[17] There are also positive interpersonal benefits of possessing shared professional identities with others. Thus, possessing a shared identity-based understanding of the roles, relationships and responsibilities of others within healthcare teams can facilitate trust in others, particularly in high-intensity situations.[18]

Having a strong sense of professional identity, however, can have its drawbacks, as illustrated by Lydia in Box 5.2. Drawbacks, often creating interprofessional dilemmas (see Chapter 12), typically arise from a strong sense of *us* (the *in-group*, which for Lydia is doctors) and *them* (the *out-group*, which for Lydia is nurses). Essentially, the stronger your identity is, the stronger you experience this *in-* and *out-groupness*.[6,19] Accordingly, there are two main interrelated consequences as we classify people into *in-* and *out-groups*. First, we have a tendency to treat *in-* and *out-groups* differently: we consider our *in-group* superior to *out-groups* and display favouritism to our *in-group*: so-called *in-group bias*.[6] Second, we tend to hold stereotypical views about both *in-* and *out-groups* (see Chapter 11, Box 11.1). Stereotypes comprise common, oversimplified, pre-conceptions about groups of people, which reduce them to a set of core characteristics overlooking human complexity, so they are neither true nor false. Stereotyped images, sometimes

---

Box 5.2 'Nurses... scary!'

'... And there's nurses standing out there [outside theatre] going, "Excuse me, you can't come out here, not with all of that blood over you," so the junior reg[istrar] and myself were like, "Nurses. Scary!"'

Lydia, female, year 3, medical student, Australia

Box 5.3 Information: stereotypes held by healthcare students about in- and out-groups

- All groups consider their own profession to be more caring than other professions or better communicators.[23–25]
- By other groups, doctors are considered to be poor team players,[26–28] the least caring and least subservient of professions.[24]
- Medical students perceive allied health professionals (AHPs) and nurses to be inferior to doctors academically, and nurses to have lower status and competence than doctors.[28,29]
- Nurses are perceived as being low in independence by a range of healthcare students (including nurse students).[26,27]

Box 5.4 Stop and do: in- and out-groups

Take a moment to consider the range of healthcare professional groups you might (or do) encounter during your learning and work. Thinking about professional identities, write down in a sentence how you view each out-group. Reflect on what you have written.

- Where does this view come from? From the media? Direct experience? Chatting with family or friends?

How different is this to how you perceive your healthcare professional group?

- If you see *in-* and *out-groups* as different, how might this affect your personal and professional relationships with out-groups?

---

coming from the media, can be either negative (e.g. 'money driven dentists' or 'lazy nurses' https://youtu.be/XsqS__jMF6w)[20] or positive (e.g. 'the healing doctor' or 'the good nurse').[21,22] See Box 5.3 for some key research findings about stereotypes held by healthcare students about their chosen profession.

Although the research findings in Box 5.3 might seem worrisome, healthcare students' perceptions of *out-groups* can improve through direct engagement with those groups, such as in the case of interprofessional learning, essentially helping students to debunk some of these stereotypes. We will cover interprofessional working and dilemmas in much greater depth in Chapter 12. For now we encourage you to work through Box 5.4.

What are Identity-related Professionalism Dilemmas?

> '...or patients saying to you stuff like, "nurse"... and you think, "I am not quite that nurse yet."'
>
> Marie, female, year 2, nursing student, UK

Through learning to become a healthcare practitioner or educator, and through the various educational transitions involved in this process of *becoming*, there are numerous ways in which your identity might cause you professionalism dilemmas. Drawing on our programme of research focussing mainly on professionalism dilemmas, we now explore some of the identity-related dilemmas we identified chronologically (i.e. those in which the narrators' identities caused the dilemma). As we do so we will examine how they are experienced, the different emotions they can evoke, alongside how learners either go along with what is happening, or how they resist certain aspects in order to maintain their professional ideals.

What Identity-related Professionalism Dilemmas Occur Across the Pre-university to Year 1 Transition?

We begin by considering the kinds of identity dilemmas typically experienced by healthcare students at the very early stages of their courses, or even prior to beginning (e.g. nursing students previously working as healthcare assistants, or pharmacy students previously working as shop assistants in community pharmacies). Other dilemmas occur at the point of transition or very soon after. Within our own research, the majority of these dilemmas were narrated by medical students. Unlike many students studying primarily academic-focused subjects (e.g. physics, psychology, geology), from the moment healthcare students begin their courses, they are expected to behave professionally both during university and workplace-based learning settings as well as outside the university setting (see Chapter 3). Here, students' identities can cause problems for them: they do not yet feel part of the profession itself and may have not yet received any formal teaching on how best to conduct themselves *professionally*. Some situations might feel reasonably easy to negotiate and cause little distress (perhaps due to the lack of professionalism education: see Pete's narrative, Box 5.5).

So we can see from Box 5.5 how Pete's identity as a male, along with the *male = doctor* stereotype thought to be held by the woman he was phoning, led to her misunderstanding that he was a doctor; a misunderstanding that Pete chose not to correct because he was getting the information he needed from her. We can see from this excerpt how this case of mistaken identity was seen as an amusing story, as indicated by multiple episodes of laughter. Although this case of mistaken identity occurred prior to medical school, this dilemma can occur at any time. The essence of the dilemma for the student or

---

Box 5.5 'Shall I tell her that I'm not a doctor?'

'… This was before medical school when I worked in the health centre… reception work… the GP had asked me to find out a bit of information about someone… he got me to phone up, I said, "I'm ringing from the health centre, have you got any information on her [patient] about her blood group" and then I sort of heard her put the phone down and shout, "Oh, has anyone spoken to a doctor from [names place] (laughter) about this lady," and I thought, "Oh God" (laughter) … then suddenly she started talking and I thought, "Shall I tell her that I'm not a doctor?" But I thought, "She's quite receptive to me at the moment so I'll leave it" (laughter) and I left it (laughter)… Looking back it probably wasn't the best thing to do, but she told me everything I wanted to know about her blood group… what she thought of her condition, I wrote it all down… gave it to the GP and I never told her that I wasn't a doctor… it got me further with her thinking I was a doctor (laughter). If I'd told her… she might have been less receptive… if she'd asked me… specifically I would have then clarified it… think she just assumed man's voice ringing from health centre.'

Pete, male, year 1, medical student, UK

Box 5.6 Stop and do: mistaken identity

Have you ever experienced a time when someone has mistaken you for being a practitioner or more experienced than you are? Thinking about this kind of scenario:

- What is the right thing to do professionally?
- What did you do?
- Would you do that now?
- If so, why?

Did you know?

In the eyes of the law, wilful misrepresentation, such as calling yourself a physiotherapist or pharmacist when you are not, is *fraud* and relates to *pecuniary advantage*. If you then also touch someone, so calling yourself a doctor and then examine them, this makes it a criminal offence.

Check out this post by the UK Crown Prosecution Service stating a precedent for misrepresentation:

http://www.cps.gov.uk/westmidlands/cps_west_midlands_news/man_pleads_guilty_of_impersonating_a_doctor_/

What is the law in your country relevant to such identity dilemmas?

---

trainee concerns what actions they should take professionally when such situations occur (see Box 5.6 for the 'stop and do' exercise).

Another common identity-related professionalism dilemma experienced by new healthcare students includes initiation ceremonies (also known as 'hazing'), involving indirect (through modelling) or direct pressure for healthcare students to over-consume alcohol.[30,31] Such ceremonies can have a strong element of hierarchy, with more experienced medical students pressurizing their younger counterparts to become over-intoxicated, sometimes with dire consequences: '[I] played pub golf [and] ended up collapsed and in hospital... [I was] ashamed. I wasted NHS resources' (year 1, medical student, UK).[31 p. 275] Medical students in our professionalism research also talked about initiation ceremonies when discussing other students' behaviours, commenting that such events could jeopardize the students' future careers as doctors, as well as bringing their universities and professions into disrepute, as illustrated in Box 5.7.

Other such alcohol fuelled professionalism lapses include a 2015 experience reported in the media of a UK medical student with his medics' rugby team on a ferry allegedly urinating on a table where a family were sitting eating (see http://www.huffingtonpost.co.uk/2015/03/19/po-ferries-ban-cardiff-un_n_6901250.html; http://cardiffstudentmedia.co.uk/gairrhydd/news/student-urinated-dinner-public/). To make this professionalism lapse worse, both the student and rugby team allegedly refused to identify the culprit, therefore failing to raise concerns as stipulated by the regulatory body (see Table 2.2 in Chapter 2). The crux of the identity matter here is that healthcare students need to be professional outside of their healthcare schools, throughout their healthcare education, including from the outset (*professionalism as integration*; see Table 2.3 in Chapter 2). As Carmen highlights (Box 5.7), while new students embody their 'student' identities, they do not yet embrace their future professional identities and this may account for much of the identity-related troubles in the early stages of healthcare education.

Box 5.7 'Our group decided to flash in front of a mosque'

PAMELA: The third-years are going around pelting first-years with eggs and stuff and… they got told off by the police and had to run away, because if you get a police caution or something then you're screwed…

FRAN: But our group decided to flash in front of a mosque with a load of people outside it… good God, I've never been so embarrassed in [my] entire life and I didn't know what to do, I was like, 'Let's all go (laughs) hope we don't get arrested'…

PAMELA: Flashing in a mosque… they're patients aren't they? At the end of the day, people in the community are potential patients and if you're going to respect patients in a hospital why wouldn't you respect them in the street… in the medical sort of professional sense of it, first-years might well not know that if you get a police caution that can affect your career…

CARMEN: Right at the beginning, although you know you're a medical student, but it hasn't quite dawned on you…

PAMELA: That you're going to be a doctor…

Pamela, Fran and Carmen, females, year 2, medical students, UK

Identity Dilemmas Across Undergraduate Healthcare Education

Healthcare students experience identity-related professionalism dilemmas both within and outside their healthcare schools beyond the initial transition period described above.[32-37] The majority of these dilemmas outside university arise due to the new ways in which healthcare students' friends and family view them, rather than how they view themselves. This includes mistaken understandings around healthcare students' levels of knowledge, such as in Gus' narrative at the beginning of this chapter, and illustrated in Box 5.8. In the early years of healthcare education, students simply do not know how to examine or interpret signs and have barely begun to assimilate their professional identity as part of themselves. In many situations, students advise others to seek assistance from their own GP: a course of action consistent with professionalism guidelines (Table 2.2, Chapter 2) around treating family and friends.

While the dilemmas reported in Box 5.8 are often laughed off, other dilemmas outside university can cause healthcare students greater distress. In our data we had various instances, for example, in which pharmacy students working in community pharmacies as shop assistants talked about being mistaken as the pharmacist, sometimes causing them to be on the receiving end of very disgruntled patients when they refused to make up prescriptions (Betsy's narrative, Box 5.9).

In terms of identity dilemmas within healthcare schools themselves, much of these are experienced as part of students' workplace learning, including their interactions with patients (sometimes as early as day 1 of healthcare school) and with other healthcare professionals. A common patient-related identity dilemma narrated by students in our research includes patients' lack of understanding of who is a student in the clinical setting (so, a case of mistaken identity) and issues such as students being introduced as practitioners, colleagues or members of the team rather than students, as illustrated in Saul's narrative (Box 5.10, section 1). Such identity dilemmas often interrelate with consent dilemmas (discussed later, Chapter 6). The crux of the matter here is students'

Box 5.8 'I've had this pain in my leg'

ANDREA: You never escape it … Even when I was travelling this summer, as soon as people find out you're a medical student they go, 'So you want to be a doctor do you, know what, I've had this pain in my leg', and you're like, 'Number one, I don't know; number two. I'm on holiday!'

WENDY: And it's always when you're eating: 'I've got this rash.' (laughter)

ANDREA: I've had that a couple of times like: 'Uncle put it away!' (laughing) 'No, no, no, I don't want to know… don't want to know about the rash!' Oh dear…

Andrea and Wendy, females, year 3, medical students, UK

Box 5.9 'Well you look like a pharmacist'

'One of the patients, he came in for methadone but he didn't come in at the time specified… I was at the counter and he kept saying to me, "Well you look like a pharmacist, just give me the methadone", and I'm like, "No, you have to wait for the pharmacist… I can't give it to you." But he got all really angry… I said, "Well you could go and come back at half past nine", which he did, but when he came back… it was quite hard to like deal with him… you have to be very professional… we were getting very, very annoyed but obviously we can't get aggressive with a patient.'

Betsy, female, year 2, pharmacy student, UK

---

responsibilities to correct such mistakes and identify themselves as 'students' versus their own desires to avoid embarrassing their seniors or confusing patients (Box 5.10, narratives 1 and 2) and their desires to obtain access to patients for the purposes of their learning, fearing access will be denied if patients realize their true 'student' status (see Chapter 6 for further discussion around tensions between patient care and student learning). In addition to students being introduced as practitioners, students sometimes narrated identity dilemmas around them acting *as if* they were practitioners, passing themselves off as doctors, dentists, physiotherapists, and so on, which could be considered deception to obtain pecuniary advantage (Box 5.6).

Another common patient-related identity dilemma comprises situations in which patients interact with students in ways that differ from how they interact with qualified healthcare professionals, often because students are 'closer' in status to patients. For example, students experience dilemmas about patients disclosing information to them, often relevant to their medical conditions, which have not been disclosed to their practitioners. Students also experience identity dilemmas when patients ask them for information and advice about their conditions, rather than asking their own healthcare providers. Sometimes they ask students for clarification following a consultation, or the patient's family tries to glean further knowledge from students (Box 5.10, narrative 3). Such dilemmas relate to the somewhat unique student-patient relationship. Students are not yet at the centre of their healthcare community of practice[4,38] – rather they are on the periphery of that community of practice – they are more similar to the patient in terms of their language and appearance, and therefore more approachable. The crux of these patient-related identity dilemmas is the issue of competence and students not going beyond their limits (e.g. by providing incorrect information or advice). While the vast majority of our participants felt happy

Box 5.10 Common identity dilemmas in the healthcare workplace

1. Mistaken identities to coerce patient consent for student involvement (see Chapter 6 also)

Narrative 1: 'my colleague'

'There was nothing particularly untoward… I've often been sat in clinics and been introduced as "my colleague"… urology in the third year, we did have clinic and it was transrectal prostate biopsy and the consultant introduced us all, "This is one of my colleagues he will be doing" or, "She will be doing the rectal examination". I don't think he ever wanted to say it was a student… he was quite ambiguous about the fact that we were third year students.'

Saul, male, year 5, medical student, UK

Narrative 2: 'I'm a student physio'

'A patient on the ward so, he was quite old, not really with it… she just said, "Know, what?", "I'm a student physio", "A what? physio?", "Oh, okay" and they don't understand like what it is, so adding 'a student' just confused things more. So like I didn't [say I was a student]…'

Gretchen, female, year 2, physiotherapy student, UK

2. Patients seeking advice from students and disclosing information to them

Narrative 3: 'on my mobile phone'

'A patient's relative contacted me seeking advice on how to care for the patient's oral health as they had recently been admitted to hospital after suffering a cerebral vascular incident. I was in the hospital at the time but was contacted by the patient's relative on my mobile phone. I gave limited advice to the relative (within my scope of knowledge) and sought further advice from a clinical teacher.… [I'm] glad that I sought advice.'

Flynn, male, year 4, dental student, UK

3. Mistaken identities of student by other healthcare professionals

Narrative 4: 'could you get the nurse?'

'The biggest problem I have encountered is not the patients mistaking you for qualified nurses but the doctors… I was looking after this patient who'd had a bleed, and there was me clutching on to her, putting pressure on her artery, and this new doctor comes along and he sort of assesses it all and said about fifteen things to me… it was Dutch! (laughs) because I understood nothing… I was on my second day ever of placement, holding this woman's hand going, "Oh" and he just shouted all these instructions and just walked off and I was like, "Ah help" (laughs) and then he came back and told me something else, I said, "Could you get the nurse" and he went, "You're the nurse" and I went, "No, the other nurse, the big tall, black haired one that is not a student" and he was like, "Oh" (laughs) … and that is obviously quite dangerous in regards to acute situations like that because the patient isn't clotting and the blood just keeps coming out…'

' Laura, female, year 2, nursing student, UK

referring patients and their families back to their practitioners for the right information, a few students reported witnessing peers going beyond their limits, thereby jeopardizing patient safety (see Chapter 7, patient safety-related dilemmas).

Finally, our participants narrated workplace identity dilemmas in relation to their interactions with other healthcare professionals, often concerning misunderstandings between nurses and medical students, medical consultants and physiotherapy students, and junior doctors and nursing students. Typical scenarios included nurses asking medical students for advice around patient care or asking students to undertake tasks that were beyond their levels of competence or abilities (e.g. signing fluid charts or writing drug charts). Occasionally, the nurses recognized their medical student roles, but believed them to be more knowledgeable than they were (particularly when medical students were in their final year nearing graduation). Physiotherapy students talked about how consultants sometimes left it to them to talk to patients about probabilities for recovery (e.g. walking) following surgery, not realizing their student identity. Another common identity-related dilemma were situations in which junior doctors (in particular) mistook nursing students for qualified nurses, asking them to undertake duties for which they were untrained (Box 5.10, narrative 4). Across all these dilemmas, physiotherapy and nursing students talked about how senior clinicians often used extensive medical jargon when conversing with them, further underscoring their misunderstandings around students' levels of seniority and therefore knowledge.

Identity Dilemmas Across Transitions into Practice

'I think it's a normal psychological aspect of thinking that we are protected here and if something happens there is always a supervisor to bail us out. That is not always going to be possible once you are finished and this scares a lot of people.'

Jessie, male, final year dental student, UK[39, p.4]

'[I feel an] increased level of anxiety because, you know, some of the responsibility of this person's health is with us absolutely... I'm suddenly a doctor. I didn't used to be a doctor...'

Skyler, female, junior doctor, two months after graduation, UK[40]

The final identity-related transition we discuss in this chapter is healthcare students moving from their student to qualified practitioner identities. This transition is inevitable and uncontrollable[41], with reports of newly-qualified doctors, dentists, nurses, physiotherapists and pharmacists finding the experience particularly overwhelming, with feelings of heightened stress around this time.[34,39,42–44] Indeed, for newly qualified nurses and doctors, their new responsibilities such as managing others and prioritizing their own time, along with administering drugs, causes the most stress.[40,43] Along with thinking about these stressors in terms of knowledge and skill deficiencies, we can also see these aspects of their new roles as identity-related. The step-change from following orders to giving them, for example, can feel strange when graduates don't *feel* like a doctor or nurse.

Within our larger body of research, we considered the relative preparedness of newly graduated doctors.[40] Along with interviewing a range of stakeholders, we asked 26 pre-registration junior doctors (at foundation year 1, so-called F1s) to record an audio diary for a period of four months in their new role. One of the main identity-related issues

---

Box 5.11 'It was a big jump'

'…Yesterday… I was asked by the nurses, effectively, to do a "do not resuscitate" form. It was quite difficult, and I didn't feel as if I was necessarily the appropriate person to do it. While I knew what the forms looked like, it was a situation where I didn't feel comfortable making – well I wasn't making the decision, the consultant on the ward round had already discussed it with the family and said, "There might not be anything else we can do for this patient, it's best that if they die, we're just going to let them die peacefully", but… all the seniors are then scrubbed in theatre leaving me as the most senior member on our team, which therefore meant it fell to me to actually do the "do not resuscitate" form, which was quite a big responsibility for me to have to do, and it's something that I didn't feel particularly confident with or happy doing. What I actually did in the end was filled it out and then took it down to my consultant who, in-between cases, signed the form for me. Because while a DNAR form can be signed by myself… it was a big jump for me to make. From feeling like an F1, that I almost follow instructions… I felt like I was having to make more of a decision than I was perhaps comfortable for…'

Walter, male, junior doctor four months post-graduation, UK

---

they frequently narrated concerned them coming to terms with their newly found responsibilities as junior doctors (see Skyler's excerpt at the beginning of this section and Walter's more detailed example in Box 5.11).

Emotional Impact and Resistance

The narratives included in this chapter illustrate keenly the emotional impact of identity-related professionalism dilemmas on students through, for example, their emotion talk (e.g. 'scary', 'ashamed', 'embarrassed', 'hard', 'anxiety', 'didn't feel comfortable', 'didn't feel particularly confident'), and through numerous episodes of laughter, probably for the purposes of narrators' coping with recounting difficult identity dilemmas.[45] However, our research has shown that identity-related professionalism dilemmas were generally less distressing than other types of dilemmas discussed in this book (e.g. patient safety and patient dignity dilemmas; discussed later in Chapters 7 and 8).

In terms of medical students in our interview study, for example, their narratives of identity-related dilemmas contained fewer 'strong' emotional words (e.g. 'disgusted', 'terrified') than other dilemmas and, also contained fewer anxiety words.[32] Additionally, in our UK questionnaire study of medical students, we found only one identity-related professionalism dilemma (i.e. 'clinician coerced patient consent for student learning by misrepresenting student identity') causing moral distress. Interestingly, although the average level of distress was mild for females (e.g. in the moment, but not lasting) and none for males, respondents did report more distress with repeated occurrences of the same event. In terms of other healthcare professionals, identity dilemmas did not feature as one of the most common dilemmas discussed in our interview study, nor did healthcare students report feelings of moral distress in relation to identity-related professionalism dilemmas.[34,40]

Such lack of moral distress for identity-related professionalism dilemmas (in comparison to other dilemmas) may partly be due to our finding that healthcare students typically report resisting identity-related professionalism dilemmas (over 70% of the time). Indeed, Flynn (Box 5.10, narrative 3) describes being 'glad' that he sought advice from his superior rather than giving possibly incorrect advice to the patient's family member. Another common act of resistance to identity-related professionalism dilemmas included students re-introducing themselves as students if a misunderstanding or misrepresentation of their identities had occurred. Nevertheless, when students went along with the 'mistaken identity' situation, this was typically because they felt the issue of their identity was unproblematic. Although mild feelings of discomfort were sometimes felt when their identities were misrepresented, they sometimes went along with this deception to save the face of their seniors and to take advantage of the additional learning opportunities it opened up to them. We encourage students, trainees and educators alike to act in accordance with both legal and ethical mandates to reduce the risk of identity dilemmas occurring, and to manage them appropriately when they arise, to protect all concerned, including the patient.

Chapter Summary

In this chapter we have discussed the various transitions that healthcare learners encounter as they become healthcare professionals and how these transitions impact on the identity-related dilemmas they experience and their developing professional identities. We have provided an overview of the benefits and drawbacks of developing strong professional identities and have discussed ways in which learners and educators can avoid and manage identity-related professionalism dilemmas. The summary points from this chapter are in Box 5.12, with suggestions for small group discussions in Box 5.13. Following these, Boxes 5.14 and 5.15 outline further learning activities and recommended reading.

Box 5.12 Chapter summary points

- Developing a strong professional identity can enhance your future career-making decisions but can also lead to the development of group stereotyping, in-group favouritism and out-group stigmatizing
- Some people find it hard to internalize their professional identities due to a lack of fit with the norms of the group
- Across learners' numerous transitions from pre-student to practitioner their student identities can be misrepresented/misunderstood, resulting in others mistaking them for being more qualified/knowledgeable than they are
- Healthcare students' behaviour outside school can compromise their future professional identities, particularly when alcohol is involved
- Newly qualified practitioners' increased responsibilities can cause them to experience identity-related dilemmas
- Identity-related dilemmas appear to cause learners less moral distress than other dilemmas, perhaps because they are more easily resolved

Box 5.13 Chapter discussion points

Check out this blog in which a medical student talks about what she does if someone calls her a doctor: http://mindonmed.com/2011/08/clinically-who-should-we-call-doctor.html

- Discuss the issues raised in this blog and your own experiences around being mistaken for or misrepresented as a healthcare practitioner

Read the article in our 'further reading' section by Adams *et al.* (2006) concerning the factors influencing the professional identities of health and social care students:

- To what extent do you think your professional identity was evident before you began your education?
- To what extent do you think that your gender, previous work experience in healthcare environments, understanding of team working and knowledge of your profession influences your own sense of professional identity?

Box 5.14 Chapter learning activities

Have you ever experienced an identity-related dilemma?

- What was the gist of it?
- When did it happen?
- Was this around a particular 'transition' in your life?
- Who was involved in the event?
- What happened? What did you do?
- What would you do if faced with this dilemma again?

Box 5.15 Chapter recommended reading

Adams K, Hean S, Sturgis P, Clark JM. Investigating the factors influencing professional identity of first-year health and social care students. *Learning in Health and Social Care* 2006;5(2):55–68.

Black LF, Monrouxe LV. 'Being sick a lot, often on each other': students' alcohol-related provocation. *Medical Education* 2014;48(3):268–279.

Hean S, Clark JM, Adams K, Humphris D. Will opposites attract? Similarities and differences in students' perceptions of the stereotype profiles of other health and social care professional groups. *Journal of Interprofessional Care* 2006;20:162–81.

Tajfel H, Turner, JC. The social identity theory of intergroup behavior. In J Jost, J Sidanius (Eds) *Political Psychology: Key Readings in Social Psychology*. New York, NY: Psychology Press, 2004: pp. 367–391.

References

1 Monrouxe LV. Identity, identification and medical education: why should we care? *Medical Education* 2010;44:40–49.

2 Monrouxe LV. Identity, self and medical education. In K Walsh (Ed.) *Oxford Handbook of Medical Education*. Oxford: University of Oxford Press, 2013: pp. 113–123.

3 Monrouxe LV. Theoretical insights into the nature and nurture of professional identities. In R Cruess, S Cruess, Y Steinert (Eds) *Teaching Medical Professionalism: Supporting the Development of a Professional Identity*, 2nd Edition. Cambridge: Cambridge University Press, 2016: pp. 37–53.

4 Wenger E. *Communities of Practice*. Cambridge: Cambridge University Press, 1998.

5 Costello CY. *Professional Identity Crisis: Race, Class, Gender and Success at Professional Schools*. Nashville, Tennessee: Vanderbilt University Press, 2005.

6 Turner J, Hogg M, Oakes P, Reicher S, Wetherell M. *Rediscovering the Social Group: a Self-Categorization Theory*. Oxford and New York: Blackwell, 1987.

7 Oakes PJ, Haslam SA, Turner JC. *Stereotyping and Social Reality*. Oxford: Blackwell, 1994.

8 Turner JC. Some current issues in research on social identity and self-categorization theories. In N Ellemers, R Spears, B Doosje (Eds) *Social Identity: Context, Commitment, Content*. Oxford: Blackwell, 1999: pp. 6–34.

9 Fiol CM. Capitalizing on paradox: the role of language in transforming organizational identities. *Organization Science* 2002;13:653–666.

10 Ajjawi R, Rees CE, Monrouxe LV. Learning clinical skills during bedside teaching encounters in general practice. *Journal of Workplace Learning* 2015;27:298–314.

11 Monrouxe LV, Rees CE, Bradley P. The construction of patients' involvement in hospital bedside teaching encounters. *Qualitative Health Research* 2009;19:918–930.

12 Rees CE, Monrouxe LV. 'Oh my God uh uh uh': laughter for coping in medical students' personal incident narratives of professionalism dilemmas. In C Figley, P Huggard, C Rees (Eds) *First Do No Self-Harm: Understanding and Promoting Physician Stress Resilience*. Oxford: Oxford University Press, 2013: pp. 67–87.

13 Roccas S, Brewer MB. Social identity complexity. *Personality and Social Psychology Review* 2002;6:88–106.

14 Savickas ML. Identity in vocational development. *Journal of Vocational Behavior* 1985;27:329–337.

15 Kroger J. *Identity Development: Adolescence Through Adulthood*, 2nd Edition. Thousand Oaks, CA: Sage, 2007.

16 McKeague T, Skorikov V, Serikawa T. Occupational identity and workers' mental health. In C. Weikert, E Torkelson, J Pryce (Eds) *Occupational Health Psychology: Empowerment, Participation, and Health at Work*. Nottingham: I-WHO Publication, 2002: pp. 113–117.

17 Berggren I, Severinsson E. Nurse supervisors' actions in relation to their decision-making style and ethical approach to clinical supervision. *Journal of Advanced Nursing* 2003;41:615–622.

18 Weick KE, Roberts KH. Collective mind in organizations: heedful interrelating on flight decks. *Administrative Science Quarterly* 1993;38:357–381.

19 Tajfel H, Turner J. The social identity theory of intergroup behavior. In J Jost, J Sidanius (Eds) *Political Psychology: Key Readings in Social Psychology*. New York: Psychology Press, 2004: pp. 367–391.

20 Wetherall C. How to stay afloat. *Nursing Standard* 2012;26:26–27.

21 Monrouxe LV. Negotiating professional identities: dominant and contesting narratives in medical students' longitudinal audio diaries. *Current Narratives* 2009;1:41–59.

22 Fealy GM. 'The good nurse': visions and values in images of the nurse. *Journal of Advanced Nursing* 2004;46:649–656.

23 Carpenter J. Interprofessional education for medical and nursing students: evaluation of a programme. *Medical Education* 1995;29:265–272.

24 Jacobsen F, Lindqvist S. A two-week stay in an interprofessional training unit changes students' attitudes to health professionals. *Journal of Interprofessional Care* 2009;23:242–250.

25 Hind M, Norman I, Cooper S, Gill E, Hilton R, Judd P, *et al.* Interprofessional perceptions of health care students. *Journal of Interprofessional Care* 2003;17:21–34.

26 Hean S, Clark JM, Adams K, Humphris D. Will opposites attract? Similarities and differences in students' perceptions of the stereotype profiles of other health and social care professional groups. *Journal of Interprofessional Care* 2006;20:162–181.

27 Ateah CA, Snow W, Wener P, MacDonald L, Metge C, Davis P, *et al.* Stereotyping as a barrier to collaboration: Does interprofessional education make a difference? *Nurse Education Today* 2011;31:208–213.

28 Tunstall-Pedoe S, Rink E, Hilton S. Student attitudes to undergraduate interprofessional education. *Journal of Interprofessional Care* 2003;17:161–172.

29 Rudland JR, Mires GJ. Characteristics of doctors and nurses as perceived by students entering medical school: implications for shared teaching. *Medical Education* 2005;39:448–455.

30 Hollmann BB. Hazing: hidden campus crime. *New Directions for Student Services* 2002;2002:11–24.

31 Black LF, Monrouxe LV. 'Being sick a lot, often on each other': students' alcohol-related provocation. *Medical Education* 2014;48:268–279.

32 Monrouxe LV, Rees CE. 'It's just a clash of cultures': emotional talk within medical students' narratives of professionalism dilemmas. *Advances in Health Sciences Education: Theory and Practice* 2012;17:671–701.

33 Monrouxe LV, Rees CE, Dennis I, Wells SE. Professionalism dilemmas, moral distress and the healthcare student: insights from two online UK-wide questionnaire studies. *British Medical Journal Open* 2015;5:e007518 doi:10.1136/bmjopen-2014-007518.

34 Monrouxe LV, Rees CE, Endacott R, Ternan E. 'Even now it makes me angry': health care students' professionalism dilemma narratives. *Medical Education* 2014;48:502–517.

35 Rees CE, Monrouxe LV. 'A morning since eight of just pure grill': a multi-centre qualitative study of student abuse. *Academic Medicine* 2011;86:1374–1382.

36 Rees CE, Monrouxe LV, Ternan E, Endacott R. Workplace abuse narratives from dentistry, nursing, pharmacy and physiotherapy students: a multi-school qualitative study. *European Journal of Dental Education* 2015;19:95–106.

37 Rees CE, Monrouxe LV, McDonald LA. My mentor kicked a dying woman's bed: analysing UK nursing students' most memorable professionalism dilemmas. *Journal of Advanced Nursing* 2015;71(1):169–180.

38 Rees C, Knight LV, Wilkinson C. 'User involvement is a sine qua non, almost, in medical education': learning with rather than just about health and social care service users. *Advances in Health Sciences Education* 2007;12:359–390.

39 Ali K, Tredwin C, Kay E, Slade A. Transition of new dental graduates into practice: a qualitative study. *European Journal of Dental Education.* 2015;20:65–72. doi:10.1111/eje.12143.

40 Monrouxe LV, Bullock A, Cole J, Gormley G, Kaufhold K, Kelly N, *et al. How Prepared are UK Medical Graduates for Practice? Final Report From a Programme of Research Commissioned by the General Medical Council.* General Medical Council, 2014. http://www.gmc-uk.org/How_Prepared_are_UK_Medical_Graduates_for_Practice_SUBMITTED_Revised_140614.pdf_58034815.pdf. (Accessed 20 January 2017).

41 Baillie L. Preparing adult branch students for their management role as staff nurses: an action research project. *Journal of Nurse Management* 1999;7:225–234.

42 Stupans I. Qualitative interviews of pharmacy interns: determining curricular preparedness for work life. *Pharmacy Practice* 2012;10:52–56.

43 Whitehead B, Holmes D. Are newly qualified nurses prepared for practice? *Nursing Times* 2011;107:20–23.

44 Thomson D, Boyle D, Legg C, Owen M, Newman M, Cole M-J. Clinical placements: the perspectives of UK physiotherapy students on how prepared they were by their university for their first clinical placements: an example of one HEI. *International Journal of Practice-based Learning in Health and Social Care* 2014;2:69–79.

45 Rees CE, Monrouxe LV, McDonald LA. Narrative, emotion and action: analysing 'most memorable' professionalism dilemmas. *Medical Education* 2013;47:80–96.

6

Consent-related
Professionalism Dilemmas

'[My dilemma was] whether or not to continue examining a patient who withdrew consent during the examination, and was then intimidated into agreeing again. [I participated in] bedside teaching with a consultant and three other students. As a group we began to examine the patient's abdomen. She began to cry so I asked the student examining to stop. The consultant then told her she'd already agreed before so we were going to examine her and asked us to continue. I refused... [because] she was clearly still in distress. She was gaining nothing from the examination, it was purely for our learning so I felt it wrong to continue. I think I did the right thing but I am still angry that I was later told off by the consultant and generally picked on for the rest of the rotation... I told my clinical advisor about this but nothing ever seemed to be done.'

Keeley, female, year 5, medical student, UK

LEARNING OUTCOMES

- To understand what consent is and why it matters in professionalism education
- To understand common myths about patient consent for student involvement in healthcare
- To discover the range of consent-related professionalism dilemmas occurring across different professions
- To discuss the impact of consent-related professionalism dilemmas
- To reflect on the various ways learners can act when faced with consent-related dilemmas

---

KEY TERMS

Consent
Consent myths
Consent-related professionalism dilemmas
Consent-related moral distress
Compliance with consent lapses
Resistance to consent lapses

Healthcare Professionalism: Improving Practice through Reflections on Workplace Dilemmas, First Edition.
Lynn V. Monrouxe and Charlotte E. Rees.

Introduction

Healthcare professionals have moral and legal obligations to involve patients wherever possible in decisions about what happens to their bodies, through informed consent. Not only is patient consent routinely requested for healthcare advice, treatment and care, but it is also required for patient involvement in healthcare research and education. Indeed, numerous bodies across healthcare stipulate that patients should know the status of students, and should be asked for their informed consent for student involvement in their care, especially when the purpose is to benefit student learning, and should have the right to refuse to take part in teaching.[1-5] However, we know from the literature, including our own research, that tensions commonly exist for healthcare students, trainees and educators between efforts to preserve patient autonomy versus efforts to help learners learn with, from and about patients in the clinical workplace.[6,7] This is illustrated starkly in Keeley's consent-related professionalism dilemma above: the consultant wilfully ignores the patient's withdrawal of consent for student teaching, leading to the patient crying and Keeley refusing to conduct the examination. Ultimately, Keeley thinks it morally wrong to continue because the examination benefits only herself and her fellow students, not the patient. In this chapter, we discuss the complexities about consent: what it is and why it matters in healthcare education and practice. We unpack several myths about patient consent for student involvement in their care, drawing on research evidence with patients, including personal experience. We then consider various consent-related dilemmas and their impact, including learners' experience of moral distress that arises when they know the *ethically correct* course of action but are thwarted in their attempts to act ethically.[8] Finally, we explore students' actions in the face of such consent-related dilemmas: do students resist or do they go along with consent lapses? We hope this chapter will help healthcare students and trainees navigate their way through consent-related professionalism dilemmas in order to protect themselves and patients.

What is Consent and Why Does it Matter?

> 'Patients have the moral and legal right to determine what will be done with and to their own person; to be given accurate, complete, and understandable information in a manner that facilitates an informed decision; and to be assisted with weighing the benefits, burdens, and available options in their treatment... They also have the right to accept, refuse, or terminate treatment without deceit, undue influence, duress, coercion, or prejudice, and to be given necessary support throughout decision-making and treatment processes.'
>
> American Nurses Association (ANA)[9, p. 2]

Informed consent, as the above quote suggests, is a patient's voluntary decision about their healthcare, made with sufficient understanding about the benefits and risks involved.[1] For consent to be valid, it must be given freely by a patient who has the capacity to consent (i.e. can make decisions due to 'normal' cognition) and in cases where patients lack capacity, decisions must be made in their best interests.[2] Specific guidance from the UK Department of Health[2] on patient consent for student involvement in their care is in Box 6.1 which highlights the conflicts students face in the clinical workplace learning environment in terms of their dual roles as students and healthcare providers.[10]

Box 6.1 Information: Department of Health guidance on patient consent for student involvement in their care

'It is particularly important that a person is aware of the situation when students or trainees carry out procedures to further their own education. Where the procedure will further the person's care – for example taking a blood sample for testing – then, assuming the student is appropriately trained in the procedure, the fact that it is carried out by a student does not alter the nature and purpose of the procedure. It is therefore not a legal requirement to tell the person that the clinician is a student, although it would always be good practice to do so. In contrast, where a student proposes to conduct a physical examination that is not part of the person's care then it is essential to explain that the purpose of the examination is to further the student's training, and to seek consent for that to take place.'[2, section 14, p. 12]

Box 6.2 Information: invalid consent[2]

1) Consent is not voluntary (i.e. coerced)
2) Consent is based on insufficient information about the nature and purpose of the intervention (e.g. for teaching, how many students are present and what they will do)
3) Inappropriate timing of consent (e.g. elicited just before or during a procedure when the patient is vulnerable)
4) Consent is elicited by a person with inadequate knowledge of the intervention
5) Consent is given by a person lacking capacity (i.e. someone unable to make decisions due to temporary/permanent cognitive disturbance)

Based on such assertions, consent can therefore be invalidated in a number of ways (see Box 6.2). Consent is an ongoing process rather than a one-off event. While verbal and even non-verbal consent (e.g. patient opening her mouth to be examined by the dental student, patient holding out his arm to have his blood pressure measured by the nursing student) may be sufficient for non-invasive, routine examinations and procedures, written consent is required for more invasive and substantial procedures, such as students conducting pelvic examinations on women under anaesthesia for the purposes of their learning (see Box 6.3).[11] Consent for student involvement in patient care can be requested by the supervising clinician, by students themselves, and also by third parties such as receptionists in general practice.[6,12,13]

What are the Ethical, Legal, Relational and Safety Bases of Consent?

Consent matters for multiple reasons. In terms of ethics, from within a principlism approach (see Chapter 2), the main ethical consideration underlying informed consent is patients having the right to bodily integrity and self-determination, as illustrated in the ANA quote above.[9] While this resonates with a Kantian perspective (see Box 6.4), a Utilitarian perspective suggests that students should be able to practise on individual patients for the ultimate benefit of future patients who will profit from well-trained

---

Box 6.3 Author's experience: 'could she conduct a vaginal examination on me to help her learn'

I was admitted to my local district hospital for surgical management of a miscarriage. I was sitting in my cubicle when one of the students from my medical school poked her head around the part-drawn curtain nervously: 'Ah, Professor Rees, I wondered whether it was you', and she paused, 'I don't think it's appropriate that I ask you my question.' Having recently published a paper on medical students conducting intimate examinations without consent, I told her to come into the cubicle and ask me whatever she was asking the other patients: educationally speaking, I was intrigued. She explained clearly her name and that she was a fourth-year medical student and that she would like to observe my procedure in theatre and if the opportunity arose could she conduct a vaginal examination on me to help her learn. I said, 'yes' without hesitation and I told her why: because she explained who she was, what she wanted to do and why, and most importantly asked my permission and that because of those two things I trusted her to respect my body while I was anaesthetized. As I signed the written consent form, my parting words to her were words I would say to every healthcare student and educator reading this book: 'Always ask the patient'.

Box 6.4 Information: Utilitarian versus Kantian perspectives (Torrance *et al.*[7])

- **Kantian:** individual patients should not be used as a means to an end (e.g. to develop the skills of the student)
- **Utilitarian:** more patients will ultimately benefit from healthcare students who practise their skills on individual patients

---

doctors. Indeed, the benefits of patient involvement in healthcare education to students include students developing and maintaining their humanism, developing their clinical and communication skills, and developing partnership relationships with patients.[14] As we can see, there is no absolute right or wrong ethical way of approaching consent, with different approaches in apparent contradiction.

From a legal standpoint, in many countries including the UK and USA, touching a patient without valid consent can comprise the criminal offence of assault and battery,[2,12,15,16] defined as: 'an intentional unpermitted act causing harmful or offensive contact with the 'person of another' (see: http://legal-dictionary.thefreedictionary.com/battery). Furthermore, patients can claim for negligence against healthcare professionals if they do not obtain valid consent for an intervention for which the patient subsequently suffers harm.[2]

From a relational standpoint, consent requests and refusals (e.g. the consultant requests that the patient give up her abdomen to allow students to learn; the patient refuses) can be considered *face-threatening acts* (*face* referring to our sense of dignity or standing in social contexts). Such acts can threaten the positive face (i.e. to maintain a positive self-image) and negative face (i.e. to have freedom of choice and from imposition) of the patient and the consultant, potentially jeopardizing the doctor-patient relationship.[6] Finally, from a safety angle, patients' involvement in decisions about their own care is associated with better healthcare outcomes.[7] Whichever way you look at it, consent matters: it protects patients and the healthcare students, trainees and professionals who serve them.

What are the Common Myths about Patient Consent for Student Involvement in their Care?

Despite there being reasonably clear guidance from regulatory bodies about patient consent for student involvement,[1-5] myths abound among healthcare students, trainees and educators about patient consent for student involvement in their care. Before continuing with this section on myths, stop and think about the issues raised in Box 6.5.

Most of the myths involve what Fretwell Wilson calls 'exaggerated fears of refusal'.[17 p. 259] That is, that patients will refuse to allow students to be involved in their care if asked, and in particular for intimate examinations and 'first-time' examinations or procedures. Research, however, has illustrated many benefits of student involvement in patient care to patients, including patients receiving more time and attention from students and clinical teachers, finding it therapeutic to talk to students, feeling empowered through helping students learn, enjoying the opportunity to influence healthcare education and appreciating the sense of giving something back to healthcare services.[14] Other myths involve the notion that consent for student involvement in patient care is unimportant in certain settings such as teaching hospitals or surgical theatres (where patients are presumed to know that students will be involved). Worryingly, such myths amongst students can actually be reinforced through their workplace learning experiences, with, for example, students' attitudes towards the importance of patient consent for their involvement in intimate examinations deteriorating after participating in obstetrics and gynaecology clerkships.[18] We examine each of these myths in turn, debunking them as we go by drawing on the research literature *with* patients.

Myth 1: Patients will Refuse Consent for Students to be Involved in their Care if Asked

'Where would we be if the patients started to say no? – that is the danger if they ask patients.'

Nurse educator from Torrance *et al.*[7, p. 94]

'We'd never get to learn how to do things 'cause everyone would just say "no, no, I want the consultant doing that, I don't want… the medical student doing that."'

Carrie, female, year 4, medical student, UK

Box 6.5 Stop and do: reflection on student involvement in patient care
• As a patient, have you ever had a healthcare student or trainee involved in your care? If so, how was this experience?
• As a patient, would you give your consent for a healthcare student or trainee to be involved in your care and why? If not, why not?
• As a healthcare learner or educator, what do you think patients want in terms of student involvement in their care? What percentage of patients do you think would allow students to be involved in routine, non-invasive procedures? What about intimate examinations? What about examinations and procedures that the student or trainee has not done before on a real patient?

Table 6.1 Patients' willingness to consent to student involvement in their care (in decreasing order).

Study	Country	Total participants	Exam type/procedure/illness/setting	Mean % would consent
*Pearce et al.[22]	UK	144	Genitourinary medicine consultations	97.1
*Koehler and McMenamin[23]	Australia	402	24 body regions including head, neck, hands and legs	96.3
*O'Flynn et al.[24]	UK	335	Chest infection, sore throat	95
Barnett et al.[25]	West Indies	210	Surgical procedures	93.3
Lynoe et al.[21]	UK	441	Range including internal medicine, psychiatry, urology and GP settings	88
Porta et al.[19]	USA	316	Elective surgical procedures	79.9
Martyn and O'Connor[11]	Ireland	222	Pelvic examinations	74
*Koehler and McMenamin[23]	Australia	402	Intimate exams	64
*O'Flynn et al.[24]	UK	335	Internal exam	50

Note: *studies examined hypothetical willingness

A common myth amongst educators and students alike is that if they ask for patient consent to be involved in their care, patients will say 'no'.[17] This misconception can then lead to a number of adverse outcomes, including not telling patients that a student is present,[19] and misrepresenting students' identities to make them appear more senior (as discussed in Chapter 5). In addition to such actions invalidating consent through lack of information and coercion (see Box 6.2), they also fly in the face of professionalism codes such as requirements to be honest and trustworthy (see Chapter 2). So how much of a myth is this? Will patients really refuse all the time? Interestingly, the research literature suggests the reverse: that patients are typically willing for students to be involved in their care. For example, a study with 137 parents and 66 child inpatients of a large New Zealand children's hospital demonstrated that they were amenable to having a medical student observe an examination, with *none* refusing to see medical students when approached by them.[20] Although fewer patients consent for students to be involved in intimate examinations, a majority still provides consent (see Table 6.1). Importantly, patients typically want consent to be sought for student involvement in their care and feel aggrieved if they are not asked.[20,21]

Myth 2: Patients will not Consent to Students Performing a Procedure on them for the First Time

'I remember the first time I took blood... the doctor's, "Oh yeah, he's done this loads and loads of times before and he's absolutely fine." (laughter)... It had the advantage of making a patient more relaxed about it, and making the whole attitude more relaxed, but it was a lie.'

Pete, male, year 3, medical student, UK

Many students and educators believe that if patients know that the student is about to perform a procedure for the first time, the patient will refuse consent. They also believe that by telling patients the truth, even if patients consent, they will be nervous, possibly making it more difficult for the student to perform well. Therefore, as seen in Chapter 5, they either lie or withhold information about their level of experience specifically for the task at hand and sometimes even about their seniority.[19,26,27] Effectively, the belief that patients will not participate in the teaching of healthcare students, if presented with a choice, means that this learning must be 'stolen' from patients by not allowing them the opportunity of providing fully informed consent.[28] Again, honesty and trustworthiness are at stake. But will patients really refuse a student's first time? For procedures like bed baths, for example, patients are often grateful for nursing students' first attempts at bathing, with patients helping students through such first-time experiences.[29] While the research evidence suggests that patients are more willing to have more senior learners involved in their care,[30] several research studies suggest that many patients are willing to consent to students doing quite invasive first-time procedures on them under supervision (see Table 6.2). Our own studies also support this (see Box 6.6 as an illustration). Importantly, patients typically want to know if it's the student's first time and state that they would be upset to discover that it was the student's first time after the event.[27]

Table 6.2 Patients' willingness to consent to student or trainees' first time (in decreasing order).

Study	Setting/ Country	Total participants	First-time procedures	Mean % would consent
Santen *et al.*[31]	USA	114	IV placement, splinting or suturing	73
*Williams and Fost[27]	USA	173	Lumbar puncture	52
*Porta *et al.*[19]	USA	316	Elective surgical procedures	45

Note: *studies examined hypothetical willingness

Box 6.6 'I need that seal of approval before I can do it'

'We'd done Venflons in clinical skills like on models… that was like a year and a half before… it was in the anaesthetics room in surgery and the ODP [operating department practitioner] said to me, "Oh, do you want to do the Venflon?"… And I said to him, "Well can we just wait for the consultant to come back in because I've not done one on a real person and I want to check?" And they were like, "Okay, that's fine whatever you're most comfortable doing." And I said to her [patient], "He's asked me to do it but I haven't done one on a patient before and I wanted to check." She was like, "Oh, no, that's fine, you've got to learn." But I felt more comfortable that she said that… because there's nothing worse than them suddenly clocking that you've not done it before and you could get really flummoxed and it just spirals… and half the time they just say to you, "Just do it anyway." But I need that seal of approval before I can do it.'

Susan, female, year 3, medical student, UK

Myth 3: Consent for Student Involvement in Patient Care is Unnecessary in Certain Settings

'It's an attitude among nurses as well, I got sent out of one consultation, a lady came and didn't want students in and this nurse outside was just ranting about, "Well they come into a teaching hospital they should expect students to be in there."'

Sally, female, year 4, medical student, Australia

We cannot assume implied consent for student involvement in patient care simply because a patient receives care from a teaching hospital.[17] In our data, practising on unconsented anaesthetised patients was one of the most common consent-related professionalism dilemmas students reported, and being in a teaching hospital was often used as an excuse for not getting patients' consent. We know that patients undergoing surgery may be unaware of the presence of students in theatres,[32,33] and are generally unaware of doctors' levels of training, including those performing their operations.[25,34] While doctors and students tend to think that patient consent for students to be present in surgery is unnecessary, overwhelmingly patients want to be asked their permission for students to be involved in their surgery.[32,33,35] Patients place more significance than students do on them observing surgery, making incisions, holding retractors, performing rectal and pelvic exams, suturing incisions and intubating.[33] Therefore, Eva's actions in Box 6.7, encouraged by her surgical team, would probably have been inconsistent with the patient's wishes.

So what is the professional thing to do? As we have seen in Box 6.1, while competent students delivering patient care do not legally speaking need to state their student status or get patient consent for their involvement in patient care, they should do these things

---

Box 6.7 'I donned some gloves and did it'

'I was forced into doing a rectal exam on an anaesthetised male patient who had not, to my knowledge, [been] consented by a consultant urologist. I was on a urology rotation in second year, and watch[ed] a procedure to stent the ureter of a man who had terminal prostate cancer that had spread to his bladder. After the procedure was done, the surgeon turned round and said, "He's got a really abnormal prostate: this would be a great one for you to feel so that you'll know what to look for in the future." I dithered, but several other surgeons were in the room and they were all saying stuff like, "Do it, you'll never learn otherwise," and, "He's out, so you're not going to hurt him"... I donned some gloves and did it. [I did so] because I felt like the ambience in the room was that this was very much the done thing, and that all the surgeons felt like it was a valuable learning experience that I'd be a fool to miss out on. Also, the comment about me never learning otherwise made me feel like I'd be seen as some kind of lightweight if I didn't step up and do it. I feel like I did the wrong thing... I now know that it is very clearly stated in our student guidebook that we are not to do these kind[s] of examinations.'

Eva, female, year 3, medical student, UK

to uphold ethics, and in the case of their involvement serving their own learning rather than patient care, then the patient needs to be fully informed about and consent to student involvement, both legally and ethically.[2] As with many areas of professionalism, consent issues are complex, with healthcare students often being simultaneously engaged in their own learning and patient care. But will patients consent if they know a student will be present? Again, the answer is probably yes. Research has found that 68% (153/225) of general surgical patients in a UK teaching hospital said they would accept student observers in theatre,[32] and 85% (97/114) of females gave written consent for students to conduct pelvic examinations on them under anaesthesia in surgery.[36] So, the take-home message here is that patients should be informed about and consent to student involvement in their care in all settings, including teaching hospitals and surgical theatres.

What are Common Consent-related Professionalism Dilemmas?

With myths abounding about patient consent for student involvement in care, it is perhaps unsurprising that we identified a multiplicity of consent-related dilemmas experienced by healthcare students across our programme of research, although such dilemmas were most commonly reported by medical students.[37-41] This difference across healthcare groups in frequency of reporting consent-related dilemmas probably reflects the different roles that students play within the workplace (see Chapter 12): medical students are often observers and primarily learners within the workplace, whereas other students (e.g. dental, nursing, physiotherapy) are also care providers.[7,42] We think medical students are therefore more likely to have problems with consent for student involvement because their healthcare interventions are often solely for the purposes of their own educational benefit (see Box 6.1). What follows is a summary of a range of consent-related professionalism dilemmas experienced by our student participants akin to those identified in Box 6.2 in three core areas: (1) students witnessing qualified colleagues not eliciting valid patient consent for healthcare interventions; (2) students' involvement in patient care activities without valid consent; and (3) students' involvement in learning activities on patients without valid consent for them to do so as students. Before moving on to the next section, work your way through Box 6.8.

Box 6.8 Stop and do: reflect on your own consent-related professionalism dilemmas

- Have you ever experienced any consent-related professionalism dilemmas?
- If so, write down your most-memorable experience: what was the gist of your dilemma, where were you and who was present, when did it take place, what happened, what did you do and why and how did you feel? Try to articulate exactly what your dilemma was at the time.
- What might you do differently if faced with a similar consent-related professionalism dilemma in the future?
- What advice would you give to one of your peers if they had this same experience?

Students Witnessing Qualified Colleagues not Eliciting Valid Patient Consent for Interventions

Students shared numerous narratives where they witnessed healthcare professionals carrying out healthcare interventions on patients without valid patient consent. Often, circumstances arose because *patients lacked capacity to consent* (see Box 6.2, point 5), either because they had temporary disturbances to their cognitive functioning as in surgical settings (e.g. severe pain, unconsciousness through anaesthesia) or more permanent and enduring disturbances to their cognition (e.g. dementia, learning difficulties, mental health problems), as commonly experienced by nursing students. In such situations, students typically discussed the appropriateness of continuing treatment without valid patient consent in the best interests of the patient. Other times, students narrated a blatant disregard for patients' autonomy and bodily integrity shown by healthcare workers who put their own needs first, such as them trying to get healthcare interventions done quickly, as illustrated in the first narrative in Box 6.9.

Students' Involvement in Patient Care Activities Without Valid Consent

Not only did students report witnessing their qualified colleagues carrying out healthcare interventions on patients without valid patient consent, but they reported doing so themselves, too. Typically such violations of consent for patient care activities occurred when it was in the patients' best interests to do so. For example, Claudia, a physiotherapy student, explains in narrative 2, Box 6.9, how she persuaded a patient needing her chest cleared to accept the suction catheter after refusing it by getting her to cough, a tactic which could be construed as *coercion* (see Box 6.2, point 1). Another concern raised by students was *patients lacking sufficient understanding of the information* (Box 6.2, point 2) provided to them to make informed decisions about their treatment, including when working with patients with English as a second language (ESL) without translators. Petra, a dental student, describes her experience of gaining patient consent for dental treatment from her patient with ESL, who she is convinced does not understand much of what she is saying, thereby invalidating consent (see narrative 3, Box 6.9).

Students' Involvement in Learning Activities on Patients Without Valid Consent for them to do so as Students

Students also explained learning on patients (e.g. practising procedures and examinations) without patient consent for them to do so as students (sometimes whilst also participating in patient care activities). Many of these dilemmas for medical students involved them observing or conducting intimate examinations and procedures on patients, often when the *patient was anaesthetised and therefore lacked capacity*.[43] Students also described how consent was often invalidated due to *patient coercion* (Box 6.2, point 1), *lack of information* (Box 6.2, point 2) and by healthcare professionals viewing *consent as a one-off event, rather than a continuous process* (Box 6.2, point 3), and therefore ignoring patients' consent withdrawals, as illustrated in Keeley's narrative at the start of this chapter (see Box 6.10 for further illustrations).

Box 6.9 Examples of consent-related professionalism dilemmas

Narrative 1: 'we had a patient who was very confused'

'We had a patient who was very confused and didn't want to be washed and very clearly refused consent, but HCA [healthcare assistant] X insisted… Our patient had variable stages of confusion, and I'd worked with her quite a bit over the past week so I knew that if you gave her time and approached her gently and at the right time, she could be coaxed into accepting a wash and a change of pad. But HCA X just wanted to get her task-list done, and when the patient refused consent she just went ahead trying to strip her anyway, saying it needed to be done regardless. I told her I was uncomfortable performing the procedure without consent, and went to tell the Sister in charge… [because] it felt very wrong… I appreciate that she needed to be cleaned and changed, but I felt that it was possible to achieve this without distressing her. I think that I was right, but I also know that it is a tricky area because when the patient lacks capacity to consent then sometimes we as nurses will need to perform procedures in their best interest without their consent, and potentially cause them distress. I worry that far too often, healthcare professionals will not have the time to spend on making sure that patients are given the time to relieve confusion and anxiety.'

Sarah, female, year 2, nursing student, UK

Narrative 2: 'either way I got my treatment and she didn't want it'

'She was you know compos mentis, completely, quite young lady, she'd just had an operation… she was ventilated and she hated having the suction done because it's uncomfortable, it's horrible to have done… I'd go to her and I'd say, "Can we clear your chest out?" and she'd usually say, "No"… I had four weeks of it to go so I just had… to take on that role [patient care] which made me feel quite uncomfortable because she didn't want it… I know it was… really in her best interests because she had so much stuff on her chest that needed clearing, it was affecting her breathing… I just felt awkward saying, "Oh well how about can I try just a few coughs instead." But then as soon as she coughs she needs the suction so either way I got my treatment and she didn't want it… there was no escaping that and I needed to do it because then that would… [be] negligence or whatever, but it was still playing at the back of my mind and… that's how I got her to consent to the treatment, she consented to one treatment, we ended up doing another.'

Claudia, female, year 3, physiotherapy student, UK

Narrative 3: 'that's not really informed consent if he doesn't really understand'

'When you've got a patient that doesn't speak English… you can't really start treatment unless you've got informed consent so… I've got a patient and I don't really know how much he understands of me because he walks in and I go, "How are you today?" and he'll go, "Yeah, yeah, yeah, good, good", and then I'll go, "Have you been in any pain at all?" And he'll go, "Yeah, yeah, yeah" (laughs)… Ooh, he doesn't know a word I'm saying (laughs)… I feel that's not really informed consent if he doesn't really understand… maybe I might do some treatment and maybe he might not agree with what I'm doing but he can't really sort of get [it] across… and he doesn't seem to bring an interpreter with him.'

Petra, female, year 5, dental student, UK

Box 6.10 Illustrations of ways in which consent was invalidated for students' involvement in learning activities with patients

---

Patient coercion (see Box 6.2, point 1)

Healthcare professionals coercing patients through misrepresenting students' identities (e.g. calling medical students 'doctors', see Chapter 5).

Insufficient information (see Box 6.2, point 2)

'There was a lady who came in [GP surgery]… she'd been told that there were students in there but I don't think she'd been told how many before she came into the room, so when she came in to find four of us in there she was like, "Oh, er, right (laughs) four of you, yes I wasn't expecting that"… Actually she didn't ask us to leave… but I think she was just a little like on edge because of it.'

Karen, female, year 1, medical student, UK

Inappropriately timed requests for consent (see Box 6.2, point 3)

'Patient seemed obliging to let us watch but… possibly felt she couldn't refuse since we were already present in the room and doctor didn't give [her the] choice of leaving if she felt uncomfortable… [we] watched procedure but tried to stay out of way, only approached when doctor encouraged us… [it was] early on in clinical experience – didn't want to voice our concerns.'

Ellie, female, year 3, medical student, UK

'Patients don't seem too fully aware or warned a student's there who would like to practise their skills… it's sort of we're in clinic discussing a case and then suddenly the examination comes along and then it's like, "Oh do you mind if Steve does an examination on you", and the woman's, you can actually see the woman sort of suddenly go a little bit shocked because it's like a little bit out of the blue.'

Steve, male, year 5, medical student, UK

Person lacks capacity (see Box 6.2, point 5)

'Patient refused consent on letting me watch their cholecystectomy, they were then anaesthetised and I was encouraged to watch by the SpR [Specialty Registrar]… I had the choice of violating [the] patient wishes without the patient knowing, or not attending and winding up the SpR for a "wasted" opportunity as he put it.'

Arthur, male, year 3, medical student, UK

What is the Impact of Consent-related Professionalism Dilemmas?

In our studies, healthcare students' consent-related dilemma narratives were littered with emotional talk, illustrating the often negative emotional impact that such dilemmas have on learners.[37–40] In particular, consent-related dilemmas contained a significant amount of anxiety talk.[39,40] As we have already seen, students express their anxieties about being placed in consent-related dilemmas using words such as 'uncomfortable', 'wrong',

---

Box 6.11 '...Only made me feel worse about medicine'

'Doctor X examined Patient Y who seemed to have learning difficulties and he required a PR [per rectal], he didn't gain sufficient consent for the PR, or for my supervision. Plus his communication was appalling. It was in a GP practice, I was in the room, there was no one else. I feel I should have decided not to observe but the doctor practically ordered me to when I hesitated, even when the patient looked upset. I carried on, which I regret. I felt I couldn't contradict my senior. [I feel] awful [about it now], the patient obviously was uncomfortable with it. I wrote about it in my portfolio and discussed it with my tutor, he then told me I shouldn't get above myself and that I should know my place, which only made me feel worse about medicine. This attitude needs to change.'

Janice, female, year 4, medical student, UK

Box 6.12 Stop and do: reflect on Steve's consent-related professionalism dilemma

Think about Steve's dilemma in Box 6.10. If you were Steve:

- Would you go along with the consent lapse? What repercussions might this have?
- Would you resist it? What repercussions might this have?
- Would you raise your concerns about the dilemma to someone? If so, who?

'worry' and 'awkward'. They talk about patients being distressed by student involvement in their care and their discontent towards their senior clinicians who they see as responsible for instigating such consent lapses. For example, Janice, a medical student, tells us how she observed a rectal examination on a patient without valid consent, and in doing so she illustrates some self-loathing (see Box 6.11).

So Janice stayed and observed the PR. Like many other students who complied with consent lapses, she talked of her regret for doing so, expressed anger, along with an erosion of how she feels about the profession: *'this attitude needs to change'*. By contrast, students in our studies who talked about resisting during consent lapses (we define resistance here as students not going along with the lapse) tended to express positive emotional talk around their resistance (e.g. 'happy', 'praised'). Our research suggests that students experience *moral distress* as a result of their consent-related dilemmas, with females reporting more distress than males for these dilemmas.[41] And while the intensity of healthcare students' moral distress increases the more they experience consent-related dilemmas (a pattern we call *disturbance*), for medical students, moral distress actually decreased in situations where clinicians instigated examinations for the benefit of student learning (a pattern we call *habituation*). This decrease in distress is likely to be because such lapses are potentially justifiable for their learning and will benefit future patients (a utilitarian perspective outlined earlier in Box 6.4).[41] In the final section of this chapter we consider the question: Should I resist, or go along with it, when faced with a consent-related dilemma? But first, work through the activity in Box 6.12.

How do Students Act in the Face of Consent-related Professionalism Dilemmas?

'I picked up a lady from an inpatient ward to have a procedure… however, I felt she was unable to consent due to a possible lack of capacity. *I was at my placement area, my mentor, two nurses and a doctor were present. I raised my concerns immediately to my mentor who spoke to the doctor, he spoke with the lady and conducted memory tests. I felt that if she didn't have capacity and we carried out the invasive procedure without proper consent we could cause this lady harm. [I feel] very happy that I spoke up for her. I was supported by the whole team and praised for speaking up.'*

Ella, female, year 1, nursing student, UK

We can see already from the narratives presented in this chapter that students either instigate consent lapses themselves, or comply or resist with lapses initiated by their clinical teachers. Our research suggests that students are more likely to report doing nothing (thereby complying) in the face of their consent-related dilemmas.[39,40] They also give many reasons for compliance, including because they are *told* to do something (e.g. examination or procedure) by their senior educators or colleagues and they fear negative repercussions if they do not comply (e.g. failing their placements as discussed in Chapter 4, or missing out on valuable learning opportunities). Sometimes they feel the interventions are in the patients' best interests or that patients have consented in some way (albeit invalid). Sometimes they are unaware of the 'right' course of action at the time, only later realizing their actions were morally dubious.

But there are things students and trainees can do when placed in a consent-related dilemma: they can resist going along with the lapse. The most common forms of resistance in our research for such situations includes acting to show concern for patients, directly challenging the instigator verbally and reporting the instigator of the lapse (see Keeley at the start of the chapter, and Sarah in Box 6.9).[39,40] While no negative repercussions were reported in Sarah's resistance narrative, Keeley reports being 'told off' and 'picked on' by the consultant for the rest of her placement. However, the outcomes of resistance are not always bad, as illustrated in Ella's narrative above, in which the whole team praised her for raising her concerns.

So, what is the *right* thing to do and *how* can we all accomplish this? Recall our analysis of the various healthcare regulators' ethical and professional policy documents in Chapter 2 in which personal and professional accountability and raising concerns feature heavily. Thus, students, trainees and educators alike are encouraged to resist consent lapses whenever possible, for the benefit of patients and learners. Although direct verbal challenges can be anxiety provoking, there are more subtle and indirect strategies that can reduce any negative repercussions.[39] For example, challenging indirectly by proactively gaining consent: tell the patient who you are, your level of experience and what you propose to do. Show concern for patients, for example, leave the room when patients have not fully consented for student observers. Report consent-related lapses appropriately. Talk with others such as peers, friends and tutors about the event in order to debrief.

It is important to think about ways of saying 'no' to clinical teachers in clear and non-confrontational ways, like those advocated in the crew resource management literature (CRM).[44] For example, performance feedback is at the heart of CRM approaches, considering both the timing and relevance of communication, along with three levels of feedback: (1) team member delivers message in brief, clear and non-blaming way

---

Box 6.13 Information: 'learning to say no to people in a non-confronting, non-combative way'

Kyle, a male medical student from Australia posted the following blog after reading an Australian newspaper article discussing our research findings around intimate examinations without consent:[43]

...I don't think it's [intimate examination without consent] a grey area, it's pretty black and white: you have to say no. The key is in not making that an awkward and uncomfortable conversation. Learning to say no to people in a non-confronting, non-combative way is pretty much a must have.

CONSULTANT: While I scrub, VE [vaginal examination] Mrs Smith.
YOU: I'm sorry, I ran out of time and wasn't able to get consent before the patient went under [anaesthetic], I'll make sure to check with the next patient though.

basically, (1) Start with an apology. You haven't done anything wrong but it makes the whole thing less combative; (2) Inform them you didn't get consent. It implies that the consultant didn't realize you didn't have consent, rather than implying they were suggesting something unethical; (3) Inform them you'll get consent on the next patient. Ends on a positive note, but more importantly is a fairly definitive end to any discussion of exams on this unconsented patient.

(See http://medstudentsonline.com.au/forum/threads/medical-students-are-performing-intrusive-exams-on-unconscious-patients.14754/)

('Dr X, I'm not sure we got consent'); (2) the message contains an important term such as *comfort* that implies value ('Dr X, I'm not comfortable with...'), and (3) if feedback is ignored, the fallback could be an appeal to halt what is happening.[44] See Box 6.13 for Kyle's suggestion to say 'no' in a non-blaming way.

Chapter Summary

This chapter has provided an overview of what consent is and why it matters within the context of healthcare professionalism. We have unpacked various myths about patient consent for student involvement and presented research evidence debunking them. We have learnt about the multiplicity of consent-related dilemmas experienced by healthcare students and trainees. We have seen how students typically go along with consent lapses because of the healthcare hierarchy (more on healthcare hierarchies later in Chapter 9), but how compliance can cause substantial upset for patients and moral distress for learners. But we have also seen positive outcomes, positive emotional reactions and better protected patients when students resist consent lapses. Furthermore, we have demonstrated how you can resist such lapses in subtle, yet powerful ways. The key take-home messages from this chapter are summarized in Box 6.14, with suggestions for small group discussions in Box 6.15. Finally, Boxes 6.16 and 6.17 outline further learning activities and recommended reading.

Box 6.14 Chapter summary points

- Consent in healthcare education and practice is complex and matters for several reasons
- Learners and educators should realize that most patients are happy for students to be involved in their care, but expect and want to be asked
- Healthcare students and trainees experience numerous consent lapses and have the option to comply or resist
- Consent lapses can be upsetting and distressing for learners, particularly if they do not resist
- Students and trainees are encouraged to resist consent lapses in subtle, less risky ways, to protect themselves and patients

Box 6.15 Chapter discussion points

- Discuss the paper 'Female identity and the vulva' by Jenny Jones, a student midwife (see recommended reading). Thinking specifically about student involvement in intimate examinations, what have you learnt from this paper that you can use to help you develop your practice?
- Discuss Kyle's suggestions about how to refuse a senior clinician's requests to be involved in patient care without patient consent (see Box 6.13). Would this work and why? What other strategies could you use?

Box 6.16 Chapter learning activities

- Find out what the policies of your school/training programme are in terms of patient consent for student/trainee involvement in their care. Is your practice and that of your peers consistent with the policy and if so/not, why?
- Find out what the policies of your school/training programme are in terms of raising concerns about consent-related dilemmas? Who should you report to and how? Is your practice and that of your peers consistent with the policy and if so/not, why?

Box 6.17 Chapter recommended reading

Carson-Stevens A, Davies MM, Jones R, Pawan Chik AD, Robbe IJ, Fiander AN. Framing patient consent for student involvement in pelvic examination: a dual model of autonomy. *Journal of Medical Ethics* 2013;39:676–680.

Jones J. Female identity and the vulva. *Midwifery Matters* 2012;135:13–16.

Leung GKK, Patil NG. Medical students as observers in theatre: is an explicit consent necessary? *The Clinical Teacher* 2011;8:122–125.

Rees CE, Knight LV. Thinking 'no' but saying 'yes' to student presence in general practice consultations: politeness theory insights. *Medical Education* 2008;42:1152–1154.

Torrance C, Mansell I, Wilson C. Learning objects? Nursing educators' views on using patients for student learning: ethics and consent. *Education for Health* 2012;25(2):92–97.

References

1 Australian Medical Council. *Good Medical Practice: A Code of Conduct for Doctors in Australia*. Kingston, Australia: Australian Medical Council, 2009.

2 Department of Health. *Reference Guide to Consent for Examination or Treatment*, 2nd Edition. London: Department of Health, 2009.

3 General Medical Council. *Good Medical Practice 2012*. London: General Medical Council, 2012.

4 NMC. *Guidance on Professional Conduct for Nursing and Midwifery Students*. NMC, London, 2010, http://www.staff.city.ac.uk/m.j.jones/PDFs/Guidance-on-professional-conduct-for-nursing-and-midwifery-students-September-2010.pdf (Accessed 2 December 2016).

5 Chartered Society of Physiotherapy. *Consent and Physiotherapy Practice*. London: CSP, 2011, http://acppld.csp.org.uk/documents/new-consent-guidance-csp (Accessed 2 December 2016).

6 Rees CE, Knight LV. Thinking 'no' but saying 'yes' to student presence in general practice consultations: politeness theory insights. *Medical Education* 2008;42:1152–1154.

7 Torrance C, Mansell I, Wilson C. Learning objects? Nursing educators' views on using patients for student learning: ethics and consent. *Education for Health* 2012;25(2):92–97.

8 Jameton A. *Nursing Practice: The Ethical Issues*. New York: Prentice Hall, 1984.

9 American Nurses Association. *Code of Ethics for Nurses*. http://www.nursingworld.org/codeofethics (Accessed 2 December 2016).

10 Hafferty FW, Franks R. The hidden curriculum, ethics teaching, and the structure of medical education. *Academic Medicine* 1994;69(11):861–871.

11 Martyn F, O'Connor R. Written consent for intimate examinations undertaken by medical students in the operating theatre – time for national guidelines? *The Irish Medical Journal* 2009;102:336–337.

12 Bartholomew K, Hooks C. Consent to student involvement in treatment – the legalities. The Royal College of Midwives, 2011, http://arro.anglia.ac.uk/295430/ (Accessed 2 December 2016).

13 Carson-Stevens A, Davies MM, Jones R, Pawan Chik AD, Robbe IJ, Fiander AN. Framing patient consent for student involvement in pelvic examination: a dual model of autonomy. *Journal of Medical Ethics* 2013;39:676–680.

14 Rees CE, Knight LV, Wilkinson CE. User involvement is a sine qua non, almost, in medical education: learning with rather than just about health and social care service users. *Advances in Health Sciences Education* 2007;12:359–390.

15 Margetts JK. Learning the law: practical proposals for UK medical education. *Journal of Medical Ethics* 2012;0:1–3; doi: 10.1136/medethics-2012-101013.

16 Tawose OM. The legal boundaries of informed consent. *AMA Journal of Ethics* 2008;10(8):521–523.

17 Fretwell Wilson R. Autonomy suspended: using female patients to teach intimate exams without their knowledge or consent. *Journal of Health Care Law & Policy* 2005; 240–263.

18 Ubel PA, Jepson C, Silver-Isenstadt A. Don't ask, don't tell: a change in medical student attitudes after obstetrics/gynecology clerkships towards seeking consent for pelvic examinations on an anaesthetized patient. *American Journal of Obstetrics & Gynecology* 2003;188:575–579.

19 Porta CR, Sebesta JA, Brown TA, Steele SR, Martin MJ. Training surgeons and the informed consent process. Routine disclosure of trainee participation and its effect on patient willingness and consent rates. *Archives of Surgery* 2012;147(1):57–62.

20 Pinnock R, Weller J, Shulruf B, Jones R, Reed P, Mizutani S. Why parents and children consent to become involved in medical student teaching. *Journal of Paediatrics and Child Health* 2011;47:204–210.

21 Lynoe N, Sandlund M, Westberg K, Duchek M. Informed consent in clinical training-patient experiences and motives for participating. *Medical Education* 1998;32(5):465–471.

22 Pearce A, Burns F, Richards M, Palmer J, Keane F. What factors influence whether a patient consents to having medical students involved in his/her sexual health consultation/examination? *HIV Medicine* 2014;15(S3):79–79.

23 Koehler N, McMenamin C. Would you consent to being examined by a medical student? Western Australian general public survey. *Medical Teacher* 2012;34:e518–e528.

24 O'Flynn N, Spencer J, Jones R. Consent and confidentiality in teaching in general practice: survey of patients' views on presence of students. *British Medical Journal* 1997;315:1142.

25 Barnett T, Cawich SO, Crandon IW, Lindo JF, Gordon-Strachan G, Robinson D, *et al*. Informed consent from patients participating in medical education: a survey from a university hospital in Jamaica. *BioMed Central Research Notes* 2009;2:252. doi: 10.1186/1756-0500-2-252.

26 Santen SA, Rotter TS, Hemphill RR. Patients do not know the level of training of their doctors because doctors do not tell them. *Journal of General Internal Medicine* 2007;23(5):607–610.

27 Williams CT, Fost N. Ethical considerations surrounding first time procedures: a study and analysis of patient attitudes toward spinal taps by students. *Kennedy Institute of Ethics Journal* 1992;2(3):217–231.

28 Gawande A. *Complications: A Young Surgeon's Notes on an Imperfect Science.* New York, NY: Metropolitan Books, 2002: pp. 11–34.

29 Wolf ZR. Nursing students' experience bathing patients for the first time. *Nurse Educator* 1997;22(2):41–46.

30 Pallin DJ, Harris R, Johnson CI, Giraldez E. Is consent 'informed' when patients receive care from medical trainees? *Academic Emergency Medicine* 2008;15:1304–1308.

31 Santen SA, Hemphill RR, Spanier CM, Fletcher ND. 'Sorry, it's my first time!' Will patients consent to medical students learning procedures? *Medical Education* 2005;39:365–369.

32 Leung GKK, Patil NG. Medical students as observers in theatre: is an explicit consent necessary? *The Clinical Teacher* 2011;8:122–125.

33 Silver-Isenstadt A, Ubel PA. Erosion in medical students' attitudes about telling patients they are students. *Journal of General Internal Medicine* 1999;14:481–487.

34 Santen SA, Hemphill RR, Prough EE, Perlowski AA. Do patients understand their physician's level of training? A survey of emergency department patients. *Academic Medicine* 2004;79(2):139–143.

35 Bray JK, Yentis SM. Attitudes of patients and anaesthetists to informed consent for specialist airway techniques. *Anaesthesia* 2002;57(10):1012–1015.

36 Broadmore J, Hutton JD, Langdana F. Medical students' experience of vaginal examinations of anaesthetised women. *British Journal of Obstetrics and Gynaecology* 2009;116(5):731–733.

37 Monrouxe LV, Rees CE. 'It's just a clash of cultures': emotional talk within medical students' narratives of professionalism dilemmas. *Advances in Health Sciences Education* 2012;17(5):671–701.

38 Monrouxe LV, Rees CE, Endacott R, Ternan E. 'Even now it makes me angry': healthcare students' professionalism dilemma narratives. *Medical Education* 2014;48:502–517.

39 Rees CE, Monrouxe LV, McDonald LA. Narrative, emotion, and action: Analysing 'most memorable' professionalism dilemmas. *Medical Education* 2013;47(1):80–96.

40 Rees CE, Monrouxe LV, McDonald LA. My mentor kicked a dying woman's bed: analysing UK nursing students' most memorable professionalism dilemmas. *Journal of Advanced Nursing* 2015;71(1):169–180.

41 Monrouxe LV, Rees CE, Dennis A, Wells S. Professionalism dilemmas, moral distress and the healthcare student: insights from two online UK-wide questionnaire studies. *British Medical Journal Open* 2015; 5:e007518.doi:10.1136/bmjopen-2014-007518.

42 Omid A, Daneshpajouhnejad P, Pirhaji O. Medical students' and physicians' attitudes toward patients' consent to participate in clinical training. *Journal of Advances in Medical Education & Professionalism* 2015;3(1):21–25.

43 Rees CE, Monrouxe LV. Medical students learning intimate examinations without valid consent: a multi-centre study. *Medical Education* 2011;45:261–272.

44 Haerkens MHTM, Jenkins DH, van der Hoeven JG. Crew resource management in the ICU: the need for culture change. *Annals of Intensive Care* 2012;2:39.

7

Patient Safety-related Professionalism Dilemmas

'[I witnessed] a surgeon not using a facemask during surgery... The patient's abdomen was being operated on, one surgeon had already opened up the patient's abdomen and another surgeon arrived to assist. This surgeon did not put on a facemask but was talking over the patient's open wound. I could see the surgeon's saliva actually going into the open wound as she talked. Serious infection control risk! I did not say anything at the time but I asked one of the nurses why the surgeon did not wear a mask, and the nurse told me the surgeon has been told on numerous occasions to put on a mask, but didn't. I didn't say anything to the surgeon myself because I felt that as the student nurse it wasn't my place to do so... I feel angry that nobody said anything but still feel that it wasn't my place to say anything.'

Ella, female, year 1, nursing student, UK

LEARNING OUTCOMES

- To understand how patient safety is defined
- To discuss factors affecting patient safety incidences in the workplace
- To understand the range of patient safety-related professionalism dilemmas experienced by learners across healthcare professions
- To consider the role of learners in developing a workplace culture of patient safety
- To reflect on the ways in which professionalism dilemmas relating to patient safety can be managed

---

KEY TERMS

Patient safety
Patient safety incident
Iatrogenic harm
Patient safety culture
Raising concerns

Healthcare Professionalism: Improving Practice through Reflections on Workplace Dilemmas, First Edition.
Lynn V. Monrouxe and Charlotte E. Rees.
© 2017 John Wiley & Sons Ltd. Published 2017 by John Wiley & Sons Ltd.

Introduction

First do no harm. These four words convey a potent reminder that every decision and action from healthcare learners and practitioners carries potential for iatrogenic (from the Greek for 'brought forth by the healer') harm, resulting from preventable (and sometime non-preventable) errors or purposeful violations of safe operating procedures.[1] Iatrogenic maltreatment is a worldwide phenomenon. Indeed, a recent study suggested that medical error is the third most common cause of death in the US.[2] In community pharmacies (through prescription error), and in dentistry, adverse events tend to reflect those found in hospital settings.[3] Patient safety is therefore intimately entwined with a number of professionalism dimensions (see Box 2.1, Chapter 2) and the ethic of non-maleficence, along with wider societal, professional and legal responsibilities to report patient safety incidents. In this chapter, we consider how patient safety and related terms have been defined and the factors influencing safety in healthcare workplaces, paying particular attention to those factors involving healthcare students and trainees. Following this, we examine the range of patient safety-related dilemmas discussed by students and trainees across our research programme, identifying ways in which students narrate patient safety-related lapses and their compliance with or resistance to those lapses (often the cause of their dilemma). Finally, the important role of healthcare students and trainees in developing a workplace culture of patient safety is addressed.

How Have Patient Safety and Associated Terms been Defined?

> *'Patient safety is the prevention of avoidable errors and adverse effects to patients associated with health care.'*[4]

There are numerous interpretations of the term *patient safety*, all of which broadly concur with that of the UK Royal College of Nursing: to minimize preventable patient harm. Leape and Berwick[5] take this further by stating that failure to treat or over-treatment also comprise patient safety. Others talk of reduction (rather than prevention) and the improvement of patient safety through best practice: 'the reduction and mitigation of unsafe acts within the healthcare system, as well as through the use of best practices shown to lead to optimal patient outcomes.'[6, p. 12] Such issues of amelioration include not only immediate care for patients, but also admissions of error (and apologizing for these), along with addressing improvements in the wider healthcare team when appropriate.[7]

Interestingly, definitions do not just focus on errors at the individual level, but include other adverse events such as accidents, violations, negligence, near-misses and complications that arise from or impact upon economic, social, cultural and organizational aspects of healthcare:[8] see Box 7.1 for some of the most common patient-safety terms and their definitions. From this perspective, the *culture* of patient safety in the workforce is emphasized rather than individual-level action.

In addition to considering patient safety as a stand-alone concept, others link patient safety with the concept of patient dignity.[11] Essentially, a positive culture of safety has a communication system based on mutual trust, shared perceptions of the importance of safety and partnership working with its major stakeholders. Consequently, the core

---

Box 7.1 Information: definitions of the most common patient-safety terms

Adverse event: 'an unintended injury or complication resulting in prolonged hospital stay, disability at the time of discharge or death and caused by healthcare management rather than by the patient's underlying disease process'.[9, p. 216]

Near miss: an event that *might* have had an adverse patient outcome, but did not.

Error: 'the unintentional use of a wrong plan to achieve an aim, or failure to carry out a planned action as intended'. [10, p. 975] A key aspect here is focus on thoughts and actions rather than outcomes (so errors might not necessarily lead to harm every time).

Violation: 'a deliberate – but not necessarily reprehensible – deviation from those practices appreciated by the individual as being required by regulation, or necessary or advisable to achieve an appropriate objective while maintaining safety and the ongoing operation of a device or system'. [10, p. 975] Again, this definition focuses on mental states and actions rather than outcomes.

Negligence: the failure to provide a standard level of care appropriate to a particular context, resulting in an adverse event occurring (so can include situations arising from all of the above).

Box 7.2 Stop and do: classifying patient safety lapses

- Have you or anyone in your group ever witnessed or participated in a situation that compromised the safety of one or more patients?
- If so, write down a list of all the different types of events you can recall.
- Try to classify them according to whether the events comprised one (or more) of the following: adverse event; near-miss; error; violation and/or negligence, and explain why.

---

values of patient safety, along with patient and family engagement, are integral to the culture within which patient dignity flourishes. Thus, the loss of dignity can be seen as an error that has adverse effects on patients.[11] However, due to the depth of discussion required for both patient safety and dignity issues, we consider the issue of patient dignity in Chapter 8.

Having outlined the various ways in which patient safety has been defined, the next section concerns the factors affecting patient safety in the workplace. Here, we adopt a human factors approach by identifying influences affecting healthcare professionals' behaviours at work. Before reading the next section, we encourage you to look at the 'stop and do' activity in Box 7.2.

What are the Factors that can Influence Patient Safety in the Workplace?

While the distinction is often made between individual, interactional, organizational and cultural levels, these are intertwined. For example, sometimes an individual error, lapse or violation has its roots within systemic or cultural factors, as illustrated earlier in Ella's narrative, with a strong hierarchical culture acting as a 'latent' factor in the surgeon's safety lapse. As such, for over 25 years, a systems approach to safety management has been adopted within high-risk organizations.[12] Reason[13] adopts a *Swiss cheese* metaphor to characterize accidents that cause harm, illustrating how errors can slip through the system despite overlapping defences and safeguards. Each slice of the cheese represents a distinct level of protection: engineered protection (e.g. alarms, physical barriers, automated shutdowns), human protection (e.g. surgeons, nurses, pharmacists), along with 'check-box' procedural safeguards and administrative controls. But despite these different layers, if the holes in the cheese line up, errors occur. Thus, while it is not always useful or desirable to lay the blame at any single layer, there are certain factors that represent the holes in the layers at the individual, interactional and cultural/organizational levels (see Box 7.3 for common risk factors across healthcare professional groups).

A powerful example of this comes from the inquiry into the Mid Staffordshire NHS Foundation Trust in the UK, with its culture of patient neglect and mistreatment leading to the unnecessary deaths of around 1200 patients in a single hospital (see Box 7.4

Box 7.3 Information: common risk factors affecting patient safety at different levels

Individual factors include:

Trainee healthcare professionals, insufficient knowledge/skills; tiredness/working long hours, gender (i.e. being male), burnout and depression.[15–21]

Interactional factors include:

Poor team communication, power hierarchies (including reluctance to raise concerns), poor interprofessional working relations, staff attitudes and behaviours, poor client/patient-practitioner communication, poor written communication (including medication errors/omissions).[15,18,20,22–25]

Organizational culture factors include:

Poor organizational communication (e.g. between workplace locations), resourcing, understaffing/excessive workload, and out-of-hours working.[15,21,25–27]

Box 7.4 Information: testimonials from patients, families and carers of substandard care received from junior doctors

'The patient went to A&E… suffering from abdominal discomfort. A junior doctor insisted it was a urine infection but the patient was certain it was appendicitis. When the patient asked to see a specialist he was ignored and discharged. The following day the patient collapsed when his appendix burst.'[28, p. 15]

'Suffering with severe vomiting and diarrhoea a diabetic woman was admitted to A&E at Stafford Hospital. She was told to drink a lot of water and was immediately discharged by a junior doctor. Her condition deteriorated further and she was readmitted to the Intensive Treatment Unit where she was sedated and given dialysis. The patient did not regain consciousness and died of a heart attack and renal failure.'[28, p. 102]

Box 7.5 Stop and do: factors behind patient safety lapses

Thinking about the events identified in Box 7.4, try to understand the factors lying behind the events, focusing on the following:

- What happened?
- Why did it happen?
- Try to classify those events according to individual, interactional and organizational cultural levels.
- Consider the ways in which these levels interact with one another.

---

for patients' testimonials of substandard care from junior doctors).[14] What was clear from this inquiry is when things go wrong, they often do so due to a complex interplay between personal, interpersonal, systemic and cultural factors. This is illustrated by Ella's narrative above, where she recounts witnessing an individual surgeon failing to adhere to hygiene standards, yet no one (including her) directly challenges the surgeon due to stark hierarchical relationships (see Chapter 9 for further discussion about healthcare hierarchies).

In addition to these common factors, there are various profession-specific factors that have negative patient safety implications. For example, there is a demonstrated increase in mortality following medical student graduates entering hospitals, [29] and working in a community pharmacy is a risk factor for malpractice allegations.[30] While workplace environmental factors have been shown to interact with individual factors (e.g. higher nurse-to-patient ratios and greater numbers of nurses with high levels of education result in lower mortality and deaths),[31] a positive workplace environment (e.g. good leadership, openness, honesty, interprofessional communication, good staffing levels) has been identified as the most important aspect affecting patient care and safety.[32] Before moving to the next section, work through the 'stop and do' activity in Box 7.5.

What Types of Patient Safety-related Dilemmas Occur Across Different Healthcare Professions?

We now outline the types of patient safety-related dilemmas narrated by healthcare professional students and trainees across our research programme. In order to examine these dilemmas, along with learners' actions, we consider them in terms of the different types of patient safety issues: errors and violations often resulting in adverse outcomes and near misses.

Dilemmas Around Patient Safety Errors

Healthcare students and trainees across our research frequently narrated witnessing healthcare practitioners breaching patient safety though a range of errors and occasionally witnessing other healthcare students' errors or admitting to making errors themselves (see Box 7.6 for an overview of the types of errors experienced across the healthcare groups in our studies).

Box 7.6 Information: overview of patient safety error types experienced across healthcare student/trainee groups

Error type	Description	Healthcare group (professional and/or student)
Commission (involving action)	Clinical procedure/surgery: mistakes	Medical, Nursing, Dental, Physio
	Communication: incorrect information/ poor handover	Nursing
	Medication: wrong dose	Medical, Nursing, Pharmacy
	Medication: wrong medication	Nursing, Pharmacy
	Medication: out of date	Nursing, Pharmacy
	Medication: wrong patient	Medical, Nursing
	Patient feeding: when nil-by-mouth	Medical, Nursing
	Wrong notes/test results	Medical
Omission (involving inaction)	Attending calls: missed or delayed	Medical, Nursing
	Medication: neglected/withheld	Medical, Nursing
	Missed diagnosis	Medical, Dental
	Patient feeding: neglected	Nursing
	Patient monitoring: neglected	Nursing, Dental
	Record keeping: neglected/omitted	Medical, Nursing, Dental

By far the most common types of errors narrated were errors of commission; specifically, students narrating witnessing healthcare practitioners breaching patient safety through making mistakes due to incompetent practice, including when undertaking practical procedures, when referring to notes and test results, and unsafe prescribing practices. These errors of commission include patients being prescribed higher doses of drugs (up to ten times the correct amount), being given drugs prescribed for another patient or being prescribed the incorrect drug for their condition (see Lysa's narrative, narrative 1, Box 7.7). Other errors include patients being given the wrong procedure (or wrong site) and procedures being carried out badly. For example, a physiotherapy graduate forgot to ask if the patient had any metal on them before she applied a pulse short-wave machine to his shoulder, but the patient had a watch on; and a nurse over-tilting the bed of a patient with an intracranial bleed (see Violet's narrative, narrative 2, Box 7.7). In surgery, narratives include patients being left with sponges inside them, and shoddy work due to time, work-related and personal pressures. Communication errors were also narrated, including nurses providing incorrect information about patients and poor handover practices.

Students narrated situations in which other students or trainees breached patient safety: including a narrative about a junior doctor who inserted a cannula in an artery instead of a vein, resulting in the patient having her arm amputated (admittedly this would be a very unusual outcome from an inadvertent arterial cannulation and other factors might be involved); a nursing student who failed many times when cannulating anaesthetised children causing them physical and emotional trauma when they woke up; and dental

Box 7.7 Students' narratives of healthcare professionals and students breaching patient safety through errors of commission

Narrative 1: 'nurses blamed pharmacy… doctors then blamed a drug allergy'

'Medical staff passed the blame for the wrong dose of an antibiotic being given to a baby around each other, [causing] adverse effects in the baby which were near fatal, [and] were put down as a drug allergy, which was not true… Nursing staff made up solution of antibiotic from an old paper they found. The dose was extremely large… nurses blamed pharmacy but pharmacy had not seen the recipe before. Doctors then blamed a drug allergy, which was not true… The pharmacist supervising me passed the information onto the lead pharmacist who dealt with the matter… [I'm] still annoyed and distressed that it was "covered up"…'

Lysa, female, year 4, pharmacy student, UK

Narrative 2: 'he died a day later'

'Nurse tilted the head of the bed down on a patient with an intracranial bleed to move him up the bed. He died a day later. I was helping in moving the patient… we are both short and I fear that she took our lack of strength into account and tilted the bed more than she should have given his clinical situation. [I did] nothing. Initially, I asked, "Should he be tilted that way?" She ignored the question… I was treated very badly on that ward and didn't feel able to convey my worry to anyone… The worry that we caused further harm will stay with me for the rest of my days I think…'

Violet, female, year 3, nursing student, UK

Narrative 3: 'that's a really, really dangerous thing to do'

'One of the girls in my group… was taking out a tooth… and she ended up… driving through the floor of the patient's mouth… there was lots of blood and… she said, "Ooh", pulled it out, and then carried on… it's not just like a little thing, that's a really, really dangerous thing to do… but we never said anything because you just don't do that, like we should have done because that's a really huge breach…'

Elissa, female, year 5, dental student, UK

Narrative 4: 'he's an arm, just get it in (laughs)'

JON: Remember that time when we were both in the ED and you were holding the old man down for me and I kept jabbing him [to insert a cannula].

HUGH: Oh yeah, that was terrible (laughter)…

JON: I went too many times… I still feel kind of pretty bad about that… so there were three of us, there was this old man who came in and he wasn't really with it… he was just sort of sleeping and like just groaning and then he smelled and he was malnourished and everything like that… so originally it was Lewis and another student and they had trouble keeping him down… I didn't know what I was thinking… I thought, 'Oh yeah, I'll have a go as well then' (laughter) and so (laughs) I got you to hold him down and… tried about five times or something… and Lewis and Stuart were telling me to stop and…

HUGH: Yeah like, 'Um I think you've had enough goes'…

JON: I thought that, you know, if he's not really with it… It was almost as if he was in the surgical frame again. So this is no longer a patient, this is just… just like, 'He's an arm, just get it in' (laughs) I sort of didn't even connect with him or anything…

Jon and Hugh, male, year 3, medical students, Australia

students carrying out poor dental work, leaving patients at risk of ulcerations and infections (see Elissa's narrative, narrative 3, Box 7.7). Some students discussed their own patient safety-related dilemmas in which they acted beyond their levels of competency, through their own volition. An example of this can be seen in Box 7.7 (narrative 4) where Jon and his medical student colleague Hugh talk about a time when they kept on trying to insert a cannula and ended up injuring the patient. In general, reasons students go ahead and undertaking these activities included them feeling the need to learn, their over-confidence and them not recognizing patients as human beings due to their drowsy or unconscious states, their illnesses (e.g. dementia) and/or them being classified as being of low social status (through appearance, personal hygiene, etc. as in Jon and Hugh's example).

Another common type of patient safety-related dilemma narrated by healthcare students comprises errors of omission. For example, students told us how they witnessed practitioners either missing or delaying calls to attend to patients for a variety of reasons, including their poor attitudes (and subsequent care) towards certain 'problem' patients, not believing students when they felt a patient was severely unwell and practitioners prioritizing teaching over patient care (Will's narrative, narrative 1, Box 7.8). Students also talked about situations in which medical and nursing staff either neglected (due to time pressures) or withheld patient medication. Overmedication was also reported in situations where doctors or nurses wished to sedate 'disruptive' patients. Time pressures also led to nursing staff neglecting patient monitoring, record keeping and sometimes feeding (e.g. a nurse knowingly omitting the testing of a diabetic patient's blood sugar because she was 'too busy'). Forgotten tests and poor record keeping were also reported in some dental student dilemmas around the actions of their peers. While there were reports of doctors missing obvious signs and symptoms in patients, dental students also reported other students overlooking key signs of mouth cancer in patients (Roslyn's narrative, narrative 2, Box 7.8). Finally, one common patient safety-related dilemma narrated by dental students was that of providing unnecessary treatment for their patients for the sake of their learning.

In addition to patient safety errors, we identified many safety violations in our data. By far the most common form of violation was *routine violations* (defined as regular shortcuts) of hygiene regulations by most types of healthcare professionals (see Talisa's and Catelyn's narratives, narratives 1 and 2, Box 7.9). The typical way in which hygiene regulations were flouted was through hand-washing failures, although failures to keep equipment clean (e.g. doctors using otoscopes to examine patients' ears without cleaning in between patients) and general unclean practices (e.g. dropping medication on the floor and then administering it to patients) were also narrated. Although medical students sometimes narrated dilemmas in which they admitted to speeding up their hand-washing practices, in our wider body of research around graduates' preparedness for practice, junior doctors also admitted to flouting hygiene rules if they felt no one would reprimand them for poor practice.

Unsafe manual handling techniques (by physiotherapy and nursing practitioners), most commonly using 'drag lifts', where the patient is literally dragged up the bed by their underarms, comprised the second most common form of routine violation in our data (See Miranda's narrative, narrative 3, Box 7.9). Other patient safety violations include senior healthcare professionals asking students to perform procedures without proper supervision, sometimes because they are busy with other patients. For example, nursing students talked about being left in charge of too many patients (sometimes an

---

Box 7.8 Students' narratives of patient safety dilemmas involving errors of omission

Narrative 1: 'page me if she starts bleeding REALLY heavily'

'History taking session in Obs and Gynae with tutor group… Doctor X, 11 medical students [present]. Doctor received a page which he answered on a nearby phone. Conversation that we heard included, "I'm with medical students right now", "How heavily is she bleeding? Okay put in an IV, I'll be down in 10–15 minutes and page me if she starts bleeding REALLY heavily." The doctor then proceeded to talk to us about the OBG history with all students, including myself, feeling rather uneasy that we were potentially taking his time from an emergency… he did not leave until about 40 minutes later. We didn't say anything, we didn't feel it would be appropriate…'

Will, male, year 3, medical student, UK

Narrative 2: 'it could be cancer'

'I assisted an Erasmus student… and I noticed something in their [patient's] mouth… an ulcer and I sort of said… quietly, not to sort of scare the patient, "Oh have you noticed this patient has like um sort of like an ulcer in their mouth?" and she's like, "Yeah it was there the last time I saw her and the time before that," so I was like, "Okay, that's worse… that makes it more serious," and I was like, "You need to tell a member of staff about this," so she went, "Okay", she went over to tell a member of staff… I was just cleaning down… when I came back the patient had gone and nobody was there and I said to her, "Oh, um, what did the clinician say about the ulcer?" and she was like, "Oh I didn't say anything", and to me that was like a really major thing… sort of life threatening, and then I said [names student], "Okay you need to get that sorted,"… the patient had already left reception… I told her it was like, "It could be cancer,"… but I mean she's like, "I'm going home tomorrow though"… I was just shocked…'

Roslyn, female, year 4, dental student, UK

Box 7.9 Students' narratives of patient safety dilemmas around rule violations

Narrative 1: not the sterile method

'Unhygienic practice was observed, not the way we were shown to do it at uni. I was observing a more senior physio in a hospital [who used the] suction – open and not the sterile method. [I] asked why they didn't use sterile open suction, it was a valid question – I thought! Didn't get a satisfactory answer from the PT ("we just don't"), so still feel confused about this…'

Talisa, female, year 4, physiotherapy student, UK

Narrative 2: did not follow correct infection control precautions

'Nurse performed male catheterization – dismissed patient's cries of pain and did not follow correct infection control precautions. At a dementia unit at a nursing home… The nurse performed a male catheterization while myself and the other student observed. The nurse did not wash her hands beforehand. She put on two pairs of sterile gloves but did not remove the first pair after cleaning the patient's genital area. She then proceeded to insert the catheter without any… gel to numb the area. The patient was very red in that area and was crying out, saying, "It's sore, it's sore". The nurse continued saying, "It's not sore, stop play acting." The old catheter was flung on the floor and the nurse did not wash her hands afterwards. [I did] nothing – just watched and then talked about it afterward with the other student nurse. I didn't feel able to question what the nurse was doing… I was also worried that there might be bad relations between me and the nursing staff for the rest of my placement…'

Catelyn, female, year 1, nursing student, UK

Narrative 3: it is illegal

'[I was] in a hospital with a healthcare assistant, she wanted to do a drag lift with a little old lady and I said, "No, we should get a slide sheet," but she said I was just being difficult and taking more time up. When I still wouldn't do it, she told the whole ward and no one would talk to me. I said "no" to doing a drag lift because it is illegal, could injure either of us health professionals and the patient. It also makes the skin "chafe"…'

Miranda, female, year 1, nursing student, UK

Narrative 4: I failed miserably

'Was asked to suture a minor injury even though I had not had any training. [I was] In A&E with consultant [who] asked me to suture a patient… I attempted to suture, though I failed miserably. Patient was not too happy about me being not so good at the sutures. I felt pressured, and also I thought I might be losing a valuable learning opportunity if I didn't go ahead….'

Donnel, male, year 5, medical student, UK

Narrative 5: not considering patient care and safety

'Labelling and dispensing methadone practice, not double checking names and addresses when handing out medication… by a pre-reg student in community pharmacy. I would be surprised if the SOP [standard operating procedure] they were following would instruct the student to follow the work pattern they were employing… [I did] nothing. I just commented on the differences between their methods and the way I perform the task at my weekend job, as I didn't want to be associated with their dangerous, and in my view, unprofessional practice….'

Gared, male, year 4, pharmacy student, UK

entire ward) due to staff shortages, and medical students frequently talked about being asked to perform procedures above their level of competency (see Donnel's narrative, narrative 4, Box 7.9). Other violations included pharmacists or pharmacy students not following safe operating practices when dispensing medication (Gared's narrative, narrative 5 Box 7.9) or concealing mistakes by destroying evidence, nurses leaving drugs unattended, and a clinician committing audit fraud (e.g. handpicking patient cases to bias results) with another making up blood pressure results.

How can Healthcare Learners' Actions and Roles Develop a Positive Workplace Culture of Patient Safety?

'... *When I've been in a room if they've [consultant's] asked me... to examine a patient... [I say], "Oh can [I] wash my hands quickly?" and then they'll go out and do it, and when I've clearly seen them not wash their hands between patients [I say], "Oh I'd better wash my hands"... one of the consultants actually said, "It's changed since the medical school opened"... our first clinical skills session is how to wash our hands, and so because we all did, they all started going "My God they wash their hands between every single person, this is terrible that we don't"... since we've been here they've implemented the whole green bottle at every door and physicians like shout at you if you walk past it and don't wash your hands... they had a whole bunch of us come through and they see us do it and they think, "Oh we should do it"...'*

Mira, female, year 3, medical student, UK

As discussed in previous sections, students and trainees report witnessing and participating in patient safety lapses. Indeed, in the narratives already presented students are distressed by these lapses, as evidenced by their negative emotional talk (e.g. 'angry', 'annoyed', 'distressed', 'worry'/'worried', 'bad'/'badly', 'terrible', 'trouble', 'uneasy', 'shocked', 'surprised', 'pressured', 'miserably', 'confused') and laughter for coping (as Jon and Hugh did earlier when they admitted to having too many attempts to insert a cannula: Box 7.7). In this section we consider students' reported actions during such lapses – both their compliance with and resistance to lapses, and the important role of students and trainees in the development of a workplace safety culture, as indicated in Mira's narrative above (for a formal definition of safety culture see Box 7.10).

There are a multitude of recommendations within the literature around how to develop a safety culture within healthcare organizations, including improvements at the individual, interactional and organizational levels. Many focus on aspects of team/organizational leadership and the development of a patient-centred and *just* culture (one that recognizes errors as systems rather than individual failures). Few, however, provide specific guidance for the healthcare student or trainee.

In Chapter 6 we introduced the concept of crew resource management (CRM) from the aviation industry, which we believe has some utility for healthcare students' and trainees' roles in strengthening the ethical climate of healthcare organizations more generally (not just where patient safety is concerned). Within CRM, communication is key. Good team communication involves having a respect for one another's roles, having direct eye-contact, introducing each other (often using first names to flatten the hierarchy), using non-judgemental words with safety as a priority rather than

---

Box 7.10 Information: definition of a safety culture

A safety culture has been defined as:

'The product of individual and group values, attitudes, perceptions, competencies and patterns of behaviour that determine the commitment to, and the style and proficiency of, an organization's health and safety management'

(Advisory Committee on the Safety of Nuclear Installations[33, p. 23]).

self-esteem or face-saving.[34] Indeed, CRM is beginning to be assimilated into healthcare settings, although to our knowledge, CRM is not an approach that has been adopted within undergraduate training contexts for healthcare students.[35] This might partly be due to the stark differences between healthcare and aviation: in aviation, junior team members are trained to speak out when they feel safety is at risk, whereas within the hierarchical healthcare culture, students and junior staff find it hard to question the behaviours and decisions made by their seniors.[36] For example, let us consider what healthcare students and trainees do in the face of patient safety lapses. Summarizing the narratives presented in this chapter we can see that they often reported doing nothing (see Ella, Lysa, Violet, Elissa, Will, Catelyn, Donnel and Gared above). Indeed, they provide numerous reasons in their narratives for doing nothing; these include hierarchy (Ella and Catelyn), loyalty towards peers (Elissa), objectification of patients (Jon and Catelyn), student learning opportunities (Donnel), low self-efficacy around challenging lapses (Lysa and Will) and high self-efficacy around beliefs of competence (Jon).

Although many students and trainees (and healthcare professionals) maintain an organizational silence around patient safety lapses,[36,37] there are those who do not. Consider other narratives presented in this chapter (e.g. Violet, Roslyn, Miranda and Mira) whereby students attempt to resist patient safety lapses. Recognizing students and trainees as leaders in their own right, drawing on communication strategies within CRM and learning from the actions of those who do resist (as illustrated by Mira at the beginning of this section) we propose the '4-Rs' approach to learners' promotion of a patient safety culture (Box 7.11).

Box 7.11 Learning activity: the '4-Rs' approach to participaing in a safety culture

Resisting: entails the refusal to go along with unsafe practice.

Role-modelling: safe practice for others to see.

Reviewing: requires that intelligent questions are asked of those who breach safe practices (including ourselves), revealing systemic, organizational and/or cultural issues that might underlie such practices and encouraging an exploration of alternative courses of action. Reviewing can include strategies drawn for CRM whereby eye-contact is made with the person who is being addressed, the person's name is used (e.g. 'Dr Jones', 'Nurse Jones'), your emotions are expressed (e.g. 'I'm anxious that', 'I'm not comfortable with this'), the problem is explicitly stated (e.g. 'Hygiene regulations are not being followed appropriately', 'This is the wrong dose of antibiotic'), what you think should be done (e.g. 'We should stop right now', 'We should double check'), ask for agreement (e.g. 'Do you agree?', 'Shall we do this?') and finally, if the situation is not resolved and patient safety is at risk, a more assertive tone might be required (e.g. 'Stop the procedure', 'Don't give her the medication'). As such, this may require persistence if the error or violation is not addressed immediately.

Reporting: involves seeking out the correct processes through which concerns can be raised, and having the courage to highlight errors or violations when witnessing their occurrences.

Learning activity: Re-read the narratives already presented in this chapter and identify any examples of these 4-Rs. In groups, enact one of the scenarios presented, using the 4-Rs approach to safety culture.

First, related to the issues of *resisting* and *reviewing*, 'speaking up' has been advocated as an assertive way of addressing breaches in situations requiring immediate action.[34,38] Indeed, research examining oncology staff communicating safety concerns found their speaking-up behaviour to be strongly related to immediate clinical safety issues such as medication errors.[39] Speaking up can be achieved through questions, opinion statements and information, and requires persistence until the error is resolved. So, within the narratives presented in this chapter, we see healthcare students indirectly challenging their seniors and peers through questioning (e.g. Violet's questioning of the nurse around the positioning of the patient and Talisa's challenge to the senior physiotherapist about them not using the sterile method). While more risky, directly challenging the protagonist is another way to break the silence. Examples above include Hugh telling Jon, 'I think you've had enough goes', and Miranda refusing to undertake a drag lift. However, resistance and (indirect) challenging can also be made 'silently' through bodily acts. Research suggests that the majority of silent acts are connected to hygiene violations, isolation and invasive procedures.[39] Similarly, within our data, students frequently narrated bodily acts of resistance in the context of hygiene breaches, akin to Mira's narrative above, in which students reported ostentatiously washing their hands in front of more senior doctors. This relates to the role modelling in the 4-Rs, where students can model appropriate behaviour, rather than directly challenging violations.

Having considered ways to resist and review medical errors and violations, and to role model good practice, we now turn to think about the last of our 'Rs', that of *reporting*. Ideally this should be in the form of incident reporting within your organization.[40] However, in situations where this is difficult (e.g. you require another person to agree and it is difficult to raise the issue directly, or they refuse) *raising concerns (whistleblowing)* indirectly with an authoritative person is the next option. Recall in Chapter 2 how improving patient safety and raising concerns is a core professionalism requirement. Amongst healthcare students and practitioners alike, however, fears abound regarding the negative consequences of raising concerns.[41] In students, amongst those fears are a sense of powerlessness and vulnerability due to the unequal hierarchies between themselves and perpetrators of the safety breaches.[42] However, students do speak out sometimes because of the clarity of professional guidelines and strong imperatives to follow them.[43] Indeed, we see this strongly in the narrative from Mirelle, a fourth year medical student in the UK (Box 7.12).

Box 7.12 'I could see that he was making up the readings'

Observed a GP… making up blood pressures for patients without performing the procedure. The GP, another student and myself [were present], before patients entered, or while in the room, the computer system had a space for the entry of the BP of patients. Doctor would simply input readings without taking blood pressures. [I] spoke to an honorary lecturer and the situation was taken higher up. Spoke to various members of clinical and university staff regarding the incident. I could see that he was making up the readings and after some consideration, and noticing that he was doing this with the majority of his patients, decided I couldn't carry it on my conscience not to pass this on. Very relieved that we whistle blew. Staff we spoke to were grateful and commended us on our professionalism and honesty, despite feeling apprehensive.'

Mirelle, female, year 4, medical student, UK

Chapter Summary

This chapter has explained what patient safety is and the factors contributing to patient safety lapses. We have examined the different types of errors and violations healthcare students and trainees experience and learners' reactions and actions in the face of patient safety lapses. We have discussed how healthcare learners can contribute to the development of a workplace culture of safety by resisting, role-modelling, reviewing and reporting. The summary points from this chapter are in Box 7.13, with suggestions for small group discussions in Box 7.14 and learning activities around the duty of candour in Box 7.15. Finally, Box 7.16 outlines some recommended reading.

Box 7.13 Chapter summary points

- Iatrogenic events occur worldwide, with the WHO asserting that up to one in ten patients suffer harm whilst receiving hospital care
- Patient safety has been variously defined to include the prevention of avoidable errors and violations and making improvements when things go wrong
- Common risk factors underlying safety lapses can be classified at the individual, interactional and organizational levels, with each level interacting
- Common patient safety dilemmas narrated by healthcare students include clinical and surgical errors, medication errors, communication errors, and violations of hygiene and safe handling regulations
- Healthcare students and trainees are central to the development of a culture of patient safety and can actively contribute through resistance, role-modelling, revealing and reporting practices

---

Box 7.14 Chapter discussion points

Discuss with your peers and educators the processes of raising concerns at your institution:

- To whom should you report?
- What responsibilities does that person have in terms of documenting your concerns?
- What other actions could you take if nothing changes?
- What safeguards are in place to protect you when you raise concerns?
- What factors impede your willingness to raise concerns?
- What changes would you make to the process of raising concerns at your institution that might address these issues?

Box 7.15 Chapter learning activities

The GMC, in association with other UK healthcare regulatory bodies, including pharmacy, dentistry and nursing, outlines a statutory duty of candour (i.e. professional responsibility for all healthcare professionals to own up to patients when something has gone wrong that has the *potential* to harm patients, offering an apology, a full explanation and remediation, see: http://www.themdu.com/guidance-and-advice/guides/statutory-duty-of-candour/statutory-duty-of-candour#sthash.DYP0TCRN.dpuf).

- What (if any) is the duty of candour (open disclosure) within your specific healthcare professional group in your own country?
- What does this duty entail for healthcare students and trainees in terms of how they should act in the face of patient safety lapses?
- Discuss the potential facilitating factors and barriers that you perceive to be present within your own learning environment and organization that might impact on your ability to carry out this duty

Box 7.16 Chapter recommended reading

King J, Anderson CM. Patient safety and physiotherapy: what does it mean for your clinical practice? *Physiotherapy Canada* 2010;62(3):172–175.

Sammer CE, Lykens K, Singh KP, Mains DA, Lackan NA. What is patient safety culture? A review of the literature. *Journal of Nurse Scholarship* 2010;42(2):156–165.

Schwappach DLB, Gehring K. 'Saying it without words': a qualitative study of oncology staff's experiences with speaking up about safety concerns. *British Medical Journal Open* 2014(5).

Seiden SC, Galvan C, Lamm R. Role of medical students in preventing patient harm and enhancing patient safety. *Quality and Safety in Health Care* 2006; 15(4):272–276.

Yamalik N, Perea Perez B. Patient safety and dentistry: what do we need to know? Fundamentals of patient safety, the safety culture and implementation of patient safety measures in dental practice. *International Dental Journal* 2012;62(4): 189–196.

References

1 Reynard J, Stevenson P. *Practical Patient Safety*. Oxford: Oxford University Press, 2009.

2 Makary MA, Daniel M. Medical error – the third leading cause of death in the US. *British Medical Journal* 2016;353.

3 Thusu S, Panesar S, Bedi R. Patient safety in dentistry – state of play as revealed by a national database of errors. *British Dental Journal* 2012;213:E3–E3.

4 World Health Organisation. http://www.euro.who.int/en/health-topics/Health-systems/patient-safety (Accessed 15 December 2016).

5 Leape LL, Berwick DM. Five years after to err is human: what have we learned? *Journal of the American Medical Association* 2005;293:2384–2390.

6 Canadian Patient Safety Institute. The Canadian patient safety dictionary. In *Institute CPS* (Ed.) Calgary: Canadian Patient Safety Institute, 2003.

7 Vincent C. *Patient Safety*, 2nd Edition. Oxford: Wiley Blackwell, 2010.

8 Yamalik N, Perea Perez B. Patient safety and dentistry: what do we need to know? Fundamentals of patient safety, the safety culture and implementation of patient safety measures in dental practice. *International Dental Journal* 2012;62:189–196.

9 de Vries EN, Ramrattan MA, Smorenburg SM, Gouma DJ, Boermeester MA. The incidence and nature of in-hospital adverse events: a systematic review. *Quality & Safety in Health Care* 2008;17:216–223.

10 Runciman WB, Merry AF, Tito F. Error, blame, and the law in health care – an antipodean perspective. *Annals of Internal Medicine* 2003;138:974–979.

11 Winokur SC, Beauregard KJ. Patient safety: mindful, meaningful, and fulfilling. *Frontiers of Health Services Management* 2005;22:17–32.

12 Reason J. Understanding adverse events: human factors. *Quality in Health Care* 1995;4:80–89.

13 Reason J. Human error: models and management. *British Medical Journal* 2000;320:768–770.

14 Francis R. Mid Staffordshire NHS Foundation Trust Public Inquiry. http://webarchive. nationalarchives.gov.uk/20150407084003/http://www.midstaffspublicinquiry.com/report (Accessed 2 December 2016).

15 Wilkins K, Shields M. Correlates of medication error in hospitals. *Health Reports* 2008;19:7.

16 Nash L, Daly M, Johnson M, Coulston C, Tennant C, va Ekert E, *et al.* Personality, gender and medico-legal matters in medical practice. *Australasian Psychiatry: Bulletin of Royal Australian and New Zealand College of Psychiatrists* 2009;17:19–24.

17 Sears K, Goodman WM. Risk factors for increased severity of paediatric medication administration errors. *Healthcare Policy = Politiques de sante* 2012;8:109–126.

18 Whang JS, Baker SR, Patel R, Luk L, Castro A, 3rd. The causes of medical malpractice suits against radiologists in the United States. *Radiology* 2013;266:548–554.

19 Aala A, Tabrizi J, Ranjbar F, Vahdati SS, Mohammadi N. Frequency of burnout, sleepiness and depression in emergency medicine residents with medical errors in the emergency department. *Advances in Bioscience and Clinical Medicine* 2014;2:6. http://www.journals. aiac.org.au/index.php/ABCMED/article/view/658 (Accessed 2 December 2016).

20 DeNoble PH, Marshall AC, Barron OA, Catalano LW, 3rd, Glickel SZ. Malpractice in distal radius fracture management: an analysis of closed claims. *The Journal of Hand Surgery* 2014;39:1480–1488.

21 Garrouste-Orgeas M, Perrin M, Soufir L, Vesin A, Blot F, Maxime V, *et al.* The Iatroref study: medical errors are associated with symptoms of depression in ICU staff but not burnout or safety culture. *Intensive Care Medicine* 2015;41:273–284.

22 Lingard L, Espin S, Whyte S, Regehr G, Baker GR, Reznick R, *et al.* Communication failures in the operating room: an observational classification of recurrent types and effects. *Quality and Safety in Health Care* 2004;13:330–334.

23 Rabøl LI, Andersen ML, Østergaard D, Bjørn B, Lilja B, Mogensen T. Descriptions of verbal communication errors between staff. An analysis of 84 root cause analysis-reports from Danish hospitals. *British Medical Journal Quality & Safety* 2011;20:268–274.

24 Mills PR, Weidmann AE, Stewart D. Hospital discharge information communication and prescribing errors: a narrative literature overview. *European Journal of Hospital Pharmacy*, 2015.

25 Stalpers D, de Brouwer BJM, Kaljouw MJ, Schuurmans MJ. Associations between characteristics of the nurse work environment and five nurse-sensitive patient outcomes in hospitals: a systematic review of literature. *International Journal of Nursing Studies* 2015;52:817–835.

26 Birkmeyer NJO, Finks JF, Greenberg CK, McVeigh A, English WJ, Carlin A, *et al.* Safety culture and complications after bariatric surgery. *Annals of Surgery* 2013;257:260–265.

27 Tan A, Thong S, Zeng A, Ng S. Analysis of critical incidents during anaesthesia in a tertiary hospital. *Anaesthesia* 2014;69:77.

28 Francis R. *The Mid Staffordshire NHS Foundation Trust Inquiry*. London: Department of Health, 24 February 2010.

29 Blakey JD, Fearn A, Shaw DE. What drives the 'August effect'? An observational study of the effect of junior doctor changeover on out of hours work. *JRSM Short Reports* 2013;4.

30 Phipps DL, Noyce PR, Walshe K, Parker D, Ashcroft DM. Pharmacists subjected to disciplinary action: characteristics and risk factors. *The International Journal of Pharmacy Practice* 2011;19:367–373.

31 Kendall-Gallagher D, Aiken LH, Sloane DM, Cimiotti JP. Nurse specialty certification, inpatient mortality, and failure to rescue. *The Journal of Nursing Scholarship* 2011;43:188–194.

32 Aiken LH, Patrician PA. Measuring organizational traits of hospitals: the Revised Nursing Work Index. *Nursing Research* 2000;49:146–153.

33 ACSNI - Advisory Committee on the Safety of Nuclear Installations, Study Group on Human Factors. Third Report: Organizing for safety. London: HMSO. 1993.

34 Kapur N, Parand A, Soukup T, Reader T, Sevdalis N. Aviation and healthcare: a comparative review with implications for patient safety. *JRSM Open* 2016;7:2054270415616548.

35 Haerkens MH, Jenkins DH, van der Hoeven JG. Crew resource management in the ICU: the need for culture change. *Annals of Intensive Care* 2012;2:39.

36 Henriksen K, Dayton E. Organizational silence and hidden threats to patient safety. *Health Services Research* 2006;41:1539–1554.

37 Morrison EW, Milliken FJ. Organizational silence: a barrier to change and development in a pluralistic world. *The Academy of Management Review* 2000;25:706–725.

38 Premeaux SF, Bedeian AG. Breaking the silence: the moderating effects of self-monitoring in predicting speaking up in the workplace. *Journal of Management Studies* 2003;40:1537–1562.

39 Schwappach DLB, Gehring K. 'Saying it without words': a qualitative study of oncology staff's experiences with speaking up about safety concerns. *British Medical Journal Open* 2014;4.

40 National Health Service. NHS Confed/NPSA briefing: *Five Actions to Improve Patient Safety Reporting*, 2008.

41 Jackson D, Peters K, Andrew S, Edenborough M, Halcomb E, Luck L, *et al.* Understanding whistleblowing: qualitative insights from nurse whistleblowers. *Journal of Advanced Nursing* 2010;66:2194–2201.

42 Cornish J, Jones A. Factors affecting compliance with moving and handling policy: student nurses' views and experiences. *Nurse Education in Practice* 2010;10:96–100.

43 Ion R, Smith K, Nimmo S, Rice AM, McMillan L. Factors influencing student nurse decisions to report poor practice witnessed while on placement. *Nurse Education Today* 2015;35:900–905.

8

Patient Dignity-related Professionalism Dilemmas

'I had been on a ward round earlier that morning and heard an elderly gentleman be told by a registrar that he had oesophageal cancer. For learning, I then went to take a history from this patient. He told me that he had never thought he would be treated as "subhuman" in a hospital. That he was unable to breathe when lying flat but that no one would get an extra pillow for him or rearrange the bed. That he had wet the bed several times because he had to wait over an hour for a bedpan. That when he did inevitably bed wet the nurses scolded him and moved him around roughly to change sheets, which gave him back pain due to his arthritis... I went and got him an extra pillow and rearranged his bed to be more upright. I then found a few urine collectors and put them on his bedside table... [I did this] because I thought the way he had been treated was inhumane and the man had just been told he had cancer so at least had the right to be in a comfortable environment. I did not tell any healthcare professionals about my concerns because I was only a third year and did not feel it was my place. That incident occurred in my first few weeks of third year and I have seen a great number of incidents like that since then, where patients are stripped of their dignity. Unfortunately I believe we become desensitized to them as you get more and more involved with the tasks on the ward. You get distracted by other jobs and you also see so many patients treated in this manner that it becomes the norm. I believe that if I witnessed the same situation now it would not distress me half as much, which I believe is a terrible thing.'

Kate, female, year 5, medical student, UK

LEARNING OUTCOMES

- To understand what patient dignity is and its relationship with professionalism
- To explore what patient dignity violations involve and how they arise
- To discover the range of patient dignity violations witnessed/enacted by healthcare students
- To discuss the impact of patient dignity violations on patients and healthcare learners
- To reflect on the various ways students, trainees and practitioners can and should act when faced with patient dignity violations

---

Healthcare Professionalism: Improving Practice through Reflections on Workplace Dilemmas, First Edition.
Lynn V. Monrouxe and Charlotte E. Rees.
© 2017 John Wiley & Sons Ltd. Published 2017 by John Wiley & Sons Ltd.

KEY TERMS
Patient dignity Communication violations Physical violations Privacy violations Dignity-related moral distress Compliance with violations Resistance to violations

Introduction

Every patient has the right to dignity and every healthcare student, trainee and practitioner has the responsibility to foster that dignity.[1] However, we know from research, including our own, that healthcare students and trainees commonly witness and/or participate in patient dignity violations.[2-6] For example, while 61% of 18,907 formal complaints made to the health service ombudsman in Australia over an 11-year period related to clinical care, a staggering 23% related to communication, including practitioners' poor attitudes and manner towards patients (15%) and inadequate quality/ quantity of information provided to patients by practitioners (6%).[7] As illustrated in Kate's narrative at the start of this chapter, patients who are acutely unwell can be treated as 'subhuman', particularly those who are most vulnerable and dependent on the care of others. As Kate explains, dignity violations are all too common; so much so that sometimes healthcare students can become immune to them as patient indignities become normalized. In this chapter, we discuss what patient dignity is and why it matters in healthcare. We explore dignity violations and how they arise through multiple factors at various levels: individual, interpersonal and organizational. We share various types of patient dignity violations articulated in key healthcare investigations and those experienced by healthcare students across our own professionalism research. We also discuss the emotional impact of these violations on students, plus their actions in the face of violations. We hope this chapter will help empower healthcare students, trainees and educators to do their best to maintain patient dignity within the healthcare workplace. Through upholding patient dignity, the dignity of *all* should be fostered: patients and staff alike.[8]

What is Patient Dignity?

What first comes to mind when you think of the word dignity? The term comes from the Latin *dignus* meaning 'worthy'.[1] Its historical trajectory is situated within three relationships: God-humanity, society-individual and freedom-determinism (see Box 8.1 for further explanation).[9] There are various definitions for dignity across the literature, with many contradictions. Dignity can be seen as: objective versus subjective, public versus private, individual versus collective, internal versus external, hierarchical versus democratic, unconditional versus contingent, static versus dynamic, descriptive versus prescriptive and so on.[9,10]

Box 8.1 Information: history of dignity as outlined by Jacobson[9]

God-humanity relationship: influenced by Biblical text, humans are thought to be made in the image of God, and are therefore sacred or worthy (e.g. 'I am worthy because I am made in the image of God').

Society-individual relationship: influenced by classical Greek ideas, humans were ascribed dignity on the basis of their standing within society (e.g. 'I am worthy because of my rank in society').

Freedom-determinism relationship: influenced by Kantian thought, dignity was viewed as belonging to all sentient human beings because of their capacity for moral freedom and determinism (e.g. 'I am worthy because I am human with free will').

Box 8.2 Information: dignity definitions

'Dignity is concerned with how people feel, think and behave in relation to the worth or value of themselves and others. To treat someone with dignity is to treat them as being of worth, in a way that is respectful of them as valued individuals.'

Royal College of Nursing[13]

'Human dignity is a principle, the value that belongs to every human being simply by virtue of being human.'

Jacobson[8, p. 1538]

'Social dignity is generated in the interactions between and among individuals, collectives and societies. Social dignity can be divided into two types: dignity-of-self and dignity-in-relation. Dignity-of-self is an individual quality of self-respect and self-worth that is identified with characteristics like confidence and integrity... dignity-in-relation refers to the ways in which respect and worth are conveyed and mirrored through individual and collective behavior... also encompasses the historical sense of dignity as adhering to status or rank.'

Jacobson[8, p. 1538]

In Box 8.2, we illustrate how the healthcare literature differentiates dignity into two types – human and social – making it clear that all patients have a right to (human) dignity but that their (social) dignity can be promoted or violated through social interactions within the healthcare setting.[9,11] While such definitions focus on the dignity of the individual, many authors stress the interdependence of dignity: by responding to another's dignity, we express and enhance our own.[8,12]

Why Does Patient Dignity Matter?

'When dignity is present people feel in control, valued, confident, comfortable and able to make decisions for themselves... When dignity is absent people feel devalued, lacking control and comfort. They may lack confidence and be unable to make decisions for themselves. They may feel humiliated, embarrassed or ashamed.'
Royal College of Nursing[13]

Box 8.3 Stop and do: reflect on whether all patients have equal worth

'Everyone has equal worth as human beings and must be treated as if they are able to feel, think and behave in relation to their own worth or value. The nursing team should, therefore, treat all people in all settings and of any health status with dignity, and dignified care should continue after death.'

Royal College of Nursing[13]

- To what extent do you agree with the above statement?
- Do you think there are certain groups of people who have less worth/value than others? Why?
- Can, for example, perpetrators of violent crimes be justifiably afforded less dignity than sick children in a healthcare context? Why?

In terms of the key professionalism documents from healthcare regulators in the four English-speaking countries identified in Chapter 2, all highlight the importance of respect, nearly all talk about patient privacy and confidentiality, and most mention patient dignity, patient rights and the importance of compassion and/or kindness. Further, in a survey of 41 countries, dignity was identified as the second most important non-clinical aspect of healthcare (the first being access to healthcare).[14]

Patients whose dignity is maintained are more likely to be satisfied with their care, and experience better healthcare outcomes, such as improved adherence to treatment.[8] Conversely, if patients are distressed over the levels of dignity afforded to them by healthcare practitioners, this can adversely affect their health and recovery.[11,15,16] Essentially, dignity is thought to serve as a barometer for the measurement of healthcare quality.[9] Before reading the next section, complete the activity in Box 8.3.

What are Dignity Violations and How do they Arise?

In some instances patients can be very unwell, to the extent that they are dependent upon the care of healthcare practitioners. Indeed, the very nature of healthcare, with its history taking, examinations and procedures, essentially works against the accomplishment of complete dignity.[1] Worldwide, there has been much public interest in patient dignity. For example, in the UK, media stories have been fuelled by high-profile healthcare investigations (e.g. 'Dying without dignity,'[17] 'Care and compassion?,'[18] 'Right here, right now,'[19] and the Mid Staffordshire NHS Foundation Trust public inquiry,[20–22] discussed in Chapter 7), which have captured both patient and public imagination and fear. Much of the literature on dignity violations focuses on the dignity of vulnerable patients such as older patients, patients within certain healthcare settings (e.g. palliative care, acute general hospital, emergency medicine, rehabilitation and mental health), women's childbirth experiences, and individuals whose life choices and/or health conditions are stigmatized.[1,9,10,15] See Box 8.4 for a list of 16 dignity violations, with examples from recent UK healthcare investigations.

Dignity violations can be brought about by factors at the level of the individual, interpersonal and organization. The individual level, for example, includes factors such as

Box 8.4 Information: Jacobson's[8] 16 patient dignity violations with illustrative examples from recent UK healthcare investigations

1) **Rudeness:** Generalized disrespect: '…One day one of the nurses came in… and she said to my Mum, "What medication have you had today?"… and my Mum said, "Sorry, what did you say?" and she snapped, "I said what medication did you have?"… I went later to find this lady and said, "Excuse me, don't treat my Mum like an elderly idiot… civility costs nothing".…'[20] p. 133/134

2) **Indifference:** Lack of consideration/care of patients, such as leaving them waiting: 'She recalled how her son had pleaded with her: "Mum please get me out of here. I'm better looked after on ward 7 when the doctor comes straight away."'[17] p. 10

3) **Condescension:** Being talked down to or spoken to like children: 'The nurse did say she had dropped her. Those were her exact words to me. She said, "Your Mum has been very naughty."'[20] p. 69

4) **Dismissal:** Having their knowledge, skills, concerns and needs ignored: 'I feel that GPs dismissed my concerns and my experiences and made me feel that I could not turn to them.'[19] p. 25

5) **Disregard:** 'Patients as invisible': 'They would carry on conversations over your head but they would never once acknowledge you… they just totally ignored me.'[20] p. 110

6) **Dependence:** Providers fostering patients' dependence around basic needs such as toileting: 'Before his admission his wife said he had been able to eat, drink, talk coherently, see to his personal care… but now he had been "turned into a zombie, a ragdoll".'[18] p. 33

7) **Intrusion:** Patients having their body boundaries transgressed (e.g. being physically exposed): 'The door was wide open. There were people walking past. Mum was in bed with the cot sides up and she hadn't got a stitch of clothing on.'[20] p. 55

8) **Objectification:** Being treated like an object rather than a person: 'They just treated him… as if he was just… a log of wood.'[20] p. 110

9) **Restriction:** Patients having limitations on their freedom: 'I heard from a number of witnesses who felt restricted in their access to patients because of visiting hours… the initial comment of the nurse which said: "We don't like you visiting during mealtimes."'[20] p. 88

10) **Labelling:** Receiving descriptive labels that suggest inferiority: 'When I rang the crisis team they called me a "bad person" for hallucinating which triggered me to self-harm for the first time.'[19] p. 56

11) **Contempt:** Treated without value: 'Because I was dressed in dossy clothes (it was cold) I think he looked at me as if to say, "She's just another scum off the street"…'[19] p. 26

12) **Discrimination:** Treated sub-optimally based on group membership: 'GP practice has marginalized her as a profoundly deaf person.'[17] p. 13

13) **Revulsion:** Treated with disgust: 'Following her husband's death his wife was spoken to by a nurse in the pub who said her, "husband was disgusting to get so fat".'[21] p. 109

14) **Deprivation:** Service access denied: 'people who were dying had extremely poor experiences in getting support outside normal working hours.'[17] p. 16

15) **Assault:** Patients' body/spirit is damaged through physical force: 'Mrs H was strapped onto a stretcher in the back of an ambulance for her safety… When Mrs H arrived at the care home, the manager noted that she had numerous injuries…'[18] p. 24

16) **Abjection:** Required to compromise beliefs/standards (e.g. hygiene): 'And this guy had got a hospital gown on… he was covered all the way down in faeces… I went down to the nurses' station, I said… "Now get up there and wash that man down and give him some dignity". That man was left 25 minutes. I thought a dog at a vet's would not be left like that and this guy has probably fought in two world wars.'[20] p. 110

Box 8.5 Information: contributory factors for dignity violations with illustrations from recent UK healthcare investigations

---

Individual

Practitioners' poor attitudes: 'Feedback from our call for evidence highlights poor staff attitudes to injuries caused by self-harm.'[19, p. 6]

Practitioners' clinical incompetence: 'In many of the cases that we reviewed, clinicians failed to recognize that the person was dying.'[17, p. 6]

Practitioners' failures to raise concerns: 'Clinicians did not pursue management with any vigour with concerns they may have had. Many kept their heads down.'[22, p. 44]

Interpersonal

Suboptimal patient-practitioner communication: 'Almost all cases we looked at highlighted failings in communication: between clinician and patients, clinicians and families…'[18, p. 12]

Practitioner-centered care: 'Patients and relatives felt excluded from effective participation in the patient's care.'[22, p. 46]

Organizational

Negative culture: 'An engrained culture of tolerance of poor standards, a focus on finance and targets, denial of concerns and an isolation from practice elsewhere… the Trust's culture was one of self-promotion rather than critical analysis and openness.'[22, p. 44]

Staff shortages: 'There was unacceptable delay in addressing the issue of shortage of skilled nursing staff.'[22, p. 45]

Complaints procedures: 'Trust management had no culture of listening to patients. There were inadequate processes for dealing with complaints.'[22, p. 44]

---

poor staff attitudes (especially towards stigmatized groups), patient dependency around basic needs (especially on unqualified staff), incompetent staff and staff failure to raise concerns (see Box 8.5).[8,10,16] The interpersonal level includes clinical and communicative interventions (e.g. taking social history, examining intimate body regions, basic care) and asymmetrical power relationships, for example between vulnerable, powerless patients and antipathetic healthcare practitioners (see Box 8.5).[1,8,10] The organizational level includes factors such as poor hospital design (e.g. open mixed-gender wards, beds close together with thin screens/curtains between preventing confidentiality and poor access to bathroom facilities) and settings characterized by 'harsh circumstances' (e.g. hierarchies, rigidity, stress/urgency, waiting times/target-focused, insufficient resources: see Box 8.5).[1,8,10,15,16] Interestingly, it is easy to see how multiple factors across different levels can interact to bring about dignity violations, such as poor staff attitudes towards vulnerable patients, coupled with asymmetric power relationships and a high stress/time urgent environment. Before moving onto the next section, complete the activity in Box 8.6.

Box 8.6 Stop and do: reflect on the relationship between dignity and the environment

- In Chapter 3, we talked about how the environment communicated to people what is and what is not valued by the institution as part of the hidden curriculum. In terms of patient dignity, Gallagher *et al.*[10, p. 8] stated: 'If we feel that the users of a facility are important people we take some trouble to ensure the accommodation is of good quality. An unsatisfactory environment of care thus implies a failure to recognize the worth or value of the patient or service user.'
- Think about a healthcare setting of your choice (e.g. hospital or community-based healthcare facility or clinic). How do the environmental features maintain or threaten the dignity of patients? Compare your thoughts with those of your peers.
- What could you do to change the physical environment to better maintain patient dignity?

Box 8.7 Stop and do: reflecting on your own experiences

- Have you ever experienced any dignity-related professionalism dilemmas?
- If so, write down your most-memorable experience: What was the gist of your dilemma? Where were you? Who was present? What happened? What did you do? Why? How did you feel? Try to articulate exactly what your dilemma was at the time.
- What might you do differently if faced with a similar dilemma again?
- What advice would you give to one of your peers if they had this same experience?

What Patient Dignity-related Professionalism Dilemmas do Healthcare Learners Witness or Participate in?

We identified numerous patient dignity-related professionalism dilemmas experienced by healthcare students across our programme of research, although medical and nursing students provided disproportionately more compared with dental, pharmacy and physiotherapy students.[2–6] These patient dignity-related dilemmas often involved the most vulnerable individuals: patients who were acutely unwell, older, those with permanent/temporary cognitive disturbances (e.g. mental health, dementia, unconscious), and those who were dying or dead. Dignity violations included both communication and physical violations, alongside both communication and physical privacy violations. Before we discuss the different violations in our data in more detail, please attempt the learning activity outlined in Box 8.7.

Communication Violations

Dignity violations typically involved communication violations (see Box 8.8) including healthcare students and practitioners talking *about* or *to* patients inappropriately. From our UK-wide questionnaire studies, such dilemmas appeared in the ten most common

---

Box 8.8 Communicative dignity violations

Narrative 1: 'I'd rather eat my own shit'

'… [I was in] a dementia and enduring mental illness care home. [Present were] myself (student nurse), 3–4 healthcare assistants, a few residents. A patient who was bedbound and had terminal cancer was calling out to staff… they all ignored him and asked if I would go and see to him because I'd been reading to him and he 'liked me'. I was about to do something else, the HCAs were all just sitting around reading magazines. I said, "He would probably like someone to read to him, he's lonely, anyone can do that, it doesn't have to be me." One of the HCAs responded in front of staff and residents, "I'd rather eat my own shit." I was shocked. I went to attend to the man… I thought attending to the resident was the best thing I could do at that time. I told my mentor and the deputy manager because I thought it was completely unacceptable to say that… they had more clout (status) than me… Had I said anything myself I would have been shunned by all the HCAs and about 85% of my placement was spent with them. I still feel angry about it, and sad for the residents…This was my first placement in my first year, I wasn't as confident then… Now I would consider complaining formally.'

Miranda, female, year 2, nursing student, UK

Narrative 2: 'bloody hell, I only cleaned you up five minutes ago'

'Witnessing a healthcare professional speak in a horrible way to a patient, while the patient was in an undignified situation. Myself, a staff nurse and the patient were present… at the patient's bed, behind closed curtains. The patient was incontinent of faeces, myself and the staff nurse started to tidy up the patient, when the staff nurse was shocked by the amount and smell of the faeces, and said, "Oh bloody hell, I only cleaned you up five minutes ago!" I was very shocked and immediately covered the patient with the bed sheet and told the staff nurse, "You can't talk to a patient like that, with which she replied, "If I knew nursing was going to be like this, I wouldn't have done it!" This she said in front of the patient. I was shocked… it was very undignified and disrespectful towards the patient and I wanted her to know I was unhappy with this. This event happened two years ago and [I] can still remember it word for word today, it has stayed with me and I probably won't forget it.'

Tilda, female, year 3, nursing student, UK

Narrative 3: 'that lady is now gone but might have been scared as she was going'

'A health professional spoke wrongly about a patient at the end of her bed as she was dying in her bed, as if the lady couldn't hear us because she was dying!?! [Present were] myself and the health professional at the end of the bed. Me and the health professional had just turned the lady in the bed. The health professional spoke about the lady in the bed while the lady was dying. She was still awake though, but unable to move. She was just saying horrible things about how she was dying and when she would pass away. [I did] nothing until I was alone out of the room. I [then] cried. I was hurt for the patient and I was disgusted. I was imagining if it was my gran in the bed. [It was] horrible, I wish I had said something to her! That lady is now gone but might have been scared as she was going.'

Jenna, female, year 2, nursing student, UK

professionalism dilemmas experienced by medical and other healthcare students.[4] One of the most common violations comprised healthcare practitioners ignoring patients by avoiding interaction with them (Box 8.8, narrative 1).

Patients were also sometimes talked down to, were questioned aggressively, were criticized (e.g. dentist telling his patient that her teeth were 'unattractive'), were teased disrespectfully, and shouted at for not cooperating with directives or complying with treatment, or for defecating (Box 8.8, narrative 2). Patients were also called derogatory names either to their face or out of earshot, sometimes using profanities (e.g. 'grumpy bastard'). Before continuing, please complete the activity in Box 8.9.

Other communication violations to patients involved healthcare practitioners giving patients insufficient information about their conditions, prognoses and treatment, and communicating badly in challenging circumstances, such as breaking bad news, death and dying. For example, a nursing student explained how a healthcare professional spoke about a dying patient's death in front of the patient as she lay conscious yet immobile in bed (Box 8.8, narrative 3). Others talked about breaking bad news to patients inappropriately: commonly these situations were rushed, with unclear information about diagnoses/management options, too much jargon and too little empathy – sometimes ignoring distress or blaming patients for their own illness (e.g. through smoking, alcohol, etc.). Other inappropriate communication narratives involved stigmatized patients – those thought personally responsible for their own health conditions, with mental health difficulties (e.g. self-harm, psychosomatic disorders, gender dysphoria, dementia, etc.) and patients with infectious diseases who are constructed as a 'risk' to practitioners (see Box 8.10).

Box 8.9 Stop and do: reflecting on derogatory terms for patients

Derogatory terms for patients, typified in medical slang, have been commonplace in healthcare practice traditionally, and have even appeared in TV dramas and medical fiction.[23–26] For example:

- FLK: funny looking kid[23,24]
- GPO: good for parts only[23,24]
- GOMER: get out of my emergency room[23,25]
- FUBAR: fucked up beyond all recognition/repair[24,26]
- PFO: pissed, fell over[24,26]
- PGT: pissed, got thumped[24,26]

Either working on your own or with colleagues, answer the following questions:

- What (if any) derogatory terms for patients have you heard? What was the context?
- What terms might you have used yourself? What was the context?
- Why might healthcare students and practitioners use such terms? Does context affect this?
- How might the use of these terms influence how students and practitioners think about patients and how they treat patients?
- How does your thinking compare with the research literature (e.g. see Fox et al.[24])

Box 8.10 Examples of commonly stigmatized patients talked *to* and *about* inappropriately

---

Drug addiction: 'addict on the floor...'

'First ever placement... had a large number of methadone addicts and there was a separate entrance for the methadone patients... they weren't allowed into the shop... I'd only just worked in the shop a couple days and all I heard was someone shout across the dispensary, "Addict on the floor, addict on the floor", and that meant an addict was in the shop... everyone in that shop, every member of staff, every patient knew that person was a drug addict...'

Donna, female, year 4, pharmacy student, UK

Sexually acquired problems: 'her dad doesn't know she takes it from behind'

'In theatres comments were made about patients... a patient with an anal fissure he [surgeon] commented on how the patient had been a naughty girl and he bets her dad doesn't know she takes it from behind...'

Peter, male, year 5, medical student, UK

Psychosomatic disorders: 'I bet she'd run out of here'

'[Patient] might have overheard... they [staff] weren't being complimentary... she was diagnosed with a stroke about 20 years ago but she cured herself of that somehow (laughter) now she's re-diagnosed with MS so they were saying that she doesn't really have anything wrong with her... like a psychogenic type of patient... putting on all these extra symptoms and they're sitting there... saying, "Oh if we put the fire alarm on... and took her wheelchair away... I bet she'd run out of here."'

Margaret, female, year 3, physiotherapy student, UK

Gender dysphoria: 'it's amusing to a lot of the staff'

'... We've got a transgender patient... there's a lot of talk about them in the shop... it's amusing to a lot of the staff... to talk about it and I must admit, I've been drawn into it as well but then I'm not the pharmacist yet...'

Richard, male, year 4, pharmacy student, UK

Dementia: 'the funny old mad man'

'...In the staff room having lunch, myself and the other student that I'd gone with... they were talking about the dementia patients in a particular derogatory way... I found that particularly offensive... talking about a specific man... "the funny old mad man" and saying he was running around the ward...'

Diane, female, year 4, pharmacy student, UK

Infectious diseases: 'double glove'

KATIE: I had a patient with hepatitis B... the clinician saw him and he took me to the side and was like 'double glove using mirrors'.

CHLOE: You're not meant to do that are you?

KATIE: No because... we should treat all patients the same... because you're telling 'they've got a blood borne disease' to everyone else...

Katie and Chloe, female, year 4, dental students, UK

Physical Violations

Sometimes healthcare practitioners' verbal annoyance at patients' non-compliance with instructions and treatment was also associated with physical aggression, for example, with one physiotherapy student recounting watching a physiotherapist grabbing a patient's walking frame and throwing it across the ward when he failed to comply with her instructions to get up and walk, and a nursing student who watched an auxiliary nurse shouting at a patient for non-compliance during bathing, and then throwing a face cloth at the distraught patient. However, possibly the most disturbing physical violations found in our data involved healthcare students being encouraged to – or of their own accord – acting to violate the bodies of dying and dead patients for their own learning. For example, a final year medical student narrated how a senior registrar suggested that she and her fellow students practise cardio-pulmonary resuscitation on a patient who had just suffered a cardiac arrest and was likely to die (see Chapter 7 for detailed discussion about students compromising patient safety by practising on patients beyond the limits of their competence). In terms of narratives around dead patients, situations include a student being asked to practise taking blood from a recently deceased patient, and more commonly patient dignity violations involving cadavers (e.g. joking around with intimate body regions as illustrated in Chapter 3, Box 3.4. and a student carving their initials into the cadaver: see Box 8.11).

Privacy Violations

We found numerous privacy violations across our data: both physical and communicative privacy. While many of the nursing students' privacy violations were physical, occurring during personal care activities like toileting, washing, feeding and lifting, medical students' narratives of privacy violations were both physical and communicative, involving confidentiality violations. Physical privacy violations included the physical exposure of patients' bodies inappropriately such as leaving patients lying naked on beds or transporting them naked to bathrooms (Box 8.12, narrative 1). Numerous narratives from students explained how patients were physically exposed for longer than necessary during routine physical examinations (Box 8.12, narrative 2).

While physical privacy could be maintained through draping and closing curtains properly around beds in the ward environment,[27] such measures did not necessarily afford communicative privacy, as illustrated earlier in Chapter 3 (Box 3.6). Students

---

Box 8.11 'A student in a different year had carved their initials into a cadaver'

'In my first years of medical school I (and the group I was working with) discovered that a student in a different year had carved their initials into a cadaver. We saw this in an anatomy session in the dissection room. There were four of us at the table, and about 30 other students and a tutor in the room. The group I was with did not want to alert the tutor to this, so I felt pressured not to, but was uncomfortable ignoring something so serious. As soon as I could after the session I emailed the head of year anonymously… it was vital that the issue was dealt with and should not be ignored, but felt more comfortable reporting this anonymously after the reaction of my group earlier. I felt I did the right thing, as something so ethically wrong had to be dealt with. I never found out for sure what happened to the student responsible, but there were a lot of rumours throughout the year that the student was expelled. I do feel guilty if I think this is true, but it was a gross misconduct… I feel I did the right thing.'

Julie, female, year 5, medical student, UK

Box 8.12 Physical privacy violations

Narrative 1: 'naked and wet on a bed'

'Healthcare assistant left a woman with late stage Parkinson's naked and wet on a bed and went off shift. [I was with] another nursing student on her first placement. We washed and dried the patient and tried to reassure them and make sure they were warm enough. I reported the healthcare assistant to the hospital authorities because it's completely unreasonable to leave a defenceless paralysed woman naked and wet for any length of time. I feel I did the right thing.'

Ruby, female, year 3, nursing student, UK

Narrative 2: 'patients were exposed inappropriately'

'An extremely busy consultant surgeon on a ward round with 50+ patients. Whole team was present, plus two students, myself and one other. Patients were exposed inappropriately, examined without proper consent, and symptoms of pain dismissed, and management plans not discussed with them. I tried to preserve the patients' dignity by coming outside the curtains during intimate examinations and helped to re-dress some patients post-examination, tried to ensure curtains were closed, etc. I was aware that the patients felt vulnerable and scared but felt unable to intervene and prevent the problem happening. I cried about it then and whenever I think about the events I feel upset that I did not do more. No one seemed bothered about the people they were seeing and the more difficult the patient (upset, elderly) the worse they were treated. I wanted to shout out, "You can't do this." I wish I had but I was not strong enough. There was a consultant, a reg[istrar], and at least three junior doctors on the round and were okay with it. I felt like I had watched a series of assaults. I discussed it with my supervising consultant and teaching fellow but am not aware if any further action was taken.'

Amelia, female, year 4, medical student, UK

Box 8.13 'Discussing the HIV and IVDU habits of a patient at the end of the bay'

'Doctor X on ward round standing at the end of the bay discussing the HIV status and IVDU [intravenous drug use] habits of a patient at the end of the bay, putting across his negative opinions loudly enough for other patients to hear. [I was] on ward round with FY1, nursing staff and another medical student. Another patient asked a question regarding the information Doctor X had been discussing to which he replied, "Oh no, we're not talking about you, we're talking about him over there". I think I just looked a bit surprised and disagreed with his comments about IVDU being a matter of patients having no self-control sufficiently for him to confront me and ask why I disagreed. [I did this on] impulse. [I am] still angry that he expressed his beliefs so loudly and compromised confidentiality and then confronted me in a relatively aggressive manner in front of the rest of the medical team. [I] felt as though I had to hold my tongue because he was a consultant.'

Grace, female, year 5, medical student, UK

Box 8.14 Stop and do: reflecting on dignity violations and your emotions

- Re-read the narratives of dignity-related professionalism dilemmas in this chapter.
- Identify which of Jacobson's[8] 16 violations are narrated within each of the stories (see Box 8.4).
- Write down your emotional reactions (if any) to reading these narratives.
- Which of these narratives most upset you and why? If none of these narratives upset you, why not? Discuss this with a peer.

---

recounted confidentiality-related dilemmas instigated by students and healthcare professionals: students talking to peers about patients in private (e.g. shared accommodation) and public spaces (e.g. public transport, or via social media: see Chapter 10 for e-professionalism dilemmas); patients revealing confidential information to students that was withheld from senior doctors causing them the dilemma of whether they should breach confidentiality and inform seniors; students witnessing healthcare practitioners sharing test results with patients' family members or talking about patients' details audibly in public spaces (wards or community pharmacies: see Box 8.13); and by filming patients inappropriately. Before reading the next section, please complete the activity in Box 8.14.

What is the Impact of Patient Dignity-related Professionalism Dilemmas?

We have already discussed the impact of dignity violations on patients in this chapter. Here we focus on the impact of patient dignity-related professionalism dilemmas on healthcare learners. In our studies, healthcare students' patient care dilemmas (i.e. dignity and safety dilemmas) contained much negative emotional talk, demonstrating that they found such violations highly distressing.[2-6] Indeed, in the above narratives we see much negative emotional talk including words like: 'shocked', 'surprised', 'angry',

---

Box 8.15 'I feel proud of my actions'

'[We were on an] acute ward and secure… mentor, patient, other student and myself [were present]. Other student, in passing, mentioned that the client had no underwear on as they could not find any in the lady's belongings. I asked why the other student had not gone to check the laundry, explained that it is unacceptable to allow the lady to be left this way. My mentor then supported my comments as I went to retrieve from the laundry some underwear and dressed the lady appropriately. Had supervision with other student and mentor at the end of the shift. The lady deserved to be shown respect and have her dignity protected by the people given the job of looking after her in her time of need. I feel that I was able to give that lady the respect and dignity that I would like to be shown to all patients if ever in this situation. I feel proud of my actions and more confident to challenge if needed. The support by my mentor was second to none and both myself and other student were given guidance and supervision before moving on.'

Jonathan, male, year 2, nursing student, UK

'disgusted', 'aggressive', 'pressured', 'sad', 'unhappy', 'cried', 'wrong/wrongly', 'horrible', 'hurt', 'difficult', 'scared', 'upset', 'uncomfortable' and 'guilty'.

Our UK-wide questionnaire studies suggest that healthcare students experience moral distress – knowing the ethical course of action but feeling unable to act[28] – as a result of their patient dignity-related professionalism dilemmas, with females reporting more distress than males and moral distress typically increasing with the more dignity violations healthcare students witness or participate in.[4] Within their narratives, healthcare students expressed more anger talk around patient care dilemmas instigated by healthcare practitioners, compared with those instigated by students,[2,3,5] and this anger may partly account for students' actions in the face of their dilemmas (see below). While students commonly expressed regret and shame for doing nothing (or not doing more) in the face of their dilemmas: 'I wish I had said something to her' (see narrative 3, Box 8.8 and narrative 2, Box 8.12), other students articulated positive emotional talk in their narratives around challenging the dignity violations they witnessed (see Box 8.11 and narrative 1, Box 8.12), with some saying they felt 'proud' of themselves for doing the 'right' thing (see Box 8.15).

How do Learners Act in the Face of Patient Dignity-related Professionalism Dilemmas?

Our research suggests that students are more likely to resist (not go along with) patient dignity violations than to go along (or comply) with them, particularly nursing students.[5,6] The most common acts of resistance in the face of patient dignity violations included showing concern for the wronged patient (see narratives 1 and 2, Box 8.8, narratives 1 and 2, Box 8.12 and Box 8.15), reporting perpetrators of violations to appropriate authorities such as academic and clinical supervisors, hospital or university management (see narrative 1, Box 8.8, Box 8.11, narrative 1, Box 8.12, and

---

Box 8.16 'He did not seem to want to rock the boat'

'Patient spoken to inappropriately on ward. X [was present], other students present. Doctors (variety of grades) close by but I don't think they heard. A patient who asked several times over around 30 minutes for help to walk to the toilet or for a commode. The nurse then telling the patient she, "Should wet the bed rather than break her leg", as the patient was trying to walk to the toilet unassisted after asking for help repeatedly and being ignored/deferred. The patient was then told she would have to have a catheter if she kept trying to walk by herself. [I] told the consultant who was concerned but said the nurses were busy. He did not seem to want to rock the boat (cause trouble). I felt very uncomfortable witnessing the incident. The patient was in the late stages of ovarian cancer and I felt it was unpleasant and unfair and was reducing her quality of life. I still feel it was unprofessional and unacceptable... I believe the nurse in question was senior which may have contributed to the [consultant's] reluctance to confront her about the incident.'

Tim, male, year 4, medical student, UK

Box 8.15), direct verbal challenges of perpetrators (see narrative 2, Box 8.8, Box 8.13, and Box 8.15) and debriefing after incidents with colleagues, peers or friends (see narrative 2, Box 8.12).

For students who either narrate complying with patient dignity violations or not challenging the perpetrators of such violations (see narrative 3, Box 8.8, and Kate's narrative at the start of this chapter), many explain their inaction to be due to healthcare hierarchies including their lowly position: 'I was only a third year' (see Kate's narrative), and their dependence on perpetrators higher in the healthcare hierarchies for good placement experiences and grades. Such healthcare hierarchies are discussed in greater detail in Chapter 9. In the above narrative (Box 8.16), a medical student also explains how despite raising his concerns about a nurse's behaviour to his consultant, his consultant does nothing. We therefore see healthcare students and trainees witness their role models failing to resist patient dignity violations.

While healthcare students may be reluctant to challenge perpetrators directly, we can see that there are numerous indirect strategies that students enact to help maintain patient dignity in the face of dignity violations.[5] As Kate explained at the start of this chapter, she was able to help partly re-instate the patient's dignity by showing him compassion: by getting him an extra pillow, re-positioning his bed and placing extra urine collectors on his bedside table. According to Jacobson,[29] 'dignity work' (i.e. purposeful acts of dignity promotion) can be affirmative (dignity promotion) or defensive (reducing dignity violations) and can be geared towards: (1) creating dignity where it does not exist; (2) maintaining it where it does exist; (3) protecting it when it is under threat; and/ or (4) reclaiming lost dignity.[29] Dignity work can be targeted at the individual level (e.g. ensuring staff are courteous towards patients, ensuring staff are appropriately trained about dignity), relationship level (e.g. ensuring patient-healthcare professional relationships are characterized by solidarity), and organizational level (e.g. ensuring accommodation is clean and private, implementing activities that give voice to patients such as advocacy groups). Think of things you could do as a healthcare student to help maintain the dignity of patients (see Box 8.17).

Box 8.17 Stop and do: how to engage in 'dignity work'

- Choose two or three of the narratives presented in this chapter.
- Identify examples of 'dignity work' that are affirmative and defensive.
- In what ways do students help to create, maintain, protect and reclaim patient dignity?
- If you were in these situations, how could you best engage in dignity work at the level of individuals, relationships and organizations?

Chapter Summary

This chapter provides an overview of what patient dignity is and why it matters. We have explored the academic literature and that from recent healthcare investigations on patient dignity violations and discussed how such violations arise within the healthcare workplace. We have discussed the dignity violations common across our programme of research (communication, physical and privacy violations) and explored how health-care learners react and act in the face of such dignity-related professionalism dilemmas. The key take-home messages from this chapter are summarized in Box 8.18, with suggestions for small group discussions in Box 8.19. Finally, Box 8.20 outlines some recommended reading.

Box 8.18 Chapter summary points

- Dignity is about the worth of people and patient dignity is key to quality healthcare
- Learners and educators must understand what dignity violations are and the multiplicity of individual, interpersonal and organizational factors that contribute to them
- Healthcare students and trainees experience numerous patient dignity-related professionalism dilemmas and have the option to resist or go along with them
- Patient dignity violations can be distressing for learners, particularly if they do not resist
- Students and trainees are encouraged to resist patient dignity violations in subtle, less risky ways, to protect themselves and patients

---

Box 8.19 Chapter discussion points

- In Kate's narrative at the start of this chapter, she talked about how healthcare students are socialized into patient dignity violations. How might students resist becoming socialized into suboptimal dignity cultures?
- One of the healthcare educators participating in our professionalism study talked about how maintaining patient safety could cause patient dignity dilemmas, such as when examining a patient safely, practitioners need to expose patients' bodies, thus breaching their dignity. In this situation, he explained that safety 'trumps' dignity. Discuss with your peers, other situations where patient safety may be more important than patient dignity. Conversely, discuss situations where patient dignity may trump safety.

> **Box 8.20 Chapter recommended reading**
>
> Fox AT, Fertleman M, Cahill P, Palmer RD. Medical slang in British hospitals. *Ethics & Behaviour* 2003;13(2):173–189.
>
> Gallagher A, Li S, Wainwright P, Rees Jones I, Lee D. Dignity in the care of older people – a review of the theoretical and empirical literature. *BioMed Central Nursing* 2008;7:11; doi:10.1186/1472-6955-7-11.
>
> Jacobson N. Dignity violation in health care. *Qualitative Health Research* 2009;19(11):1536–1547.
>
> Lin YP, Watson R, Tsai YF. Dignity in care in the clinical setting: A narrative review. *Nursing Ethics* 2012;20(2):168–177.

References

1 Whitehead J, Wheeler H. Patients' experiences of privacy and dignity. Part 1: a literature review. *British Journal of Nursing* 2008;17(6):381–385.

2 Monrouxe LV, Rees CE. 'It's just a clash of cultures': emotional talk within medical students' narratives of professionalism dilemmas. *Advances in Health Sciences Education* 2012;17(5):671–701.

3 Monrouxe LV, Rees CE, Endacott R, Ternan E. 'Even now it makes me angry': healthcare students' professionalism dilemma narratives. *Medical Education* 2014;48:502–517.

4 Monrouxe LV, Rees CE, Dennis A, Wells S. Professionalism dilemmas, moral distress and the healthcare student: insights from two online UK-wide questionnaire studies. *British Medical Journal Open* 2015;5:e007518. doi:10.1136/bmjopen-2014-007518.

5 Rees CE, Monrouxe LV, McDonald LA. Narrative, emotion, and action: analysing 'most memorable' professionalism dilemmas. *Medical Education* 2013;47(1):80–96.

6 Rees CE, Monrouxe LV, McDonald LA. My mentor kicked a dying woman's bed: analysing UK nursing students' most memorable professionalism dilemmas. *Journal of Advanced Nursing* 2015;71(1):169–180.

7 Bismark MM, Spittal MJ, Gurrin LC, Ward M, Studdert DM. Identification of doctors at risk of recurrent complaints: a national study of healthcare complaints in Australia. *British Medical Journal Quality and Safety in Health Care* 2013;0:1–9. doi:10.1136/bmjqs-2012-001691.

8 Jacobson N. Dignity violation in health care. *Qualitative Health Research* 2009;19(11):1536–1547.

9 Jacobson N. Dignity and health: a review. *Social Science & Medicine* 2007;64:292–302.

10 Gallagher A, Li S, Wainwright P, Rees Jones I, Lee D. Dignity in the care of older people – a review of the theoretical and empirical literature. *BioMed Central Nursing* 2008;7(11): doi:10.1186/1472-6955-7-11.

11 Lin Y-P, Tsai Y-F, Chen H-F. Dignity in care in the hospital setting from patients' perspectives in Taiwan: a descriptive qualitative study. *Journal of Clinical Nursing* 2011;20:794–801.

12 Pullman D. The ethics of autonomy and dignity in long-term care. *Canadian Journal on Aging* 1999;18(1):26–49.

13 Royal College of Nursing. *The RCN's definition of dignity*. London: RCN, 2008, http://www.rcn.org.uk/__data/assets/pdf_file/0003/191730/003298.pdf (Accessed 1 December 2016).

14 Valentine N, Darby C, Bonsel GJ. Which aspects of quality of care are most important? Results from the WHO's general population surveys of 'health system responsiveness' in 41 countries. *Social Science & Medicine* 2008;66(9):1939–1950.

15 Whitehead J, Wheeler H. Patients' experience of privacy and dignity. Part 2: an empirical study. *British Journal of Nursing* 2008;17(7):458–464.

16 Lin Y-P, Watson R, Tsai Y-F. Dignity in care in the clinical setting: a narrative review. *Nursing Ethics* 2012;20(2):168–177.

17 Parliamentary and Health Service Ombudsman. *Dying Without Dignity. Investigations by the Parliamentary and Health Service Ombudsman into Complaints about End-of-life Care*. London: Parliamentary and Health Service Ombudsman, 2015, http://www.ombudsman.org.uk/__data/assets/pdf_file/0019/32167/Dying_without_dignity_report.pdf (Accessed 1 December 2016).

18 Parliamentary and Health Service Ombudsman. *Care and Compassion? Report of the Health Service Ombudsman on Ten Investigations into NHS Care of Older People*. London: Parliamentary and Health Service Ombudsman, 2011, https://www.gov.uk/government/uploads/system/uploads/attachment_data/file/247493/0778.pdf (Accessed 1 December 2016).

19 Care Quality Commission. *Right Here, Right Now. People's Experiences of Help, Care and Support During a Mental Health Crisis*. Gallowgate: Care Quality Commission, 2015, http://www.cqc.org.uk/sites/default/files/20150630_righthere_mhcrisiscare_full.pdf (Accessed 1 December 2016).

20 Francis R. *Independent Inquiry into Care Provided by Mid Staffordshire NHS Foundation Trust, January 2005–March 2009*. Volume 1. London: The Stationery Office, 2010, http://webarchive.nationalarchives.gov.uk/20130107105354/http://www.dh.gov.uk/prod_consum_dh/groups/dh_digitalassets/@dh/@en/@ps/documents/digitalasset/dh_113447.pdf (Accessed 1 December 2016).

21 Francis R. *Independent Inquiry into Care Provided by Mid Staffordshire NHS Foundation Trust, January 2005–March 2009*. Volume II. London: The Stationery Office, 2010, http://webarchive.nationalarchives.gov.uk/20130107105354/http://www.dh.gov.uk/prod_consum_dh/groups/dh_digitalassets/@dh/@en/@ps/documents/digitalasset/dh_113069.pdf (Accessed 1 December 2016).

22 Francis R. *Report of the Mid Staffordshire NHS Foundation Trust Public Inquiry. Executive Summary*. London: The Stationery Office, 2013, https://www.gov.uk/government/uploads/system/uploads/attachment_data/file/279124/0947.pdf (Accessed 1 December 2016).

23 Coombs RH, Chopra S, Schenk DR, Yutan E. Medical slang and its functions. *Social Science & Medicine* 1993;36:987–998.

24 Fox AT, Fertleman M, Cahill P, Palmer RD. Medical slang in British hospitals. *Ethics & Behaviour* 2003;13:173–189.

25 Shem S. *The House of God*. London: Bodley Head Ltd, 1979.

26 Mercurio J. *Bodies*. London: Jonathan Cape, 2002.

27 Wilson N, Hopkins-Rosseel D, Lust C, Averns H, Hopman W. Draping education to promote patient dignity: Canadian physiotherapy student and instructor perceptions. *Physiotherapy Canada* 2012;64(2):157–166.

28 Jameton A. *Nursing Practice: The Ethical Issues*. New York, NY: Prentice Hall, 1984.

29 Jacobson N. *Dignity and Health*. Nashville: Vanderbilt University Press, 2012.

9

Abuse-related Professionalism Dilemmas

'[I] couldn't find the medicine Kardex [medication administration record] for pre-op patient... [the] staff nurse that was supervising me said she had not seen it, so I had to call the duty doctor to ask him to rewrite the pre-op prescription... [the] duty doctor arrived on ward to re-write prescription and when he approached me the staff nurse said, "Oh, is it this Kardex you are looking for?"... I apologized to the doctor for... basically wasting his time and took the Kardex to organize the pre-op meds for the patient, which were overdue. Later I asked the staff nurse about why she had said she had not seen the Kardex and she laughed and said, "What can you do about it anyway?"... It seemed to be a power thing. It is sad that power games may have detrimental effects on patient care and that there is nothing you can do really... it wasn't a one-off incident in the ward... and seemed to be all part of the ward culture. Everyone knew the staff nurses who caused animosity and hassle but they were left unchecked by senior staff and peers... no one wanted to tackle the ward culture thing and I was only there for a short time so I guess I opted out a bit because you have enough stress getting through placements without causing yourself more hassle.'*

Morag, female, year 3, nursing student, UK

LEARNING OUTCOMES

- To understand what workplace equality, diversity and dignity are and why they matter in professionalism education
- To discuss what workplace abuse is and its relationship with power
- To understand the causes and consequences of workplace abuse
- To discover the range of abuse-related professionalism dilemmas occurring across different healthcare professions
- To reflect on ways in which workplace abuse can be prevented and managed

---

Healthcare Professionalism: Improving Practice through Reflections on Workplace Dilemmas, First Edition.
Lynn V. Monrouxe and Charlotte E. Rees.
© 2017 John Wiley & Sons Ltd. Published 2017 by John Wiley & Sons Ltd.

KEY TERMS
Equality, diversity and dignity at work Workplace abuse and bullying Power and hierarchy Abuse-related professionalism dilemmas Prevention and management of workplace abuse

Introduction

Individuals, teams and organizations in healthcare have moral and legal responsibilities to uphold equality, diversity and dignity at work for *all* healthcare students, trainees and practitioners.[1-5] However, we know from the literature, including our own research, that healthcare students and trainees experience all too commonly a multiplicity of workplace abuses (work-related, person-related and physical intimidation), either directly or indirectly through witnessing the abuses of others.[6,7] Such abuses are perhaps unsurprising given the innumerable hierarchies in healthcare, with hierarchies relating to levels of training, specialties, and healthcare professions. Such hierarchies can breed abuses of power, as illustrated by Morag's narrative above. In her narrative, Morag implies that the staff nurse wields power over her by withholding information, which she refers to as a power game indicative of that specific ward's culture. With her lowly standing in the healthcare hierarchy, Morag believes she can do nothing to resist such power games and seemingly neither do other ward staff, which serves to sanction such negative workplace behaviours. As Morag suggests, not only does the staff nurse's behaviour impact negatively on Morag and her doctor colleague whose time is wasted, but it also has detrimental effects on patient care. In this chapter, we discuss the complexities around workplace equality, diversity and dignity: what these are and why they matter. We try to unpack workplace abuse and bullying and its relationship with power. We then consider the causes and consequences of workplace abuse at various levels: *individual, interactional, work and organizational.* We then share various types of abuse-related professionalism dilemmas experienced by healthcare students and trainees in our programme of research, including learners' reactions and actions in the face of such abuse. Finally, we discuss key abuse/bullying prevention and management approaches. We hope this chapter will help healthcare students and trainees better negotiate healthcare hierarchies and navigate their way through inevitable experiences of workplace abuse, to protect themselves, their colleagues and ultimately patients.

What are Equality, Diversity and Dignity at Work and Why Do They Matter?

Equality, diversity and dignity at work have both moral and legal bases and are principles that have been embraced by healthcare professions across the globe (see Box 9.1 for definitions). In the UK, for example, the Equality Act 2010 identifies nine 'protected characteristics' (age, disability, race, religion and belief, sex, sexual orientation, gender reassignment, marriage and civil partnership, and pregnancy and maternity).[9] Although

---

Box 9.1 Information: defining equality, diversity and dignity

Equality: 'challenging discrimination, removing barriers faced by people from different groups, and creating a fairer society where everyone can participate and has the same opportunities to fulfil their potential' (General Medical Council).[1, p. 1]

Diversity: 'recognizing, respecting and valuing the differences that everyone has, as well as leveraging the opportunities that different people bring to the work that we do' (General Medical Council).[1, p.1]

Dignity: 'concerned with how people feel, think and behave in relation to the worth or value of themselves and others. To treat someone with dignity is to treat them as being of worth, in a way that is respectful of them as valued individuals' (Royal College of Nursing).[8]

Box 9.2 Stop and do: reflect on 'protected characteristics' in a country of your choice

- Think of a non-UK country of your choice. This may be the country of your birth or that of your parents, where you currently live, or where you might desire to live and work in the future.
- Does this country have 'protected characteristics' like the UK? If not, find out more about their approach to equality and diversity. If they do have protected characteristics, what are they?
- How do the protected characteristics of your chosen country compare with those of the UK?
- Which of the protected characteristics are you most and least comfortable with and why?
- How might your levels of comfort influence how you interact with colleagues with those protected characteristics?

---

not a protected characteristic as such, public bodies are also meant to show due regard to socio-economic considerations.[9] Indeed, the UK National Health Service often considers social class because of its close relationship with health inequalities. It is essentially through legislation like the Equality Act 2010 that healthcare employers and regulators as public service providers have duties to promote equality amongst workers with and without protected characteristics, eliminate unlawful discrimination and harassment, take positive action to include people with protected characteristics, determine and publish equality objectives, and publish information demonstrating compliance with the Equality Act.[2,3] Underpinned by such law, all healthcare regulators in the UK voice their commitment to dignity at work through publication of their equality and diversity strategies.[1-5] Before reading the next paragraph, attempt the activity in Box 9.2.

In terms of healthcare regulators' professionalism documents from English-speaking countries (see Chapter 2, Table 2.2), all talk about the importance of practitioners being respectful (specifically respecting dignity and diversity), although much of this talk is directed at practitioners' relationships with patients rather than each another (see Chapter 8 for in-depth coverage of patient dignity). In terms of what these key professionalism documents say about workplace equality, diversity and dignity, there are more similarities across the healthcare professional groups and countries than differences.[10–29] For example, all documents talk about the need to respect colleagues and most identify the importance of educating colleagues and working collaboratively with them. Furthermore, various documents highlight the need for professionals to avoid bullying, harassing or discriminating against their colleagues (more common in Australian, UK and USA documents) whilst others advocate supporting colleagues' health and well-being (particularly notable in the UK documents) and resolving any conflicts with colleagues (more common in Canadian, UK and USA documents). There were, however, some notable differences between the healthcare professions: dentistry was the only group to talk about dentists needing to treat colleagues fairly in financial transactions.[16]

So, why do workplace equality, diversity and dignity matter beyond moral ideals and legal compliance? In short, they matter because of patient care. First, patient populations are typically diverse and the workforce needs to reflect that diversity in order to best meet the needs of *all* patients.[1] For example, sometimes patients with 'protected characteristics' such as gender and ethnicity (e.g. Hispanic females) prefer to be treated by healthcare professionals with those same protected characteristics.[30] Second, healthcare students, trainees and practitioners need to enact consistent behaviours and talk in the workplace to treat *all* people equally and with dignity: colleagues and patients alike (see Chapter 8 on patient dignity). If, for example, practitioners repeatedly discriminate against colleagues with certain protected characteristics (such as those who self-identify as lesbian, gay, bisexual or transgender), they might also discriminate against patients with those same characteristics, either directly or indirectly through patients witnessing acts of colleague-colleague discrimination (see Box 9.3 for one patient's perspective on witnessing colleague-colleague verbal abuse). Third, we know that when students, trainees and practitioners feel undermined and bullied by their colleagues, they often avoid interacting and communicating with them, thereby impairing effective teamworking.[31] They are less likely to raise concerns about perceived bullies' suboptimal healthcare practices or seek help when faced with difficulties beyond their competence, plus they are more likely to commit serious medical errors themselves.[31–34] Altogether, such situations open the door to safety lapses (see Chapter 7), jeopardizing patient care.[31] Finally, equality, diversity and dignity at work also matter because students and trainees

---

Box 9.3 'If I were him I'd smack him in the face'

'The last time I was in hospital… which was about three weeks back, I was only in overnight, but there was a junior doctor, young chap he was, and we could see he was dying on his feet… I don't know what he [the consultant] was saying to him because… he [consultant]… was foreign, now they don't speak very good English for us to understand and if you've got someone who's really tired… they're trying to listen to someone who's not speaking very well, expecting you to know everything I don't think that's fair… several times I've said to my husband if I were him [junior doctor] I'd smack him [consultant] in the face… because the way he was spoken to, the young doctor I felt really sorry for him… I'm not saying all doctors are like it but think I'd say nine out of ten that I've come across they're [junior doctors] treated like underlings… subservient… "You're here to do my bidding" sort of thing.'

Mary, female patient representative from GMC study[35]

who feel bullied and undermined are more likely to be dissatisfied with their training and learning and this can influence workforce retention.[31]

What is Workplace Abuse and its Relationship with Power?

A multiplicity of terms exist and are sometimes used interchangeably across the research literature and policy documents like those mentioned above: bullying; undermining; harassment; discrimination; hostility; incivility; mobbing; abuse and so on (see Box 9.4 for key definitions). We have previously employed the term 'abuse' in our research rather than 'bullying' because 'bullying' has a narrow definition based on frequency, intensity, duration and power disparity.[42] We think 'bullying' can therefore miss one-off abusive events experienced by healthcare students as part of their short clinical placements.[6,33] Einarsen *et al.*[43] talks about three clusters of bullying and harassment behaviours in the workplace: work-related (e.g. being given tasks with unreasonable deadlines); person-related (e.g. receiving offensive remarks about your personality); and physical intimidation (e.g. threats of, or actual physical abuse: see Box 9.5). Students can experience these directly or indirectly through witnessing the abuse of their peers or healthcare professionals. Essentially, all can be seen to involve abuses of power within the hierarchical structures and cultures of the healthcare workplace.

Healthcare has innumerable hierarchies both within and across different healthcare professions.[44] Before reading on, complete the activity in Box 9.6. Within each healthcare profession, higher-ranked practitioners (e.g. consultant or nurse consultant) are thought to assume more authority and power over more junior staff (e.g. registrar or staff nurse). Furthermore, prestige hierarchies are thought to exist within medicine with specialties, with active, specialized, biomedical and technological characteristics such as surgery being afforded higher levels of prestige than specialties with opposite qualities such as psychiatry.[45] Across different healthcare professions, medical practitioners are thought to be at the top of the healthcare hierarchy, while other professionals (e.g. nurses) are considered to be lower.[32,46,47]

Box 9.4 Information: defining abuse, bullying, harassment, authority, power and prestige

Abuse: unwanted harmful, injurious or offensive acts directed at someone by another.[36,37]

Bullying: 'Repeated and persistent negative actions towards one or more individual(s), which involve a perceived power imbalance and create a hostile work environment'.[38, p. 1214]

Harassment: 'the act of systematic and/or continued unwanted and annoying actions of one party or a group, including threats and demands' (http://legal-dictionary.thefreedictionary.com/harassment).

Authority: refers to the right, or perceived right to exercise power.[39]

Power: 'that capacity or potential to influence'.[40, p. 9]

Prestige: a measure of regard or esteem eliciting positive, neutral or negative evaluations shared among individuals.[41]

Box 9.5 Illustrations of different types of abuse

Work-related abuse

'In a clinic a consultant told me to take blood pressure, I felt out of practice and uncertain of the equipment so said I was uncomfortable taking it and asked for some help, I was shouted at and refused help, [and] told to get on with it.'

Dawn, female, year 4, medical student, UK

Person-related abuse

'The patient referred to myself as a refugee, told me to go back to my own country and proceeded to make derogatory comments about my country.'

Nadia, female, year 2, nursing student, UK

Physical intimidation

'[I was] physically pushed out of the way of the computer by pharmacist on a number of occasions.'

Suzanne, female, year 2, pharmacy student, UK

Box 9.6 Stop and do: reflect on healthcare hierarchies

- Write the following healthcare roles on separate slips of paper. Here, we list them in alphabetical order: dentist, dental hygienist, dental nurse, dental student, general practitioner, medical student, mental health nurse, nursing student, pharmacist, pharmacy student, physician, physiotherapist, physiotherapy student, psychiatrist, registered nurse, specialist nurse practitioner, surgeon.
- Working on your own or with your peers, arrange the slips of paper in a manner that you think best represents healthcare hierarchies.
- Reflect on why you have put them in the order that you have.
- What (if any) disagreements did you have with your peers about the order and why?

Box 9.7 'It's a very female environment'

'It can be quite tricky for a man going into a pharmacy because… it's a very female environment… you're quite often the only man in the shop with a whole team of women around you… I found that in the shop when I went into it there was a male pharmacist who was the manager there… he was the big baddie and all the females sort of united against him… they'd all talk… behind his back… then I could see how it is quite tricky for a man to go into a pharmacy.'

David, male, year 4, pharmacy student, UK

All of these different hierarchies imply ingrained power asymmetries between those in superordinate and subordinate positions, with the former perceived as being power-*full* and the latter being power-*less*.[46] Power is often considered at a macro level such as exploring structural inequalities,[48] as illustrated in Box 9.7. However, power is also considered at micro (interactional) levels (as illustrated in Box 9.5). Interestingly, from a Foucauldian perspective, power is not necessarily something that is held and wielded by superordinates (e.g. consultants) but is instead something that can be enacted throughout healthcare encounters by subordinates too (e.g. patients), as illustrated in the second quote in Box 9.5.[46,49,50] Power can also be resisted by subordinates.

What are the Causes of Workplace Abuse?

A multiplicity of factors at numerous levels are thought to contribute to abuse and bullying in the healthcare workplace.[6,51] Organizational psychology approaches typically focus on the complex interplay between multiple factors at different levels: individual, interactional, work and organizational levels.[6,51] In terms of the individual level, both recipient (e.g. low assertiveness and higher neuroticism) and perpetrator characteristics (e.g. low social competence and higher aggressiveness) have been found to contribute to abuse.[6,51] At an interactional level, the recipient-perpetrator relationship contributes to abuse through things like personality and identity clashes, including out-group denigration (see Chapter 5), interpersonal conflicts, reciprocal attacks, and so on.[6,51] At the work level, high workload, understaffing, role ambiguity and time pressures, and suboptimal physical environments (such as noisy, hot and cramped) can also contribute to abuse.[6,51] Finally, at the organizational level, hierarchical and competitive cultures, organizational change (such as financial and staff cuts, role conflicts and job insecurity), authoritarian and laissez-faire leadership approaches and lack of disciplinary action for bullying have also been found to contribute to abuse.[6,51] In Box 9.8, we present a range of contributory factors across these levels by way of illustration.

Box 9.8 Illustrations of different contributory factors for abuse at different levels

Individual

Perpetrator's emotional state: 'Patient swore and implied I was deliberately hurting him [during dental treatment] in an aggressive tone… Patient was clearly worked up and nervous.'

Letitia, female, year 5, dental student, UK

Perpetrator's personality: 'I was given an inappropriately low mark for placement by a domineering supervisor.'

Megan, female, year 3, physiotherapy student, UK

Interpersonal

Recipient-perpetrator disagreement over patient management: 'The foetal heart rate was increasing so the midwife assessed the situation and… wanted the doctor to prescribe some drugs… the doctor looked at the foetal heart rate and disagreed with the midwife… the midwife came in with another midwife to "back her up" against the doctor and bullied the doctor in front of the patient, rolling their eyes at the doctor and undermining her.'

Lisa, female, year 4, medical student, UK

> **Work**
>
> **Cramped physical environment:**
>
> LINDA: Another thing is that pharmacies are very, very small spaces and you spend a lot of time brushing past, you'll say, 'I'm sorry'… 'cause you accidentally you're there so confined a space if one of you is dispensing and one of you is say, like putting the order away, or doing trays, you constantly brush past each other…
>
> SARAH: I've worked with a male pharmacist who… you don't really want someone like him, you know, they get a bit too close to you… that can quite easily happen in a close space…
>
> Linda and Sarah, female, year 4, pharmacy students, UK
>
> **Organization**
>
> **Hierarchical ward culture and lack of disciplinary action:** 'It seemed to be a power thing… it wasn't a one off incident in the ward… and seemed to be all part of the ward culture… no one wanted to tackle the ward culture thing.'
>
> Morag, female, year 3, nursing student, UK (see full narrative at the start of this chapter)

What are the Consequences of Workplace Abuse?

There can be various adverse consequences of abuse, again at the level of individuals, relationships, work and organization. The consequences for the recipients of abuse include emotional upset and moral distress, anxiety and depression, self-medicating through drinking alcohol, physical health problems, sleep disturbances, cynicism about the profession and low self-confidence.[6,51–53] In terms of consequences for relationships, as mentioned above, abuse can result in recipients and bystanders avoiding perpetrators, which in turn can reduce team communication, including raising concerns, adversely influencing team performance.[31] Also discussed above, the consequences of abuse on medical work include abuse recipients being less likely to seek help and more likely to make mistakes, influencing patient safety.[51] Finally, in terms of consequences for the organization, abuse can lead to increased staff absenteeism and turnover and therefore understaffing, plus reduced organizational productivity and low morale.[51] In Box 9.9, we present a range of consequences across these levels by way of illustration.

What Abuse-related Professionalism Dilemmas do Healthcare Learners Experience?

The healthcare workplace is notorious for its high levels of abuse and bullying, with medical student abuse being researched now for over 30 years.[49,52,53] Prevalence rates for healthcare workplace bullying and abuse differ depending on the measurement methods used (e.g. self-labelled bullying or rating negative behaviours) and durations adopted.[51,55] They also vary according to the concepts explored (e.g. bullying or abuse) and the study participants (i.e. healthcare professional group, level of training etc.). This variation is illustrated neatly in Table 9.1, which includes a few recent examples of studies from Western cultures with larger (n > 500) sample sizes.

Box 9.9 Illustrations of different consequences of abuse at different levels

Individual

Abuse affecting the recipient's well-being: 'In the clinician's office… [I was] yelled at for asking for advice… [and] received consistent, indirect poor treatment on the ward (e.g. being ignored)… I thought that the clinical sub-dean should be aware of the treatment I received and the ill-effects afterwards (…depressive episodes… persistent rumination).'

Tom, male, year 3, medical student, UK

Interpersonal

Student abuse affecting student-patient relationship: 'A healthcare assistant came over to me when I was treating a patient, he said, "Oh, why are you wearing gloves?" directly in front of the patient… and he said, "Well you don't need to wear gloves for every patient you're just wasting money." When he walked away the lady I was treating said, "Well he clearly knows loads more than you, why are you treating me?"'

Elle, female, year 3, physiotherapy student, UK

Work

Student abuse affecting delivery of patient care: 'I think she's [supervisor] scary… she's a little bit nasty and she makes me feel uncomfortable and you just don't think logically when you're with a patient because you're worried what she's going to say… I had a patient a… while ago now for a crown prep so… I needed a double appointment for it and… he phoned an hour late said he's stuck in traffic but by the end of that I only had like an hour to actually complete this crown prep… that combined with having this particular supervisor I just said, "I'll treat you another day"… if I'd had another supervisor maybe I would have seen him.'

Lisa, female, year 4, dental student, UK

Organization

Abuse affecting student absenteeism: 'Doctor X's favourite line was, "Humiliation is the best way of learning", hence every time I got something wrong there was shouting and unpleasant remarks (i.e. "If you did this when you are qualified you would be struck off")… at the time I was severely affected by Doctor X to the extent I was unable to go into school for several days from fear…'

Kelly, female, year 4, medical student, UK

You will see from Table 9.1 that the vast majority of healthcare students participating in our two UK-wide surveys stated that they had experienced abuse in the last 12 months (over 70% of males and 80% of female students).[52] These prevalence figures are much higher than the other two UK surveys presented in Table 9.1 because: (1) we asked participants to say whether they had experienced a range of negative workplace behaviours (labelled 'abuse'); (2) our participants were students (and thus most subordinate and least socialized into the healthcare hierarchy); and (3) our timeframe was longer. We were not surprised by these high figures given that we had already identified large numbers of abuse narratives in our previous qualitative research.[58–61] In fact, over one fifth ($n = 410/2033$,

Table 9.1 Recent prevalence figures for bullying and abuse in the healthcare workplace.

Authors	Sample and duration	Concept	Duration	Prevalence
Miedema *et al.*[56]	774 members of the College of Family Physicians of Canada	Abuse	Career	39% (severe) 75% (major) 98% (minor)*
Iglesias and De Bengoa Vallejo[57]	538 Spanish nurses	Bullying	Past 6 months	17%
Carter *et al.*[33]	2950 UK NHS staff (nurses, doctors, dentists, AHPs, HCAs, administrators)**	Bullying	Past 6 months	19.9%
GMC[31]	49,994 UK medical trainees	Bullying	Current rotation	8%
Monrouxe *et al.*[52]	2397 UK medical students	Abuse	Past 12 months	80.4% (female) 71.5% (male)
Monrouxe *et al.*[52]	1399 UK dental, pharmacy, physiotherapy and nursing students	Abuse	Past 12 months	83.3% (female) 71.3% (male)

Note: *minor abusive incidents included disrespectful behaviour, verbal anger and threats, major abusive incidents included physical aggression and sexual harassment, and severe abusive incidents included physical and sexual assaults; **AHPs: allied health professionals, HCAs: healthcare assistants

---

Box 9.10 Stop and do: reflect on your abuse-related professionalism dilemmas

- Have you ever experienced any abuse-related professionalism dilemmas?
- If so, write down your most-memorable experience: what was the gist of your dilemma, where were you and who was present, when did it take place, what happened, what did you do and why and how did you feel? Try to articulate exactly what your dilemma was at the time.
- What might you do differently if faced with a similar abuse-related professionalism dilemma in the future?
- What advice would you give to one of your peers if they had this same experience?

20.2%) of our professionalism dilemmas presented across these qualitative papers were about healthcare students being the recipients or bystanders of workplace abuse. Before reading the next paragraph, complete the activity in Box 9.10.

Across our oral and written narratives elicited from our interview and survey studies respectively, we found that healthcare students' abuse-related professionalism dilemmas were mostly recounted in the hospital setting for nursing, physiotherapy, and medical students, and the community setting for dental and pharmacy students, and most were perpetrated by clinical teachers from the same profession (although some healthcare groups such as nursing/pharmacy experienced numerous abuse dilemmas with patient perpetrators). Covert status-related abuse was most commonly narrated in our data. Akin to the work-related abuse illustrated in Box 9.5, covert, status-related abuse included subtle forms related to healthcare hierarchies, such as students: (1) being ignored and excluded from learning opportunities; (2) being asked repeated questions in intimidating ways and beyond their levels of competence for their stage of training; (3) having information withheld from them (as in Morag's narrative at the start of this chapter); (4) receiving critical feedback unconstructively and destructively (see Chapter 4); and (5) being given unpleasant or menial tasks inappropriately.[6,7] Such covert, status-related abuses are illustrated in the following narrative by Helen (see Box 9.11, narrative 1).

Box 9.11 Illustrations of covert, status-related, verbal and physical abuse

Narrative 1: 'I was ignored and laughed at'

'As a new nursing student I was placed on a ward where I was greeted with hostility and suspicion. I was told to perform obs[ervations] for 28 patients who I knew nothing about because the "staff" would not let me near the patients' notes or files. When I tried to make conversation I was ignored and laughed at. I was later warned by my "mentor" not to "get in the way" of the HCAs [healthcare assistants] that ran that particular ward or he would make trouble for me… I went home and cried, thought about what happened and reported it to my programme leader… [I am] still apprehensive and sad that this has happened. Student nurses are feeling unwelcome, unwanted and unsupervised both on the ward and out in the community.'

Helen, female, year 1, nursing student, UK

Narrative 2: 'watching consultant shout and swear loudly'

'[I was] watching a consultant shout and swear loudly in the middle of the ward at one of his juniors. I was on attachment with a urology consultant present with my placement partner. We were on ward round (I think) and happened to be there mid-afternoon during visiting hours… The consultant needed to check up on a patient and then started shouting about changes made to the medication. He rounded on his junior and shouted loudly along the lines of, "For fuck's sake, why the bloody hell did you do that?" He went on for a while and I would regard it as a rant. [I did] nothing. Wanted a hole to open up in the ground as it was in the centre of the ward at the nurses' station. Both my partner [and I] shared worried looks and didn't know where to put ourselves. You don't point out to a consultant who is already visibly seething that he is being unprofessional. [I am] embarrassed still. I genuinely wished I had the confidence to stand up to him. Would I do so now? Probably not but if he was shouting at me then I would definitely make a complaint.'

Greg, male, year 4, medical student, UK

Narrative 3: 'the patient hit me when I lent in to talk'

'A confused dementia patient became very angry and aggressive and hit me on entering the side room. I was alone on entering the room but the nurse saw what happened from the nurses' station. I only went in to offer the patient breakfast. The patient hit me when I lent in to talk [so I] just removed myself from the side room and reported [it] to my mentor. [I] thought it was the best thing to do for my own safety. [I now] feel fine, just more aware about confused patients becoming aggressive. I was [not] angry or upset as the patient was unaware of their actions.'

Susan, female, year 3, nursing student, UK

Another common type of abuse experienced and witnessed by students was verbal abuse. Such verbal abuse could be person-related such as students being called derogatory names (e.g. plank, grasshopper, stupid, etc.) or work-related such as students being admonished in front of patients and colleagues and verbally threatened with punishments such as low grades (see Chapter 4). Such verbal abuses can be seen in Greg's narrative, in which he recounts witnessing the verbal abuse of a junior doctor by a consultant in the middle of a ward round in front of colleagues and patients (see Box 9.11, narrative 2).

Another common person-related abuse experienced by healthcare students included discrimination and harassment involving those protected characteristics set out in the Equality Act 2010 (see Box 9.12). Particularly common were students experiencing or witnessing the sexual harassment and gender discrimination of female students, racial discrimination of ethnic minority students, and age discrimination of

---

Box 9.12 Examples of discrimination and harassment involving protected characteristics

Narrative 1: Gender: 'you should be an erotic dancer'

'[I received] inappropriate sexual and sexist remarks from a consultant/module leader. [I was in the] hospital, one particular rotation, same consultant repeatedly. Other medical students and junior staff usually present. The consultant repeatedly made sexual remarks about my appearance and also derogatory remarks about women to me (e.g. you should be an erotic dancer, not a doctor…). [I] tried to laugh them off, make them seem less serious. I didn't want to challenge the consultant, who was also module lead. Some staff are just power-driven bullies. I was embarrassed and offended at the time, but since then I've been okay, as the consultant lost respect, not me.'

Karen, female, year 5, medical student, UK

Narrative 2: Age: 'he was 18 at the time'

'I've been on a placement where the other person was much younger, he was 18 at the time and the educators did treat me and him differently, which is quite interesting. And I can understand to a certain degree because, as an older student, you do pick up a few simple life skills but then, on the flipside, what he was good at, I don't think the educator picked up on. His academic stuff was really, really strong, something that I was trying to learn from him… I don't think that's really a fair judgement.'

Mike, male, year 3, pharmacy student, UK

Narrative 3: Religion and spiritual beliefs: 'they would laugh at my beliefs'

'A psychiatrist verbally bullied my spiritual beliefs and made my placement hell. I was in a mental health community team, there were social workers and nursing staff and other psychiatrists. They would laugh at my beliefs… belittle me and humiliate me, I would try to make a joke of it but it became too upsetting [so I] took a lot of sick days because I was scared to face the team… [I was] sad and upset that she [psychiatrist] could do that.'

Aysha, female, year 3, nursing student, UK

Narrative 4: Race and religion: 'I haven't been subjected to racial comments before'

'It seemed people looked at my religion and had their own idea of who I am rather than seeing me for my abilities. I was at an endoscopy unit at X Infirmary. I had a few incidents where I was told by nurses not to talk about my religion. I spoke to another nurse and my friends for advice. I wanted to complain to the university about the behaviour of the nurses towards me at the unit but was afraid they may fail me on my assessment. I feel awful, I haven't been subject to racial comments before and to be looked down because I have a different religion to the staff was heartbreaking. I felt betrayed by professionals whom are meant to respect diversity and recognize individuality… This has made me insecure, every time someone walks past me I feel they are thinking the same as the nurse and once again judge on my religion and race rather than the person I am.'

Pippa, female, year 1, nursing student, UK

Narrative 5: Sexual orientation: 'the registrar began to gossip about a colleague'

'I was in a consulting room waiting for the consultant to arrive for clinic. The registrar began to gossip about a colleague who had just "come out" as gay. He then made comments about being uncomfortable and disgusted by homosexual men. I had a quiet word to his consultant about the inappropriate behaviour and views displayed. His comments made me uncomfortable and angry. He should have kept his views to himself and certainly not shared them in front of patients. [I am now] less distressed than at the time but still annoyed.'

Sasha, female, year 5, medical student, UK

Narrative 6: Disability: 'he verbally discriminated against me due to my specific learning disability'

'On a number of occasions he [professionalism tutor] verbally discriminated against me due to my specific learning disability… and threatened me with Fitness To Practise regarding issues which I have since found out are more than acceptable (my assistance of a scribe in examinations). He has disrespected many of the organizations who assist dyslexic pupils and caused me great distress over my last year through threats regarding this issue. I looked into the acceptable adjustments allowed in postgraduate exams for disabled students and have since found that it is more than acceptable for me to have a scribe… Therefore his threats were unfounded and caused me great distress, through both the fear and the direct upset caused by his behaviour. I was worried that his threats were true and that I could not expect the assistance I had required. It still causes me distress to think about it; however, I am less worried as I now know it will not affect my clinical career even if he is threatening me.'

Fred, male, year 2, medical student, UK

Narrative 7: Pregnancy and maternity: 'everyone joked and said it was because she was pregnant'

'I had a history I needed to present to a doctor, and one of the female SHOs said to come back in the afternoon because she'd be free, so I did. When I did come back she was still really busy and instead asked if I'd like to take another history in the meantime… eventually

I ended up going to A&E to find something to do, and I bumped into the same doctor but she was listening to someone else's history… I asked him [other student] how he managed to get her to listen to his history when I had chased her all day. He then said, "It's a dog eat dog world", and then when she heard she started shouting at me in front of everyone saying I had no enthusiasm for medicine… it still upsets me when I think back; everyone just joked and said it was because she was pregnant…'

Sally, female, year 4, medical student, UK

younger healthcare students by clinical colleagues and patients. Sometimes students recounted discrimination on the basis of their intersecting personal identities such as race and religion. Although we have examples of students experiencing or witnessing the discrimination of other protected characteristics (e.g. sexual orientation, disability and pregnancy), these abuses were less frequent in our data.

Finally, less frequent in our data were examples of physical intimidation in which healthcare students reported being hit, nearly hit or threatened physical violence by patients or colleagues (note that medical students reported fewer incidents of this than other healthcare students such as nurses).[52] Students also reported witnessing the physical abuse of healthcare professionals in the workplace, typically by patients. Such physical abuse from patients can be seen in Susan's narrative (see Box 9.11, narrative 3). Although Susan excuses the patient hitting her due to their condition (confusion, dementia), she is clearly cognizant of the threat to her own safety posed by this patient.

How can Workplace Abuse be Prevented and Managed?

Although some healthcare students do nothing in the face of abuse (see narrative 2, Box 9.11), healthcare students in our research typically did something, with common responses including challenging or reporting perpetrators (see narrative 2, Box 9.11, and narrative 5, Box 9.12), debriefing with supportive people such as friends and peers (see narrative 4, Box 9.12) and bodily acts of resistance such as leaving the site of the abuse (see narrative 3, Box 9.11). What we also see from the narratives above is that abuse recipients sometimes downplay the abuse at the time by trying to laugh it off or make jokes (see narratives 1 and 3, Box 9.12), possibly using laughter/humour as a coping strategy.[62] However, what is clear from these narratives is that abuse-related professionalism dilemmas have a huge emotional impact on students, as discussed in the previous section on consequences. It causes them real psychological upset, evidenced in their narratives through their anxiety (e.g. 'apprehensive', 'worried', 'embarrassed', 'upset', 'scared', 'afraid', insecure', 'uncomfortable', 'fear', 'distress') and anger talk (e.g. 'offended', 'hell', 'angry', 'annoyed').[58–61] It is important, therefore, that healthcare workplace abuse is better prevented and managed.

Numerous abuse/bullying prevention and management interventions targeted at different levels (individual, team and organizational: see Box 9.13) have been reviewed in recent literature syntheses.[51,55] While there is considerable variability in the effectiveness of these individual interventions, interventions classed as participatory (e.g. those including active participants from all levels of the organization) and those receiving supportive leadership were most likely to be successful.[49,53] Indeed, Illing *et al.*[51] recommend that preventive approaches need first to target leaders and managers, leaders

---

Box 9.13 Bullying prevention and management strategies (Illing *et al.*)[51]

Individual level

Training, coaching and mentoring individuals
Informal support for individuals
Therapeutic approaches and counselling for individuals

Relationship level

Team building and training
Conflict management training
Mediation between recipients and perpetrators of bullying
Multisource feedback
Bystander interventions (e.g. staff being expected to challenge negative workplace behaviours)

Organizational level

Work climate (e.g. positive climate)
Work design/environment (e.g. increased time, autonomy)
Leadership/management (e.g. leaders that are good role models and committed to tackling bullying)
Codes of conduct, policies and legislation (e.g. anti-bullying policies)
Employee selection (e.g. well-designed selection systems)
Monitoring of organizational data (e.g. bullying prevalence and staff absenteeism/satisfaction/turnover)
Formal investigations/grievance procedures/punitive measures and rewards

---

Box 9.14 Stop and do: how should you manage abuse in your own institutional context?

- Thinking about your own institutional context and regulatory body, how should you act in the workplace to maintain equality, diversity, and dignity at work? What should you do if you are the recipient or bystander of workplace abuse/bullying?
- The GMC[31] outlines three ways that trainees can report bullying: (1) through the annual GMC national training survey; (2) through local systems; (3) through GMC/local confidential helplines. Thinking about your own institutional context and regulatory body, how should you report workplace abuse/bullying?

---

and managers need to support bullying interventions when they are introduced, anti-bullying organizational policies should be established, there is pro-active monitoring of organizational 'bullying' data and effective formal and informal training should be developed and implemented to prevent and manage bullying.

Things for healthcare students, trainees and educators to consider include learners having opportunities to: (1) reflect on their own and others' workplace behaviours; (2) better understand equality, diversity and dignity at work; and (3) develop communication and conflict management skills through rehearsing how to challenge workplace incivility.[51] Before reading the summary of this chapter, work through the activity in Box 9.14.

Chapter Summary

This chapter has provided an overview of what equality, diversity and dignity at work are and why there matter within the context of healthcare professionalism. We have explored workplace abuse and bullying and its relationship with healthcare hierarchies and power. We have learnt about the multiplicity of abuse/bullying causes and consequences at various levels, and have discussed various workplace abuses experienced by healthcare students and trainees. We have discussed how healthcare learners act and react in the face of abuse and considered key prevention and management strategies. The key take-home messages from this chapter are summarized in Box 9.15, with suggestions for small group discussions in Box 9.16. Finally, Box 9.17 outlines some recommended reading.

Box 9.15 Chapter summary points

- Learners and educators need to understand what workplace equality, diversity and dignity are and why they matter in healthcare education and practice
- Learners and educators must understand what workplace abuse and bullying are and understand their relationship with healthcare hierarchies and power
- Healthcare students and trainees experience various workplace abuses directly and indirectly
- Healthcare students and trainees need to find ways of coping with abuse within the broader context of organizational policies and practices for preventing and managing abuse

---

Box 9.16 Chapter discussion points

- How might you uphold equality, diversity and dignity at work when some protected characteristics may seem at odds with one another? For example, how might you simultaneously respect the rights of females alongside those holding patriarchal cultural beliefs?
- Think about the different types of abuse experienced by healthcare learners in this chapter. Focusing on a student narrative of your choice, discuss how you might deal with such abuse when perpetrated by different people: clinical teacher, peer or patient. Discuss the different challenges that may exist depending on who the perpetrator is.

Box 9.17 Chapter recommended reading

Carter M, Thompson N, Crampton P, *et al.* Workplace bullying in the UK NHS: a questionnaire and interview study on prevalence, impact and barriers to reporting. *British Medical Journal* 2013;3:e002628. doi:10.1136/bmjopen-2013-002628.

Rees CE, Monrouxe LV. 'A morning since eight of just pure grill': a multi-school qualitative study of student abuse. *Academic Medicine* 2011;86(11):1374–1382.

Rees CE, Monrouxe LV, Ternan E, Endacott R. Workplace abuse narratives from dentistry, nursing, pharmacy and physiotherapy students: a multi-school qualitative study. *European Journal of Dental Education* 2015;19:95–106.

Wright W, Khatri N. Bullying among nursing staff: relationship with psychological/behavioural responses of nurses and medical errors. *Health Care Management Review* 2015;40(2):139–147.

References

1 General Medical Council. *Equality and Diversity Strategy* 2014-2017. Manchester: GMC, 2014, http://www.gmc-uk.org/Equality_and_diversity_strategy_2014_17.pdf_54829092.pdf (Accessed 1 December 2016).

2 Nursing & Midwifery Council. *Nursing and Midwifery Council Equality and Diversity Strategy*. London: NMC, 2011, https://www.nmc.org.uk/globalassets/siteDocuments/Annual_reports_and_accounts/NMC_Equality-and-diversity-strategy-2012.pdf (Accessed 1 December 2016).

3 General Dental Council. *General Dental Council Equality and Diversity Strategy*. GDC, 2014, http://www.gdc-uk.org/Aboutus/Equalityanddiversity/Documents/Equality%20and%20Diversity%20Strategy.pdf (Accessed 1 December 2016).

4 Health Professions Council. *Equality and Diversity Scheme*. London: HPC, 2007, http://www.hpc-uk.org/assets/documents/100021B1HPCEqualityandDiversityScheme.pdf (Accessed 1 December 2016).

5 General Pharmaceutical Council. *Equality, Diversity and Inclusion Scheme*. GPhC, 2012, https://www.pharmacyregulation.org/sites/default/files/GPhC%20Equality%20Diversity%20and%20Inclusion%20Scheme%202012%20-%202014.pdf (Accessed 1 December 2016).

6 Rees CE, Monrouxe LV. 'A morning since eight of just pure grill': a multi-school qualitative study of student abuse. *Academic Medicine* 2011;86(11):1374–1382.

7 Rees CE, Monrouxe LV, Ternan E, Endacott R. Workplace abuse narratives from dentistry, nursing, pharmacy and physiotherapy students: a multi-school qualitative study. *European Journal of Dental Education* 2015;19:95–106.

8 Royal College of Nursing. *The RCN's Definition of Dignity*. London: RCN, 2008, http://www.rcn.org.uk/__data/assets/pdf_file/0003/191730/003298.pdf (Accessed 1 December 2016).

9   The Stationary Office. *Equality Act*. London: The Stationary Office, 2010, http://www.legislation. gov.uk/ukpga/2010/15/pdfs/ukpga_20100015_en.pdf (Accessed 1 December 2016).

10 Australian Medical Council. *Good Medical Practice: a Code of Conduct for Doctors in Australia*. Kingston, Australia: Australian Medical Council, 2009, http://www.health.nt.gov.au/ library/scripts/objectifymedia.aspx?file=pdf/39/02.pdf (Accessed 1 December 2016).

11 Royal College of Physicians and Surgeons of Canada. *The Draft CanMEDS 2015 Physician Competency Framework*. Ottawa: Royal College of Physicians and Surgeons of Canada, 2015, http://www.royalcollege.ca/portal/page/portal/rc/common/documents/ canmeds/framework/framework_series_1_e.pdf (Accessed 1 December 2016).

12 General Medical Council. *Good Medical Practice*. Manchester: General Medical Council, 2013, http://www.gmc-uk.org/Good_medical_practice___English_1215.pdf_51527435. pdf (Accessed 1 December 2016).

13 American Board of Internal Medicine Foundation-American College of Physicians-American Society of Internal Medicine-European Federation of Internal Medicine. Medical professionalism in the new millennium: a physician charter. *Annals of Internal Medicine* 2002;136:243–246.

14 Australian Dental Council. *Professional Attributes and Competencies of the Newly Qualified Dentist*. Melbourne: Australian Dental Council, 2013, http://www.adc.org.au/ documents/Professional%20Competencies%20of%20the%20Newly%20Qualified% 20Dentist%20-%20February%202016.pdf (Accessed 1 December 2016).

15 Royal College of Dental Surgeons of Ontario. *Code of Ethics*. Toronto: Royal College of Dental Surgeons of Ontario, 2004, http://www.rcdso.org/Assets/DOCUMENTS/Professional_ Practice/Code_of_Ethics/RCDSO_Code_of_Ethics.PDF (Accessed 1 December 2016).

16 General Dental Council. *Standards for the Dental Team*. London: General Dental Council, 2013, http://www.gdc-uk.org/Newsandpublications/Publications/Publications/ Standards%20for%20the%20Dental%20Team.pdf (Accessed 1 December 2016).

17 American Dental Association. *ADA Principles of Ethics and Code of Professional Conduct*. Chicago: American Dental Association, 2012, http://www.ada.org/~/media/ADA/ Publications/Files/ADA_Code_of_Ethics_2016.pdf?la=en (Accessed 1 December 2016).

18 Australian Nursing and Midwifery Council. *Code of Professional Conduct for Nurses in Australia*. Melbourne: Australian Nursing and Midwifery Council, 2008, http://www. nursingmidwiferyboard.gov.au/Codes-Guidelines-Statements/Professional-standards.aspx (Accessed 1 December 2016).

19 Canadian Nurses Association. *Framework for the Practice of Registered Nurses in Canada 2015*. Ottawa: Canadian Nurses Association, 2015, https://www.cna-aiic.ca/~/media/cna/ page-content/pdf-en/framework-for-the-pracice-of-registered-nurses-in-canada.pdf?la=en (Accessed 1 December 2016).

20 Nursing and Midwifery Council. *The Code: Standards of Conduct, Performance and Ethics for Nurses and Midwives*. London: Nursing and Midwifery Council, 2015, https:// www.nmc.org.uk/globalassets/sitedocuments/nmc-publications/nmc-code.pdf (Accessed 1 December 2016).

21 American Nurses Association. *Code of Ethics for Nurses*. Silver Spring, MD: American Nurses Association, 2015, http://www.nursingworld.org/codeofethics (Accessed 1 December 2016).

22 Australian Physiotherapy Association. *Australian Standards for Physiotherapy*. Canberra: Australian Physiotherapy Association, 2006, https://physiocouncil.com.au/

media/1021/the-australian-standards-for-physiotherapy-2006.pdf (Accessed 1 December 2016).

23 National Physiotherapy Advisory Group. *Essential Competency Profile for Physiotherapists in Canada*. National Physiotherapy Advisory Group, 2009, http://www. physiotherapyeducation.ca/Resources/Essential%20Comp%20PT%20Profile% 202009.pdf (Accessed 1 December 2016).

24 Chartered Society of Physiotherapy. *Code of Professional Values and Behaviour*. London: Chartered Society of Physiotherapy, 2011, http://www.csp.org.uk/publications/code-members-professional-values-behaviour (Accessed 1 December 2016).

25 American Physical Therapy Association. *APTA Guide for Professional Conduct*. Alexandria, VA: American Physical Therapy Association, 2010, http://www.apta.org/ uploadedFiles/APTAorg/Practice_and_Patient_Care/Ethics/GuideforProfessionalConduct. pdf (Accessed 1 December 2016).

26 Pharmaceutical Society of Australia. *Code of Ethics for Pharmacists*. Deakin, ACT: Pharmaceutical Society of Australia, 2015. https://www.psa.org.au/download/codes/ code-of-ethics-2011.pdf (Accessed 1 December 2016).

27 National Association of Pharmacy Regulatory Authorities. *Model Standards of Practice for Canadian Pharmacists*. Ottawa: National Association of Pharmacy Regulatory Authorities, 2009, http://napra.ca/Content_Files/Files/Model_Standards_of_Prac_for_ Cdn_Pharm_March09_Final_b.pdf (Accessed 1 December 2016).

28 General Pharmaceutical Council. *Standards of Conduct, Ethics and Performance*. London: General Pharmaceutical Council, 2012, https://www.pharmacyregulation.org/ sites/default/files/standards_of_conduct_ethics_and_performance_july_2014.pdf (Accessed 1 December 2016).

29 American Pharmacists Association. *Code of Ethics for Pharmacists*. American Pharmacists Association,1994, http://www.pharmacist.com/code-ethics (Accessed 1 December 2016).

30 Bender DJ. Patient preference for a racially or gender-concordant student dentist. *Journal of Dental Education* 2007;71(6):726–745.

31 General Medical Council. National Training Survey 2014. *Bullying and Undermining*. Manchester: GMC, 2014, http://www.gmc-uk.org/NTS_bullying_and_undermining_ report_2014_FINAL.pdf_58648010.pdf (Accessed 1 December 2016).

32 Eisler R, Potter T. Breaking down the hierarchies. *Nursing Management* 2014;21(5):12. doi: 10.7748/nm.21.5.12.s13.

33 Carter M, Thompson N, Crampton P, Morrow G, Burford B, Gray C, *et al.* Workplace bullying in the UK NHS: a questionnaire and interview study on prevalence, impact and barriers to reporting. *British Medical Journal* 2013;3:e002628. doi: 10.1136/ bmjopen-2013-002628.

34 Monrouxe LV, Bullock A, Cole J, Gormley G, Kaufhold K, Kelly N, *et al. How Prepared are UK Medical Graduates for Practice?* Final Report from a programme of research commissioned by the General Medical Council, May 2014. http://www.gmc-uk.org/about/ research/25531.asp (Accessed 1 December 2016).

35 Wright W, Khatri N. Bullying among nursing staff: relationship with psychological/ behavioural responses of nurses and medical errors. *Health Care Management Review* 2015;40(2):139–147.

36 Silver HK, Glicken AD. Medical student abuse. Incidence, severity and significance. *Journal of the American Medical Association* 1990;263:527–32.

37 Wilkinson TJ, Gill DJ, Fitzjohn J, Palmer CL, Mulder RT. The impact on students of adverse experiences during medical school. *Medical Teacher* 2006;28:129–135.

38 Salin D. Ways of explaining workplace bullying: a review of enabling, motivating and precipitating structures and processes in the work environment. *Human Relations* 2003;56:1213–1232.

39 McKimm J, Swanwick T. Educational leadership. In T. Swanwick (Ed.) *Understanding Medical Education. Evidence, Theory & Practice*. Oxford: Wiley-Blackwell, 2010: pp. 419–437.

40 Northouse PG. *Leadership. Theory and Practice*, 6th Edition. Los Angeles: Sage, 2013.

41 Grue J, Johannessen LE, Rasmussen EF. Prestige rankings of chronic diseases and disabilities. A survey among professionals in the disability field. *Social Science & Medicine* 2015;124:180–186.

42 Lutgen-Sandvik P, Tracy SJ, Alberts JK. Burned by bullying in the American workplace: prevalence, perception, degree and impact. *Journal of Management Studies* 2007;44:837–861.

43 Einarsen S, Hoel H, Notelaers G. Measuring exposure to bullying and harassment at work: validity, factor structure and psychometric properties of the Negative Acts Questionnaire-Revised. *Work & Stress* 2009;23(1):24–44.

44 Walton MM. Hierarchies: the Berlin Wall of patient safety. *Quality & Safety in Health Care* 2006;15:229–230.

45 Norredam M, Album D. Prestige and its significance for medical specialties and diseases. *Scandinavian Journal of Public Health* 2007;35:655–661.

46 Rees CE, Ajjawi R, Monrouxe LV. The construction of power in family medicine bedside teaching: a video observation study. *Medical Education* 2013;47:154–165.

47 Yeh M-Y, Wu SM, Che HL. Cultural and hierarchical influences: ethical issues faced by Taiwanese nursing students. *Medical Education* 2010;44:475–84.

48 Dennis A, Martin PJ. Symbolic interactionism and the concept of power. *British Journal of Sociology* 2005;56:191–213.

49 Mills S. *Michel Foucault*. Abingdon: Routledge, 2003.

50 Rees CE, Monrouxe LV. 'I should be lucky ha ha ha ha': the construction of power, identity, and laughter within medical workplace learning encounters. *Journal of Pragmatics* 2010;42(12):3384–3399.

51 Illing JC, Carter M, Thompson NJ, Crampton PES, Morrow GM, Howse JH, *et al.* Evidence synthesis on the occurrence, causes, consequences, prevention and management of bullying and harassing behaviours to inform decision making in the NHS. Final report. NIHR Service Delivery and Organisation Programme, 2013, http://www.nets.nihr.ac.uk/__data/assets/pdf_file/0006/85119/FR-10-1012-01.pdf (Accessed 1 December 2016).

52 Monrouxe LV, Rees CE, Dennis A, Wells S. Professionalism dilemmas, moral distress and the healthcare student: insights from two online UK-wide questionnaire studies. *British Medical Journal Open* 2015;5:e007518. doi:10.1136/bmjopen-2014-007518.

53 Loerbroks A, Weigl M, Li J, Glaser J, Degen C, Angerer P. Workplace bullying and depressive symptoms: a prospective study among junior physicians in Germany. *Journal of Psychosomatic Research* 2015;78:168–172.

54 Silver HK. Medical students and medical school. *Journal of the American Medical Association* 1982;247:309–310.

55 Quinlan E, Robertson S, Miller N, Robertson-Boersma D. Interventions to reduce bullying in health care organizations: a scoping review. *Health Services Management Research* 2014;27(1–2):33–44.

56 Miedema B, Hamilton R, Lambert-Lanning A, Tatemichi SR, Lemire F, Manca D, *et al.* Prevalence of abusive encounters in the workplace of family physicians. *Canadian Family Physician* 2010;56:e101–8.

57 Iglesias MEL, De Bengoa Vallejo RB. Prevalence of bullying at work and its association with self-esteem scores in a Spanish nursing sample. *Contemporary Nurse* 2012;42(1):2–10.

58 Monrouxe LV, Rees CE. 'It's just a clash of cultures': emotional talk within medical students' narratives of professionalism dilemmas. *Advances in Health Sciences Education* 2012;17(5):671–701.

59 Monrouxe LV, Rees CE, Endacott R, Ternan E. 'Even now it makes me angry': healthcare students' professionalism dilemma narratives. *Medical Education* 2014;48:502–517.

60 Rees CE, Monrouxe LV, McDonald LA. Narrative, emotion, and action: analysing 'most memorable' professionalism dilemmas. *Medical Education* 2013;47(1):80–96.

61 Rees CE, Monrouxe LV, McDonald LA. My mentor kicked a dying woman's bed: analysing UK nursing students' most memorable professionalism dilemmas. *Journal of Advanced Nursing* 2015;71(1):169–180.

62 Rees CE, Monrouxe LV. Laughter for coping: medical students narrating professionalism dilemmas. In CR Figley, P Huggard, CE Rees (Eds). *First Do No Self-Harm: Understanding and Promoting Physician Stress Resilience*. New York: Oxford University Press, 2013: pp.67–87.

10

E-professionalism-related Dilemmas

'Outside of the workplace, I was involved in writing crude and salacious comments on a forum. It was a [sporting] club [online] forum with around 20–25 members. We thought it was an anonymous forum but a member of the public complained and subsequently I sat a fitness to practise hearing for misconduct behaviour. [I] apologized and showed remorse because I had made a mistake and I wanted to rectify the problem. I learnt a big lesson about probity and acting professionally outside the workplace.'

Edward, male, year 4, medical student, UK

LEARNING OUTCOMES

- To understand what comprises online social networks (OSNs) and what the benefits and challenges are for OSN use in terms of learning professionalism (e-professionalism)
- To discover the range of e-professionalism-related dilemmas occurring across different healthcare professions
- To understand the various psychological, social and technological factors that impact on why we engage with OSNs in the way we do
- To reflect on ways in which e-professionalism can be maintained and managed whilst engaging with online activities

---

KEY TERMS

E-professionalism
Web 2.0
Online social networks
Boundary crossing
Self-disclosure
Self-presentation

Healthcare Professionalism: Improving Practice through Reflections on Workplace Dilemmas, First Edition.
Lynn V. Monrouxe and Charlotte E. Rees.

Introduction

Avatars, cookies, connectivity, followers, lurkers, surfing, networking and viral. The likelihood is that the meanings of these words have changed dramatically over your lifetime: as well as retaining their original sense, all of these, and many more words, have a specific meaning when used in connection with the Internet. The Internet itself has developed over time. Originally it comprised a repository for information sharing (so-called Web 1.0), for which the vast percentage of users were simply acting as consumers of content.[1] However, with the advent of the Web 2.0 platform in the early 2000s, users were able to participate in content *creation*. Such creation brought forth *social media*: 'a group of Internet-based applications that build on the ideological and technological foundations of Web 2.0, and that allow the creation and exchange of User Generated Content'.[2, p. 61] These online social network (OSN) applications enable us to share information, experiences, beliefs, photographs, video/audio clips, and so on, and include social networking sites (e.g. Facebook, LinkedIn), blogs (e.g. WordPress, Tumblr), microblogs (e.g. Twitter, Snapchat) and content-sharing websites (e.g. YouTube, Instagram). Some people seem to enjoy this creative and expressive side of the Internet. Indeed, recent figures show that around one million of us use Snapchat every day, 316 million actively use Twitter every month and Facebook has 1.49 billion users,[3] with 90% of 18–29-year-olds using some form of online social network.[4] So every day, millions of people are publicly sharing their photographs, videos, daily events and even their innermost emotions with the world. Some of us are more *digitally savvy* than others.[5] Rather than belonging to a specific generation (Millennials, Net Generation, etc.), digitally savvy people tend to come from media-rich households, and reach to the Internet as a preference for information, banking, shopping and so on. In this chapter we consider how things have changed since the advent of the Internet and what this means for professionalism: including the importance of e-professionalism, the types of e-professionalism lapses healthcare learners commit and the associated repercussions, the psychological, sociological and technological factors associated with social media use and regulatory bodies recommendations for the prevention and management of e-professionalism lapses.

What are the Benefits of OSNs for Professionalism?

We can be anywhere; so long as there is Internet, we are *connected* to the world. From thousands of miles away, our friends, family and acquaintances can contact us through a variety of OSNs. We can see their photographs and videos within moments of events occurring. As a consequence of this, the world appears to shrink the more connected we become. The versatility of the Web 2.0 technologies therefore opens up exciting opportunities for sharing information and collaboration with others across the globe, providing an easy and efficient way of organizing people for events and tasks. And not just connecting with friends and family: communication between educators and students, within our peer groups, across professional networks, and communicating information more generally to the *outside world* is commonplace. This ability changes the way in which we view and act in the world.

It has been demonstrated that OSNs have the potential to keep us up to date with the most recent advances in medicine and to enhance our learning.[6] Learning is enhanced because of the rich visual and aural content, frequently requiring us to participate in communicative activities. Such interactive learning is thought to be a preference for today's students.[7] More than ever before, learners are engaging with novel forms of education that promote agency, autonomy and engagement across a multitude of real and virtual learning spaces connecting physical, geographical, institutional and organizational boundaries.[8]

What are the Challenges of OSNs for Professionalism?

Along with the creativity and freedom in learning and communicating, OSNs also facilitate greater and freer expression of our internal world, to anyone and everyone who happens to pass by. We can send jpegs, animated gifs and emoji across a variety of social media platforms: for example, on WhatsApp alone there are over 800 different emoji, each with a unique meaning, and an online emoji database with thousands of examples (http://emojipedia.org/). The immediacy and creativity with which social media enables us to share our thoughts and feelings so readily with the world is alluring and often fun and we frequently engage in this sharing seamlessly across our social, educational and workplace environments. In short, the line between our private and professional lives is blurring. Arguably, it is this seamless engagement with others via OSNs that creates a range of e-professionalism challenges for healthcare professionals and students, ultimately leading to some people committing professionalism lapses online.

Consider Edward's narrative at the beginning of this chapter. The boundary between his workplace and his personal space was crossed through his participation in an online forum. What for some people might be considered 'typical banter' between male sporting colleagues when conducted in a relatively private space (e.g. same-sex changing rooms)[9] was in fact conducted online. The 'crude and salacious' conversation between Edward and his sporting fellows was written down for all to see and for all to identify those concerned. It was documented. Subsequently reported by a member of the public, Edward faced a fitness to practise hearing for professional misconduct.

However, Edward is not alone. A 2012 national survey of 48 US state medical boards (responsible for medical licensure and discipline) asked the executive directors about eight specific online violations of professionalism by doctors.[10] They found that over 90% of the boards had to deal with at least one of the violations. Most commonly issues around boundary crossing and honesty were cited: inappropriate online communication with patients (e.g. sexual misconduct 33/48; 69%), using the Internet for inappropriate practice (e.g. Internet prescribing without established clinical relationship 30/48; 63%) and online misrepresentation of credentials (29/48; 60%). Healthcare students have also been found to breach professionalism codes when online.[11] For example, a recent survey of 682 healthcare students (including medicine, nursing, pharmacy, physical therapy and dentistry) found that while the majority believed that posting drug-use (94%), criminal behaviour (91%), obscenities (including inappropriate nudity and sexual content: 72%), patient/client information (99%) and criticizing others (69%) was unprofessional, 27% admitted to posting such material themselves.[11] Before we move on to consider how e-professionalism has been defined and the various types of e-professionalism lapses that might occur whilst using OSNs, please engage with the 'stop and do' exercise in Box 10.1.

> **Box 10.1 Stop and do: reflect on your right to *free speech* and *freedom to act* as a healthcare student or practitioner**
>
> 'If patients and clients have the right to have their personal lives and information kept from being disclosed, then me being a health professional – I also have a personal life. One that is enjoyed and should be able to be enjoyed freely without interference or judgement.'[11, p. 4]
>
> To what extent do you agree with this statement? How can you maintain a sense of self (including your sexual, gendered and political identities) without interference or judgement? Think back to the notion of 'professionalism as segregation' (Chapter 2, Table 2.3), how does the statement above relate to this within an online environment?

What is E-professionalism and Why is it Important?

'I'm rubber and you're glue. Anything you say bounces off of me but sticks forever in cyberspace.'
http://ericksonbarnett.com/blog/detail/quote-of-the-week-the-internet-never-forgets/

There are surprisingly few explicit definitions of what comprises e-professionalism. While policy documents tend to prioritize the protection of patients when discussing online behaviour, they also urge healthcare students and professionals to take great care to uphold professionalism values when using electronic communication and social networking sites.[12] Thus, apart from breaches of patient confidentiality and illegal behaviours, there is no real consensus about what comprises an e-professionalism lapse.[13] The most succinct definition across the literature comes from Cain and his colleagues, who specifically define e-professionalism as: 'the attitudes and behaviours (some of which may occur in private settings) reflecting traditional professionalism paradigms that are manifested through digital media.'[14, p. 67] Thus, e-professionalism does not extend beyond the concept of professionalism itself, rather it merely addresses professionalism within the online world.

E-professionalism is greater than ensuring one's online communications (e.g. email, discussion boards, etc.) are suitably worded: so-called *netiquette*. E-professionalism entails that we construct and maintain an online professional persona across all personal and professional media platforms within which we engage, or within which we are associated. Any kind of digital representation (e.g. group affiliations, photographs, videos as well as social acts of *tagging, liking, favouriting, friending, following*, etc.) can be seen as a means through which we signal our persona: *who we are.*[15] They reveal subtle, and not so subtle, clues to our underlying attitudes, our behaviours (or potential behaviours) and have the potential to blur the boundaries around aspects such as private versus public lives and what comprises a *relationship.*[16] Furthermore, due to the limitations of privacy online, others can easily access information about us. This wider online presence, beyond any single media use, gives out further clues to who we might be, from which other people can extrapolate who *they think* we are, and who they think we are in relation to them. Finally, that the public (and therefore patients) can access such information at any time (as the opening quote to this section suggests) means that this could comprise a form of *self-disclosure.* Too much self-disclosure by healthcare practitioners is typically considered to be a boundary violation in terms of the patient-practitioner relationship, particularly by patients themselves who have a lower threshold for students' inappropriate online personas.[17]

Box 10.2 Stop and do: who are you online?

Using the web-browser of your choice, try searching for yourself online (if you have recently done this you might need to delete the cookies stored on your machine to get the most up-to-date results).

Now, imagine you are a member of the public and you have been searching the Internet to find out about you. Looking at your results, answer *yes*, *maybe* or *no* to the following questions:

- Are you identifiable as a healthcare student or trainee?
- Would you feel comfortable having 'you' involved in your healthcare?
- Would you feel happy to have 'you' present as a learner when consulting your health-care practitioner?
- Would you trust 'you' to know your personal details?

If your answer to any of the above questions is *no* or *maybe*, what is it about 'you' that makes you hesitant? What do you think you can do to change your response to *yes*? What about the issue of identifiability: how do you feel about using an avatar? Do you self-identify as a healthcare student or trainee? What are the issues around self-identification in this way and the use of avatars? (check the guidance, e.g. in the UK the GMC states that if you identify as a doctor you must also use your own name).[24]

Considering the wider online presence that we have, e-professionalism-related dilemmas can have a wide ranging impact: they can affect specific individuals (e.g. the person interacting with the OSN), certain relationships (e.g. student-student, student-patient, student-teacher), organizations (e.g. hospitals, universities) and professional groups (e.g. doctors, physiotherapists, nurses) to which we belong. For example, reconsider our opening narrative. Edward's online behaviour certainly affected him personally in that he was required to attend a fitness to practice hearing for his misconduct. However, because a member of the public discovered and reported his behaviour to the medical school, we can infer that somehow he was identified as being a student of that particular organization. Edward's behaviour therefore has the potential to harm the reputation of both his medical school and his university (which might prove very costly).[18] Further, it is likely that other members of the public would have seen this posting, or heard about it. They might have even linked this specific action to other profession-specific lapses they have read or heard about.[19,20] As such, Edward's e-professionalism lapse could provide further confirmatory evidence that medical students (and doctors) are a 'bad bunch' and therefore is likely to reflect poorly on the medical profession as a whole. Indeed, researchers and professional bodies recognize that e-professionalism lapses can easily erode the social contract between healthcare professionals and society.[21,22] Had Edward been caring for a patient, that patient might well have lost trust and terminated their relationship (patients have been known to request a different physician due to questionable behaviours on OSNs).[23]

While we have presented an extreme scenario of the possible damage that Edward's behaviour might incur, it is worth reflecting on these issues as you read our next section concerning the range of e-professionalism-related dilemmas experienced by healthcare students and practitioners across our programme of research. Before continuing, however, we urge you to work through the 'stop and do' exercise in Box 10.2, designed to get you thinking about your own online persona.

What E-professionalism Lapses do Healthcare Learners Commit?

'For digital natives, the idea that some of this information should remain private, or that it might impact the patient-doctor relationship, seems strange. They have grown up in a "hyperpersonal" world, in which it feels comfortable to digitally expose oneself online.'[25], multimedia Appendix[1]

It has been suggested that because today's students and trainees have grown up in a *hyperpersonal* world, they do not feel restricted in terms of what and how they post online.[25] However, a great deal of research examining students', trainees' and healthcare practitioners' OSN presence appears to suggest that healthcare students and professionals *at all ages* are at risk of e-professionalism lapses.[10,26,27] Indeed, there are a number of e-professionalism lapses specifically engaged in by healthcare practitioners (e.g. using the Internet to practice inappropriately, Internet prescribing and misrepresentation of credentials).[10] Here we focus on common lapses across healthcare students, trainees and practitioners according to the wider healthcare literature, whilst considering what policy-related documents have to say about the issues and how to mitigate them. While this is not intended as a definitive list, key lapses commonly found are: maintaining confidentiality, privacy and dignity, boundary-crossing, lack of respect for others and maintaining honesty/transparency. We now consider each one in turn.

Maintaining Confidentiality, Privacy and Dignity

Confidentiality refers to the safeguarding of patient information and is closely associated with the concept of privacy that relates to the patient's right to be treated with dignity and respect (as discussed in Chapter 8).[28] In brief, policymakers' confidentiality and privacy concerns include problems around the use of OSNs for: discussing patients' cases with patients (or their families), communication about patient cases with other doctors or students, revealing identifying information about a patient to a specific group of people – such as 'friends' on Facebook – or to the public (e.g. via blogging sites).[12,29–32] Furthermore, the use of photography online is also a concern: guidelines stipulate that clinical photography can be justified, used and even published to an audience not directly involved in patients' treatment for medical education and research purposes (so-called secondary use of clinical photography).[33]

These concerns are not unfounded. Consider Robyn's narrative (Box 10.3, narrative 1) about her peer who discussed an embarrassing incident with a patient on their Facebook page, potentially revealing the identity of the patient to the majority of her classmates. Furthermore, Kristen's narrative (Box 10.3, narrative 2) of a peer who posted a photograph of a patient's operative report on Facebook suggests that confidentiality and privacy can be violated in a range of ways online. These narratives echo findings from the wider literature in which healthcare students' online violations of patient confidentiality, privacy and dignity have been identified.[11,34–39] Such violations include posting pictures of cadavers, dying or dead patients and deriding patients online.[11,36,38,39]

Boundary-crossing

Professional boundaries have been defined as the limits that protect the space between the professional's power and the recipient's vulnerability.[41] Boundaries can also be seen in terms of the space between one's personal and professional lives. Thus, when patients and professionals interact as if their relationship is a social rather than a professional

---

Box 10.3 Narratives of e-professionalism lapses by healthcare students

---

Narrative 1: 'making her patient easily identifiable'

'Another student breaching confidentiality on Facebook. About 75% of my year probably saw this online breach; she discussed embarrassing things that had happened during her OSCE making her patient easily identifiable. I emailed her privately and told her to take it off because I was thinking about the man in question and how he would feel knowing he was being discussed like this. I wish I had gone to the authorities but I didn't. This person has since come close to breaches again and I feel she is clinically unfit. The first instance may have ended in her expulsion had I had the bravery to report her. I think whistleblowing should be encouraged and an easy way of doing it for students should be in place.'

Robyn, female, year 2, medical student, UK

Narrative 2: 'for everyone's eyes to see'

'Patient confidentiality and data protection. At home with a fellow medical student house-mate, we were on Facebook. Another student had taken a photograph of part of a patient's operative report and posted it on Facebook (although it did not contain the patient's name or any identifying details). I commented on the photo asking if it should really be on Facebook for everyone's eyes to see. I would have whistle blown but it may have become a fitness to practise matter and I did not want it to ruin their career. So I hinted that it might just be a tad inappropriate… They took the photo down. Quite honestly I was disgusted at their attempt to appear "cool" by compromising patient confidentiality.'

Kristen, female, year 2, medical student, UK

Narrative 3: 'most of the girls were 'pretty'

'Member of staff adding female students on Facebook, [I was] with friends… on Facebook. I observed it happen with a few students. [My] housemate let me look at his [staff member's] Facebook page after she was added. Saw most of the girls were "pretty"… He never talked to them on Facebook that I could see. [I] talked to another senior member of staff about it, mentioning no names. As it wasn't bothering any of the people involved and I wasn't directly involved only observed it, then we thought it best to leave it. [I reported it because] I thought it was the responsible thing to do. [I was] relieved afterwards as I feel I did something about it. [I] was terrified when bringing it to the staff member's attention.'

Nathan, male, year 4, dental student, UK

Narrative 4: 'I do fear slightly for patient safety'

'A particular student posts very unprofessional statements about the course on his Facebook page regularly… they have spoken about planning on seeing patients hung-over, a video urinating through a letterbox, putting a dead hamster in a condom and chasing people, taking pictures and putting them on[line] of other students being physically sick over themself… has turned up drunk… to a lab session and told stories of beating up a young boy and of driving well over the speed limit and crashing his car. I took some print screens of some Facebook posts with a thought of going to say something about it but have not actually done so. I feel that if I say anything it may backfire on me… that will vastly decrease my popularity within the entire medical school. I still feel very unhappy about this student studying medicine here. I do not think he is in any way fit to practice and I do fear slightly for patient safety.'

Chris, male, year 2, medical student, UK

Narrative 5: 'this was on Bebo'

'Student A and B started having a little tit for tat comments to each other on Bebo… they'd wrote … that we were sitting in a pharmacology lesson and she'd learnt that aspirin kills unborn babies, and her comment was, "Maybe the NHS should try these, there's a lot of people…" girls [then] approached me from the course asking if I'd seen Student A's Bebo page [they said], "Think you should go and read it"… [she was] commenting, it's amazing how much I have in common with [names serial killer nurse]… I had to take this to the school… [they] suspended her for two weeks… before she was due to come back… I'd got 18 messages on my mobile, and 20 phone calls on the house phone… I went on my Bebo page and there was a short story from her… there was one about the young lad who's no longer here, about how he comes into class still drunk from the night before, suffering the effects from the pills he's taken the night before… then a little bit about Student B and a bit about myself which was, "Behaves inappropriately towards girls in the classroom young enough to be his daughter" and that's embarrassing for me…'

Corey, male, year 2, nursing student, UK

Narrative 6: 'people were cheating'

'People cheating by texting their friends in later groups what the cases are. I told the examiner I believed people were cheating and asked the examiner if we could all please hand our phones in and then sign them out once every group had done the OSCE. I was enraged that they were cheating – and thought I could stop it. [I'm] still very angry that it goes on. I would never tell anyone about it – as although it makes me angry, I think it would be too harsh to tell considering the consequences. Also I have direct proof.'

Basil, male, year 4, medical student, UK

relationship, a 'boundary violation' arises. Here, boundaries are important for the individual professional (who is more than just a nurse, a dentist, etc.), but also for the institution for whom they work and for the profession. Such boundaries ensure that identities do not become diffused (i.e. while a representative, the individual is not the profession as a whole). In this era of OSNs, new dilemmas are presented around what comprises an appropriate boundary for people working and learning within various power-relationships and across institutional and professional domains, particularly as even so-called personal OSN postings are very often publically accessible.

The importance of maintaining boundaries across OSNs is a common feature across healthcare social media policy documents, although primarily focusing on the professional boundary between healthcare practitioners and patients/clients.[12,29–31,42,43] However, as we can see in Nathan's narrative (Box 10.3, narrative 3) boundaries between students and staff are also important.

Although research suggests that faculty members and the public tend to be more conservative around what is acceptable behaviour on OSNs than students,[17] not all groups are homogenous. Consider, for example, Chris' narrative in Box 10.3 (narrative 4). Here, Chris highlights a number of online (and offline) professionalism lapses of a peer, some

---

Box 10.4 Stop and do: should photography in clinical settings be prohibited?

Read the two scenarios below and answer the following questions:

- Should you take and post the picture in Scenario 1? In Scenario 2?
- How do these scenarios differ?

Scenario 1

Nyangeni *et al.*[36] reported on nurse students' use of OSNs in the Eastern Cape. They found that student nurses sometimes had a strong desire to tell others about their patients' illnesses, for example: 'Those babies with congenital defects, people with extensive side effects like in psychiatry when they do those hallucinations and they don't really know where they are. And also if maybe you are cleaning patient's wound or how it is then you take a picture and send…'[36, p. 4]

Scenario 2

'Suppose that you are the only one working the late night shift in a remote rural clinic when someone enters with what appears to be a poisonous spider bite that is causing her a lot of pain. You cannot identify the bite, which is necessary for giving the appropriate treatment… if you take a picture and post it in a tropical medicine Facebook group (that is only used by academics and physicians) someone might give you an answer.'[40, p. 67]

---

of which resonate with findings from the wider healthcare literature in which a variety of online boundary violations have been identified, including: inappropriate relationships (e.g. requesting patient friendships; having relations and posting them on OSNs),[34,36] posting sexually suggestive/explicit content (e.g. provocative personal photographs, sexually suggestive talk),[11,34,35,37–39,44] intoxication (e.g. pictures of self and others drunk, holding alcoholic beverages),[11,34,35,37–39,44] drug use (e.g. pictures of self engaging in drug taking, drug paraphernalia)[11,34,38] and criminal behaviour.[35] Whilst the majority of these e-professionalism lapses occur on personal pages (e.g. Bebo or Facebook) they can also been seen in other online spaces such as blogs. Before we continue outlining key e-professionalism lapses, we suggest you undertake the 'stop and do' exercise in Box 10.4.

Lack of Respect

Respecting patients, colleagues, the workplace and the profession are also key issues across many healthcare social media policy documents and are closely linked with the issue of defamation.[12,28–31,42,43] Cooperative working with colleagues, including communicating appropriately via social media, is emphasized.[31] Thus, warnings against 'cyber-bullying' that includes harassing or threatening others, inciting hatred or discrimination, swearing, using sexually explicit, racial or homophobic language, encouraging violence or self-harm and making gratuitous comments online about employers or co-workers are commonly mentioned across these documents.[12,28,31] Such actions are thought to constitute *lateral violence*, negatively affecting not only individuals but also team-based care, with the potential to create patient-safety situations (see Chapters 7 and 9 for related issues).[28]

Defamation of individuals, institutions and of professions online is also of concern. Making unsubstantiated, unsustainable comments and even repeating or replaying words spoken by another, all comprise acts of defamation.[29,42] Defamation can lead to expensive civil law cases, often involving sizeable payouts for compensation.[29] Even

---

Box 10.5 Stop and do: boundaries, where to draw the line?

Go online and find a blog written by individuals from your profession: in what way (if any) do you think this blog crosses the professionalism threshold for you?

Where do you draw the line?

- How many swear words, sexual or racial references does it take to cross the line?
- How many cues to alcohol or drug abuse before an online persona is considered to be an e-professionalism lapse?

---

simply expressing everyday frustration regarding your current job through social media is warned against.[28,43] Not only does this portray you as having poor professional judgement, but it might also be construed as defamation of your employer's character.[43] Humour is also considered to be problematic due to the paucity of contextual information in online communication. Thus the portrayal of patients, vulnerable socioeconomic groups, and other healthcare professionals (e.g. during end-of-year variety shows) is thought to be inappropriate for publication.[32]

Corey's narrative in Box 10.3 (narrative 5) succinctly summarizes some of the issues highlighted across these policy documents – the actions of 'Student A', not only constitute cyber-bullying of Corey and some of his fellow classmates, it also brings into disrepute the nursing profession itself, with references to a male nurse serial-killer. Corey's narrative reflects issues found within the wider literature around lack of respect online including reports of profanity (e.g. swearing about peers, educators, rotations, courses or university),[11,34,35,37,39,45] lack of respect for educators/school,[38] cyberbullying,[46,47] and discriminatory language use (racist, sexist, homophobic).[34,35,37–39] Such acts are often picked up and reported in online newspapers so that damage to the patient and profession is frequently exacerbated.[48–50] We suggest you pause here and go to the 'stop and do' exercise in Box 10.5.

Honesty and Transparency

Ensuring honesty in an online environment often requires transparency on the part of the user. Across the policy-related documents, the three main areas emphasizing honesty and transparency are: advice-giving, advertising and conflicts of interest.[12,22,31,43] In terms of student honesty, the use of OSNs for plagiarism, cheating prior to or during exams is also mentioned.[32] This latter issue resonates with Basil's narrative (Box 10.3, narrative 6) in which he talks about his peers cheating via texts during an OSCE exam. Although academic dishonesty occurs within healthcare professional education, there have been no studies to our knowledge that have specifically examined so-called 'cyber-cheating'. However, studies conducted with other student groups (e.g. science students) about plagiarism involving the Internet suggests there is wide student-acceptance around using the Internet for undertaking academically dishonest behaviours.[51]

What are the Repercussions for E-professionalism-related Lapses?

For healthcare professionals, e-professionalism lapses have serious repercussions, including termination of employment and deregistration from professional boards.[48,52–54] For students, a range of disciplinary actions have been reported, including: total dismissal, temporary suspension, formal warning, remediation, mentoring, informal warning, mental health evaluation and sometimes no actions taken.[34,55,56] However, as well as these direct repercussions, indirect repercussions for e-professionalism lapses have been identified: specifically, employers have begun to use information gathered via OSNs – so-called *cyber-vetting* – to evaluate job candidates when making hiring decisions. In this context studies have shown that candidates with OSN postings that emphasize drinking are deemed unprofessional, less attractive, less likely to attract a job interview and more likely to be offered a lower salary if hired.[57,58]

Of the above repercussions, one that stands out as being particularly unusual is the referral of students for mental health evaluation. We now consider the interaction between psychological, social and technological aspects of OSNs use when we try to understand why we behave as we do in this environment. It is this interaction that might lie at the root of some of the seemingly strange online behaviour undertaken by health-care practitioners and students. We believe that a better understanding of these issues might facilitate a reduction in e-professionalism lapses.

What are the Psychological, Social and Technological Factors Associated with Social Media Use?

'I think it's [interacting via OSNs] really difficult for us because like other people talk about their daily life, but that is our daily life. And we are facing patients like all the time. And that is our topic. We want to discuss the cases either for academic use or just release our emotion.'

Tung-Hsu, male, year 4, medical student, Taiwan

Having outlined key issues concerning e-professionalism from the perspective of healthcare regulators' codes of conduct and current research, we now take a step back to attempt an understanding of why some people behave the way they do online: ways they would consider to be unthinkable in a face-to-face environment. The impact that OSNs have on our lives is much debated. We can think of OSNs, and the apparatus that connects us, as mediating communication tools between others and ourselves. But what motivates us to use these tools in the first place? What mediating factors – in terms of specific platform attributes or social processes – do they facilitate? And what do we get back from engaging with OSNs that facilitates further engagement (or disengagement)? It is important that we think about these issues to understand what is *really* happening psychologically, socially and technologically as we interact via OSNs in order to understand why e-professionalism lapses might occur.

There is a range of personal and social factors that motivate people to engage with OSNs. From an individual perspective, OSN use can be seen as meeting our needs around interpersonal/intergroup relations (e.g. to feel part of a family or group) and knowledge/creativity. Consider Tung-Hsu's narrative at the beginning of this chapter where he talks about his needs for academic engagement and personal support when interacting via OSNs. In terms of how these needs might be met, there are a number of different factors that interact (see Box 10.6 for an overview of the psychological, social and technological factors discussed below).

First, we are motivated to present ourselves to others in a favourable light to gain acceptance and affection.[59] We continually give off conscious and unconscious messages as we disclose aspects of who we are (or who we want to be). Via OSNs we create expressions of our *self* through pictures, video and text, displaying our clothes, our language, our entertainment preferences and even the food we eat. We also engage in verbal self-disclosure as we tell people, even strangers, our innermost thoughts and feelings. Such self-disclosure is thought to foster reciprocal disclosure by others and ultimately feelings of friendship.[60] Some of us disclose a lot, others very little. For example, some of us are more sociable, agreeable and less volatile than others (see the *Big 5* in Box 10.6). Whether these really are stable traits or different states that fluctuate across time and situation is debatable. The point is, we all recognize that we have different preferences for interacting in particular situations.

Face-to-face communication is faster and easier than online communication as it represents a *high social presence*, with rich verbal and non-verbal cues and immediate feedback, enabling the reduction of ambiguous messages and unintended meanings. When someone is *perceived* as being present, we can better understand their characteristics, qualities and inner feelings and therefore interaction is often smoother. Online interaction is mediated via technology, so is asynchronous, often with low social presence.[61] Furthermore, online, the other(s) are *many* (not just one) and interactions can become confused. This produces a feeling known as *deindividuation* (loss of self-awareness).[61] When this occurs we might treat our audience as an homogenous group, with similar values and thoughts to ourselves. This loss of self-awareness can also lead us to communicate in a *hyperpersonal* manner, often increasing our level of self-disclosure. OSN platforms differ in the amount and swiftness of feedback that interacts with aspects such as deindividuation and willingness to self-disclose (e.g. Twitter vs. Facebook). There is also a tendency to believe that *information overload* online results in very few people attending to our disclosures, making us less guarded in what we say.[62] Further, the absence of authority figures in the online environment and the facilitation of equality, also contributes to our lack of inhibition online.[61] In short, online behaviour depends on a complex interaction between individual needs, desires and personalities, the degree to which specific media supports a feeling of social presence, along with our psychological responses to this and beliefs about the online world (see Box 10.6. for a summary).

Box 10.6 Information: some psychological, social and technological factors in OSN use

Psychological/social factors

Self-presentation: we are motivated to manage others' impressions of ourselves driven by individual goals (e.g. the need to be liked, to bolster or maintain self-esteem).[59]

Self-disclosure: self-presentation is achieved through self-disclosure: our revelation – consciously or unconsciously – of intimate thoughts, emotions and personal preferences consistent with how we wish others to see us. Reciprocal self-disclosure creates a *climate of trust*, even between strangers. We have conflict between self-disclosure and privacy: the *privacy paradox*.[63]

Big-5 personality traits: *openness to experience*: imagination, curiosity, aesthetics, emotional sensitivity and tolerance; *conscientiousness*: organized versus spontaneous approach; *extraversion*: seeks stimulation in the external world, company of others, and expresses positive emotions; *agreeableness*: extent of focus on maintaining positive social relations; *neuroticism*: level of emotional stability.

- High neuroticism: greater OSN use, more general self-disclosure, emotional disclosure (e.g. venting and personal dramas), and self-presentation.[64,65]
- High extraversion: high OSN use to communicate/socialize, high number of friends, high faux pas (e.g. lapses).[64,66]
- High agreeableness: high levels of interaction to communicate and connect, low attention-seeking, low faux pas.[64,67]
- High conscientiousness: high number of 'friends', low attention-seeking, low faux pas [64,66,67]

Uses and gratifications: social media use is directed towards 'need gratification' according to five goals:[68] education/information, identification with others, entertainment, social interaction enrichment and escapism.

Technological factors

Social presence: OSNs represent a low-social presence situation due to the asynchronous nature of communication and an absence of the 'other' in the physical presence (a kind of invisibility).[61]

Anonymity: online people can manipulate and change or choose not to reveal their identity and this can lead to a lack of inhibition.[61]

Media richness: media facilitates differing amounts of information – immediacy of feedback, number of cues, potential for natural language and personalization. Our goal when communicating is uncertainty reduction. Some media are more effective than others in facilitating this (e.g. Skype versus Snapchat).[69]

Interactions between psychological and technological factors

Deindividuation: visual anonymity leads to loss of awareness of our own and others' individuality. When this occurs, there is an illusion of communicating with like-thinking people.[69]

Solipsistic introjection: the sense that our mind has merged with that of another (e.g. the person we are communicating with online). Without the nuances of face-to-face interactions we fill in the gaps of who the other is, often mixing fantasy with reality and holding imagined text-like conversations in our minds with the 'other'.[61]

Hyperpersonal: when communicating online, greater levels of self-disclosure and more personal questions are asked of others than in face-to-face discussions.[69]

Dissociative imagination: the process of disassociating oneself from our online persona during our offline life: any indiscretions or faux pas are put aside as if another person committed them.[61]

What are the Regulatory Recommendations for the Prevention and Management of E-professionalism Lapses?

Having considered the psychological, social and technological issues around why we behave the way we do online, we now consider the 'dos and don'ts' approach to prevention and management of e-professionalism lapses as adopted by healthcare regulators and education providers. It is also worth noting that increasingly more and more universities are developing their own regulations regarding appropriate online behaviour and we encourage you to explore yours.

Maintaining Patient Confidentiality, Privacy and Dignity

To maintain patient confidentiality, it has been specified that no patient-related images, information or comments should be posted on OSNs.[28,30] In the case of anonymous patient-case discussions via OSNs for education or to highlight best practice, patients must be informed and provide their consent (acknowledged online), the sum of online information must not identify them and pseudonyms, referencing old cases or changing a few irrelevant facts is deemed insufficient.[12,28,31,32,42,43]

Boundary-crossing

In terms of boundary violations, precautionary actions, such as removing pictures, postings, tags, increasing security settings and even entirely deleting OSN personal profiles are often recommended.[13,70] However, these precautions can sometimes be ineffective for a variety of reasons. For example, although avoiding the acceptance of 'friend' requests from patients is the recommended advice to avoid boundary violations,[29–31,42,43] we believe that even greater caution should be taken. Be careful who you friend: a survey of 721 million Facebook users found that 92% of them were connected by only four degrees of separation,[71] meaning that you are connected to everyone else by only four other people. A friend of your friend could be your patient, employer or future employer.[27] Furthermore, with posts being freely shared between friends, images and text travel fast and cannot be easily deleted.

Honesty and Transparency

In terms of honesty and transparency, when offering general medical advice – such as participating in discussion boards or commenting on websites – identifying yourself as a healthcare practitioner (or student), your name, credentials and who you are representing is commonly seen as 'best practice'.[12,22,31,43]

Raising Concerns

The issue of raising concerns has been highlighted as another way of preventing or managing e-professionalism lapses.[28–31] Essentially, if a healthcare professional colleague is harming their own reputation via OSNs, then you should politely let them know, but if they are breaching patient confidentiality or privacy, then most policy recommendations specify that they should be reported.[28–31]

Chapter Summary

In this chapter we have examined the use of online social networks (OSNs) by health-care students and professionals. Having briefly acknowledged positive ways of engaging with OSNs (e.g. education), we have mainly focused on challenging issues around e-professionalism in an attempt to understand what the issues are, why they occur and ways of preventing them. We have learnt that healthcare professionals and students commit a range of e-professionalism lapses via OSNs around issues such as: maintaining confidentiality, privacy and dignity, boundary-crossing (including friending patients, posting sexualized images, alcohol use and profanity), lack of respect for others and maintaining honesty and transparency. We have also seen how a moment of rashness, can have a rippled effect, affecting: individuals (e.g. deregistration, job losses, being removed from the course, temporary suspension, would-be employers vetting them); institutions (e.g. damaged reputations, legal actions), interpersonal relationships (e.g. specific therapeutic relationships) and the profession as a whole (e.g. loss of trust).

We have tried to understand why people sometimes commit certain acts of indiscretion online: things they would never consider doing in a face-to-face environment. As such we have learned that there are various psychological, social and technological factors that interact that enable these lapses to occur more readily in this context. Finally, we have considered a range of *dos and don'ts* that various healthcare regulatory bodies stipulate in order for us to regulate and prevent e-professionalism lapses. The key take-home messages from this chapter are summarized in Box 10.7, with suggestions for small group discussions in Box 10.8 and chapter learning activites in Box 10.9. Finally, Box 10.10 outlines some recommended reading.

Box 10.7 Chapter summary points

- E-professionalism relates to the same dimensions as professionalism but within an online environment
- Common lapses include boundary crossing, confidentiality and privacy breaches, lack of respect, honesty and transparency, and the issue of raising concerns
- The relative anonymity that OSNs afford, means certain personal characteristics and beliefs can impact on the likelihood of someone committing e-professionalism lapses
- By understanding why e-professionalism lapses occur, along with heeding to the recommended *dos and don'ts*, we might mitigate and even avoid committing e-professionalism lapses

---

Box 10.8 Chapter discussion points

Think about your most-memorable e-professionalism lapse and about what you have learnt in this chapter:

- Would this have occurred in a face-to-face environment?
- Can this be explained in terms of the psychological, social and technological issues highlighted above?
- Would knowledge of the recommendations by healthcare regulators have prevented this from occurring?

Box 10.9 Chapter learning activities

Thinking about OSN use:

- Where are the private spaces? Can these really be protected?
- Is it ethical for future employers to judge prospective employees on social media posts when others may not use it? Hence, you are not comparing people evenly.
- Is it ethical to judge someone's social media persona if that person took steps to keep it private? So, perhaps someone with access to it shared it with others who normally wouldn't have access to it.
- What about your identity? Would it ever be appropriate to use a pseudonym online?

Take a look at the range of YouTube videos below with varying levels of anonymity:

- How appropriate are these to have online?
- How identifiable are people?
- What, if any, repercussions might these have at the level of the individual, interpersonal, institutional and profession?

Medicine: https://www.youtube.com/watch?v=61carCsPOsc
Dentistry: https://www.youtube.com/watch?v=-sATYhkz2jU
Physiotherapy: https://www.youtube.com/watch?v=BlQha5yRAas
Pharmacy: https://www.youtube.com/watch?v=3Cvv5uFbjfM
Nursing: https://www.youtube.com/watch?v=GxCR9mLMEjQ

Box 10.10 Chapter recommended reading

An example of professional use of social media:

http://www.justice.vic.gov.au/utility/social+media/social+media+policy
Video for staff of the Department of Justice (Victoria, Australia) explaining the key elements of their social media policy

https://www.ncsbn.org/347.htm
Video from the National Council of State Boards of Nursing (USA) in which the key points of their guidelines are summarized with narratives of potential scenarios of inappropriate social media use

Excellent medical blog: http://www.kevinmd.com/blog/

References

1 Balachander K, Graham C. Key differences between Web 1.0 and Web 2.0. *First Monday* 2008;13, http://firstmonday.org/article/view/2125/1972 (Accessed 2 December 2016).
2 Kaplan AM, Haenlein M. Users of the world, unite! The challenges and opportunities of Social Media. *Business Horizons* 2010;53:59–68.

3 DMR. http://expandedramblings.com/index.php/resource-how-many-people-use-the-top-social-media/ (Accessed 2 December 2016).

4 Pew Research Center. *Social Media Usage: 2005–2015*. 2015, http://www.pewinternet.org/2015/10/08/social-networking-usage-2005-2015/ (Accessed 2 December 2016).

5 Brown C, Czerniewicz L. Debunking the 'digital native': beyond digital apartheid, towards digital democracy. *Journal of Computer Assisted Learning* 2010;26:357–369.

6 Cheston CCMD, Flickinger TEMDMPH, Chisolm MSMD. Social media use in medical education: a systematic review. *Academic Medicine* 2013;88:893–901.

7 Platt A. Teaching medicine to millennials. *Journal of the Physician Assistant Education Association* 2010;21:42–44.

8 McLoughlin C, Lee MJW. Personalised and self regulated learning in the Web 2.0 era: international exemplars of innovative pedagogy using social software. *Australasian Journal of Educational Technology* 2010;26:28–43.

9 Adams A, Anderson E, McCormack M. Establishing and challenging masculinity: the influence of gendered discourses in organized sport. *Journal of Language and Social Psychology* 2010;29:278–300.

10 Greysen SR, Chretien KC, Kind T, Young A, Gross CP. Physician violations of online professionalism and disciplinary actions: a national survey of state medical boards. *Journal of the American Medical Association* 2012;307:1141–1142.

11 White J, Kirwan P, Lai K, Walton J, Ross S. 'Have you seen what is on Facebook?' The use of social networking software by healthcare professions students. *British Medical Journal Open* 2013;3:e003013 doi:10.1136/bmjopen-2013-003013.

12 Federation of State Medical Boards. Model Guidelines for the Appropriate Use of Social Media and Social Networking in Medical Practice. https://www.fsmb.org/Media/Default/PDF/FSMB/Advocacy/pub-social-media-guidelines.pdf (Accessed 2 December 2016).

13 Chretien KC, Goldman EF, Beckman L, Kind T. It's your own risk: medical students' perspectives on online professionalism. *Academic Medicine* 2010;85(10) Supplement: S2068–S2071.

14 Cain J, Romanelli F. E-professionalism: a new paradigm for a digital age. *Currents in Pharmacy Teaching and Learning* 2009;1:66–70.

15 Donath J. Signals in social supernets. *Journal of Computer Mediated Communication* 2008;13:231–251.

16 van Dijk J. *The Culture of Connectivity: a Critical History of Social Media*. Oxford: Oxford University Press, 2013.

17 Jain A, Petty EM, Jaber RM, Tackett S, Purkiss J, Fitzgerald J, *et al*. What is appropriate to post on social media? Ratings from students, faculty members and the public. *Medical Education* 2014;48:157–169.

18 Henderson J. Dalhousie dentistry school's Facebook scandal has cost $650 K. CBC News 2015. http://www.cbc.ca/news/canada/nova-scotia/dalhousie-dentistry-school-s-facebook-scandal-has-cost-650k-1.3187543 (Accessed 2 December 2016).

19 Kennedy I. *Learning from Bristol: the Report of the Public Inquiry Into Children's Heart Surgery at the Bristol Royal Infirmary 1984–1995*. Bristol Royal Infirmary Inquiry, 2001.

20 Baker R. Implications of Harold Shipman for general practice. *Postgraduate Medical Journal* 2004;80:303–306.

21 Neville P, Waylen A. Social media and dentistry: some reflections on e-professionalism. *British Dental Journal* 2015;218:475–478.

22 American Society of Health-System Pharmacists. ASHP statement on use of social media by pharmacy professionals: developed through the ASHP pharmacy student forum and the ASHP section of pharmacy informatics and technology and approved by the ASHP Board of Directors on April 13, 2012, and by the ASHP House of Delegates on June 10, 2012. *American Journal of Health-System Pharmacy.* 2012;69:2095–2097.

23 Farnan JM, Paro JA, Higa JT, Reddy ST, Humphrey HJ, Arora VM. Commentary: the relationship status of digital media and professionalism: it's complicated. *Academic Medicine* 2009;84:1479–1481.

24 General Medical Council. Doctors' use of social media. http://www.gmc-uk.org/Doctors__ use_of_social_media.pdf_51448306.pdf (Accessed 2 December 2016).

25 Gholami-Kordkheili F, Wild V, Strech D. The impact of social media on medical professionalism: a systematic qualitative review of challenges and opportunities. *Journal of Medical Internet Research* 2013;15:e184.

26 Osman A, Wardle A, Caesar R. Online professionalism and Facebook – falling through the generation gap. *Medical Teacher* 2012;34:e549–556.

27 Cain J, Scott DR, Tiemeier AM, Akers P, Metzger AH. Social media use by pharmacy faculty: student friending, e-professionalism, and professional use. *Currents in Pharmacy Teaching and Learning* 2013;5:2–8.

28 National Council of State Boards of Nursing. A *Nurse's Guide to the Use of Social Media.* https://www.ncsbn.org/NCSBN_SocialMedia.pdf (Accessed 2 December 2016).

29 Australian Medical Association Council of Doctors-in-Training, New Zealand Medical Association Doctors-in-Training Council, New Zealand Medical Students' Association, Association. AMS. *Social Media and the Medical Profession: a Guide to Online Professionalism for Medical Practitioners and Medical Students.* https://ama.com.au/sites/ default/files/Social_Media_and_the_Medical_Profession_FINAL.pdf (Accessed 2 December 2016).

30 General Dental Council. *Guidance on Using Social Media.* http://www.gdc-uk.org/ Dentalprofessionals/Standards/Documents/Guidance%20on%20using%20social% 20media.pdf (Accessed 2 December 2016).

31 Nursing and Midwifery Council. *Guidance on Using Social Media Responsibly.* In Nursing and Midwifery Council (Ed.) https://www.nmc.org.uk/globalassets/sitedocuments/nmc-publications/social-media-guidance.pdf (Accessed 2 December 2016).

32 Canadian Federation of Medical Students. *CFMS Guide to Medical Professionalism: Recommendations For Social Media.* http://www.cfms.org/files/internal-policy-bylaws/ CFMS%20Guide%20to%20Social%20Media%20Professionalism.pdf (Accessed 2 December 2016).

33 General Medical Council. *Making and Using Visual and Audio Recordings of Patients: Contents.* http://www.gmc-uk.org/Making_and_using_visual_and_audio_recordings_of_ patients_2011.pdf_40338254.pdf (Accessed 2 December 2016).

34 Chretien KC, Greysen SR, Chretien JP, Kind T. Online posting of unprofessional content by medical students. *Journal of the American Medical Association* 2009;302:1309–1315.

35 MacDonald J, Sohn S, Ellis P. Privacy, professionalism and Facebook: a dilemma for young doctors. *Medical Education* 2010;44:805–813.

36 Nyangeni T, Du Rand S, Van Rooyen D. Perceptions of nursing students regarding responsible use of social media in the Eastern Cape. *Curationis* 2015;38:E1–9.

37 Kjos AL, Ricci DG. Pharmacy student professionalism and the internet. *Currents in Pharmacy Teaching and Learning* 2012;4:92–101.

38 Henry RK, Molnar AL. Examination of social networking professionalism among dental and dental hygiene students. *Journal of Dental Education* 2013;77:1425–1430.

39 Thompson LA, Dawson K, Ferdig R, Black EW, Boyer J, Coutts J, *et al*. The intersection of online social networking with medical professionalism. *Journal of General Internal Medicine* 2008;23:954–957.

40 Palacios-González C. The ethics of clinical photography and social media. *Medicine, Health Care and Philosophy* 2015;18:63–70.

41 Peterson M. *At Personal Risk: Boundary Violations in Professional-client Relationships*. New York: WW Norton & Co, 1992.

42 Royal College of Nursing Australia. Social Media Guidelines for Nurses. http://www.ota.org.au/data/Documents/SocialMediaRCNA.pdf (Accessed 2 December 2016).

43 Canadian Physiotherapy Association. Social Media Guidelines. https://physiotherapy.ca/social-media-guidelines (Accessed 2 December 2016).

44 Walton J. What's on YOUR Facebook profile? Evaluation of an educational intervention to promote appropriate use of privacy settings by medical students on social networking sites. Medical Education Online 2015; 20: 10.3402/meo.v20.28708.

45 Clauson KA, Ekins J, Goncz CE. Use of blogs by pharmacists. *Journal of the American Society of Health-System Pharmacists* 2010;67:2043–2048.

46 Qureshi Z, Mason K. Cyberbullying: the impact on trainee doctors. *Clinical Teacher* 2015;12:214–217.

47 Farley S, Coyne I, Sprigg C, Axtell C, Subramanian G. Exploring the impact of workplace cyberbullying on trainee doctors. *Medical Education* 2015;49:436–443.

48 Boroff D. Portland nursing assistant sent to jail after posting dying patient's buttocks on Facebook, 2012, http://www.nydailynews.com/news/national/portland-nursing-assistant-jail-posting-dying-patient-buttocks-facebook-article-1.1035207 (Accessed 2 November 2016).

49 Wyke T. Young medical student could be kicked off her course after she took a selfie of herself smiling next to a seriously ill woman in Mexico, 2015, http://www.dailymail.co.uk/news/article-3192508/Young-medical-student-kicked-course-took-selfie-smiling-seriously-ill-woman-Mexico.html (Accessed 2 December 2016).

50 Beckford M. Online medics reveal secret names for patients and colleagues. *Telegraph* 17 September 2011, http://www.telegraph.co.uk/news/health/news/8768876/Online-medics-reveal-secret-names-for-patients-and-colleagues.html (Accessed 2 December 2016).

51 Szabo A, Underwood J. Cybercheats: is information and communication technology fuelling academic dishonesty? *Active Learning in Higher Education* 2004;5:180–199.

52 American Society of Registered Nurses. When Facebook goes to the hospital, patients may suffer, 2010, http://www.asrn.org/journal-nursing/786-when-facebook-goes-to-the-hospital-patients-may-suffer.html (Accessed 2 December 2016).

53 Cain J. Online social networking issues within academia and pharmacy education. *American Journal of Pharmaceutical Education* 2008;72:10.

54 Greysen SR, Kind T, Chretien KC. Online professionalism and the mirror of social media. *The Journal of General Internal Medicine* 2010;25:1227–1229.

55 Ziring D, Danoff D, Grosseman S, Langer D, Esposito A, Jan MK, *et al*. How do medical schools identify and remediate professionalism lapses in medical students? A study of US and Canadian medical schools. *Academic Medicine* 2015;90:913–920.

56 CTV News. Dalhousie University announces more penalties for dentistry students, 2015, http://www.ctvnews.ca/canada/dalhousie-university-announces-more-penalties-for-dentistry-students-1.2180907 (Accessed 2 December 2016).

57 Bohnert D, Ross WH. The influence of social networking websites on the evaluation of job candidates. *Cyberpsychology, Behavior and Social Networking* 2010;13:341–347.

58 Weathington BL, Bechtel AR. Alternative sources of information and the selection decision making process. *Journal of Behavioral and Applied Management* 2012;13:108–120.

59 Goffman E. *The Presentation of Self in Everyday Life*. London: Penguin, 1990.

60 Sprecher S, Treger S, Wondra JD, Hilaire N, Wallpe K. Taking turns: reciprocal self-disclosure promotes liking in initial interactions. *Journal of Experimental Social Psychology* 2013;49:860–866.

61 Suler J. The online disinhibition effect. *Cyberpsychology and Behavior* 2004;7:321–326.

62 Moll R, Pieschl S, Bromme R. Trust into collective privacy? The role of subjective theories for self-disclosure in online communication. *Societies* 2014;4:770.

63 Taddicken M. The 'Privacy Paradox' in the social web: the impact of privacy concerns, individual characteristics, and the perceived social relevance on different forms of self-disclosure. *Journal of Computer-Mediated Communication* 2014;19:248–273.

64 Seidman G. Self-presentation and belonging on Facebook: how personality influences social media use and motivations. *Personality and Individual Differences* 2013;54:402–407.

65 Correa T, Hinsley AW, Zúñiga HGd. Who interacts on the Web?: The intersection of users' personality and social media use. *Human Behavior in Computers* 2010;26:247–253.

66 Amichai-Hamburger Y, Vinitzky G. Social network use and personality. *Human Behavior in Computers* 2010;26:1289–1295.

67 Stoughton JW, Thompson LF, Meade AW. Big Five personality traits reflected in job applicants' social media postings. *Cyberpsychology, Behavior, and Social Networking* 2013;16:800–805.

68 McQuail D. *Mass Communication Theory: an Introduction*. London: Sage Publications, 2010.

69 Walther JB. Computer-mediated communication: impersonal, interpersonal, and hyperpersonal interaction. *Communication Research* 1996;23:3–43.

70 Strausburg MB, Djuricich AMMD, Carlos WGMD, Bosslet GTMD. The influence of the residency application process on the online social networking behavior of medical students: a single institutional study. *Academic Medicine* 2013;88:1707–1712.

71 Backstrom L, Boldi P, Rosa M, Ugander J, Vigna S. Four degrees of separation. *Proceedings of the 4th Annual ACM Web Science Conference*. ACM, Evanston, Illinois, 2012;33–42.

11

Professionalism Dilemmas
Across National Cultures

Co-authored by Lynn Monrouxe, Charlotte Rees,
Ming-Jung Ho and Madawa Chandratilake

I saw the patient in the palliative care center and... the patient didn't know he had cancer but the families knew. And the families, they signed the agreement for the DNR, do not resuscitate. However the patient... had clear consciousness but we cannot talk to him. We cannot talk about: "Oh you have cancer and do you want to receive DNR if you are in... danger situation"... if his disease goes to the end stage and he become like, um, coma... then his family, his son and daughter, they sign about the DNR agreement... But that doesn't make sense because we should let the patient know that he will receive the DNR. But I think in Taiwanese culture, this situation is really common, yeah.'

Chang-Chi, male, year 7, medical student, Taiwan

LEARNING OBJECTIVES

- To explore what culture is and how it can affect our professionalism behaviours
- To recognize that professionalism definitions and guidance are culturally bound
- To understand different dimensions of professionalism values and behaviours found across national cultures
- To discover the range of professionalism dilemmas that occur within different cultural contexts
- To appreciate the importance of looking beyond our own cultural frame of reference to understand how professionalism dilemmas might be alternatively interpreted
- To develop strategies for effectively engaging in intercultural interactions when facing professionalism dilemmas across different cultural contexts

---

KEY TERMS

Cultural dimensions
Cultural and intercultural competence
Intercultural professionalism dilemmas
International health electives

Healthcare Professionalism: Improving Practice through Reflections on Workplace Dilemmas, First Edition.
Lynn V. Monrouxe and Charlotte E. Rees.
© 2017 John Wiley & Sons Ltd. Published 2017 by John Wiley & Sons Ltd.

Introduction

We all live, learn and work within our own cultural spaces, comprising shared rituals, social scenarios and everyday practices. To an ever-increasing degree, healthcare students' and professionals' work involves interaction and cooperation with patients and other healthcare practitioners whose cultural backgrounds differ from their own. Furthermore, international health electives, often in developing countries, are common within healthcare students' curricula. Thus, cultural difference is everywhere. But what do we mean by culture and what does this mean to you as you learn or teach within the healthcare workplace? This chapter is concerned with developing an understanding of different cultural approaches to professionalism. In doing so, at times it might seem like we are simplifying the complexity of culture, running the risk of *thinking nationally* or making statements about any specific grouping. As such we would like to acknowledge from the start that we believe that differences *within* country cultures may occasionally be greater than differences *between* country cultures and so would like to guard against classifying and stereotyping individuals. Indeed, consider Chang-Chi's narrative that opens this chapter. His own cultural perspective differs to that of others within his own country setting. It is for this reason that we specifically draw upon the notion of inter-cultural capability[1] in this chapter as we explore how different cultures are thought to encompass a set of inter-related dimensions that might be similar or different to other cultures. We also consider the concept of different cultural spaces, and the different types of professionalism dilemmas that might occur within them. Finally, we consider how situations might be culturally interpreted as we explore some of the intercultural dilemmas experienced by Western students during their international health electives.

What is Culture?

Culture has been defined as: 'the total range of activities and ideas of a group of people with shared traditions, which are transmitted and reinforced by members of the group' (http://www.collinsdictionary.com/dictionary/english/culture). So, culture is created in institutions (families, religion, our governments and so on) through which we are social-ized. Culture is maintained within and across those institutions by way of role models and explicit or implicit rules that limit what we can and cannot do, defining opportuni-ties and fostering our patterns of interaction.[2] Cultural values and practices are primar-ily derived from the larger philosophical bases within which different people live. And culture is dynamic rather than static. Within any culture, new ideas, discoveries and experiences with other cultures create change. For example, and focusing more specifi-cally on the issue of national culture, culture has been further defined as: 'shared beliefs, attitudes, norms, roles, and values found among speakers of a particular language who live during the same historical period in a specified geographic region.'[3, p. 6] So, culture includes the *values* (how we should do things) and *practices* (how things are done) in the *here and now*. Culture also includes our internal psychological functioning in terms of our independence from or interdependence with others. Finally, it is culture that gives us a sense of identity – both individual and group identities – as it provides us with a sense of *belonging* and a moral compass that guides us towards 'right' ways of thinking and behaving, ways which differ across cultures.

Practices therefore arise from the interaction between values from the different cultures we are exposed to. Although each and every one of us develops our own set of values as we interpret explicit/implicit messages around us, there is also a set of typical values that can be associated with specific cultures. Furthermore, we are not always aware of our own cultural worldviews. Much of what we learn about the nature of the world remains invisible: like a *cultural iceberg*, with our visible behaviours often being mere reflections of what lies beneath.[4] As such, only a small proportion of our values are manifested as practices. To add another layer of complexity to the issue of culture, the values, beliefs and attitudes that lie beneath our visible behaviours can sometimes contradict one another. Rather than being a coherent set, our internalized culture has been described as *a loose network* of knowledge, categorically structured, along with a set of implicit theories about the world.[5, p. 710] This is because, as we go through life, we experience many different institutional settings that do not always convey the same cultural messages (see Chapter 3 earlier, where we talk about the hidden curriculum). So, we can think of ourselves as possessing a *cultural repertoire*, comprising different ways of interpreting the world, from which we can construct various strategies for acting, depending upon the contextual nuances of any given situation.[6] This concept of cultural repertoire is important, and we will refer to this throughout this chapter; by thinking of ourselves in this way we can see how our collection of cultural understandings can be expanded to enable us to deal more effectively when encountering *inter*cultural professionalism dilemmas. Having provided a brief overview of what culture is, we now consider different types of culture: the range of values individuals possess and how individuals understand and behave in the social world.

What Different Cultural Dimensions are there?

Although stereotyping of others should be avoided (Box 11.1), it is useful for us to have an understanding of the common, reasonably stable, characteristics and values across different cultures. Through this understanding we might better recognize how these affect our own values and practices (so which ones are present in our cultural repertoire) and how they might impact on those of others around us (as part of their cultural repertoires). In order to provide some insight into these factors, in Box 11.2 we present Maleki and de Jong's[7] nine (overlapping) *clusters* of cultural dimensions developed from a synthesis of around 30 years of research in this area (see further reading at the end of this chapter).

Box 11.1 Information: ethnocentrism and stereotyping

Ethnocentrism: the imposition of your own cultural values and beliefs onto others, often devaluing the culture of the 'other'. Your own worldview is seen as *the* 'right' way: anything else is deemed invalid or incorrect.

Stereotyping: reducing groups of people to a set of core characteristics or *types* rather than viewing individuals as possessing a range of unique and personal characteristics. Stereotypes can be positive or negative, but by overlooking the complexity of human beings, they are neither true nor false.

Box 11.2 Information: nine clusters of cultural dimensions (Maleki and de Jong[7])

1. Individualism vs. collectivism

Focuses on the interrelatedness between individuals, such as whether they have autonomy and are judged by *what they do*, as in individually achieved attributes (so individualism) or are instead embedded within a group and are judged by *who they are*, as in ascribed relational attributes (so collectivism). This also relates to the degree to which meaning within interactions is inferred from the settings in which communication occurs (high-context) or from the words themselves (low-context).

2. Power distance

Characterizes *acceptable* hierarchical relations and therefore the distribution of power between, for example, leaders and followers. So, the power distance between leaders and followers in egalitarian relationships would be accepted less than the power distance in hierarchical relationships.

3. Uncertainty avoidance

Focuses on the extent to which people feel uncomfortable with situations that are uncertain, unknown or unstructured. So, uncertainty-avoidant cultures typically like rules, future-planning and performance orientation.

4. Mastery vs. harmony

Highlights the degrees of competitiveness, achievement and self-assertion vs. the striving for consensus, equity and harmony. This includes an element of external (mastery) vs. internal (harmony) control.

5. Traditionalism vs. secularism

Comprises aspects of religiosity, humanity and a temporal focus on the past (as in traditionalism) as opposed to a secular orientation and flexibility.

6. Indulgence vs. restraint

Focuses on the extent to which the gratification of one's desires and feelings are free and people express emotions openly (indulgence) or such gratification is restrained and people control such emotional expression (restraint).

7. Assertiveness vs. tenderness

Considers the extent to which one is assertive/aggressive versus kind and tender in both social relationships and communication styles.

8. Gender egalitarianism

Focuses on gender equality, which is typically expected in individualistic cultures with low power distance. However, there are still some modern societies today with strong gendered role divisions and therefore greater power distance between men and women.

9. Collaborativeness

Encompasses the extent to which teamwork is valued within a culture, with cultures either focusing on individual goals or precedence of group acceptance, loyalty and group interest. This dimension, however, differs from the *individualism vs. collectivism* dimension above in that there are individualistic cultures which are high in teamworking (e.g. Nordic countries) and collectivistic cultures in which teamworking is not prioritized (e.g. Iran, Colombia).

Box 11.3 Stop and do: reflecting on your own intercultural encounters

Think about a recent or 'most memorable' situation when you felt as if another person you were with held different values to your own?

Thinking about that time, can you identify which of Maleki and de Jong's[7] cultural dimensions might be relevant to describe these differences?

How did the differences manifest themselves during the event?

Identify which dimensions reside within your own cultural values and behaviours. What contradictions (if any) do you have and why?

So, as you go through your daily activities of working with patients and healthcare practitioners, there are a number of key issues about cultures that you can reflect on. For example, consider the opening narrative from Chang-Chi, a Taiwanese medical student who talks about a dilemma he experienced when a patient he was attending had not been consulted about his DNR status. Here, we see an intersection between the culture of the younger student – learning medical education in Taiwan drawing on a Western biomedical culture (including the cultural dimension of individualism); and living alongside younger/urbanite Taiwanese friends who, as a whole, are ever-increasingly influenced by Western values – and the older patient (and his family) whose culture has been strongly influenced by Eastern cultural dimensions of collectivism in which the patient is fully embedded within his family and the group is the primary unit. This situation occurs despite both the student and the patient growing up and living in the same country. It is this intersection of differing cultures, along with the context in which the situation occurs (a Taiwanese hospital), that creates the professionalism dilemma for this young student. In addition, Chang-Chi's dilemma demonstrates some of the complexities of culture: it not being fixed in time or place. And it is within this very complexity that you (as a healthcare student or practitioner) are learning and working. Box 11.3 guides you through some reflective questions about your own intercultural experiences.

What are *Eastern* and *Western* Cultural Spaces?

It is important to understand that *East* is not synonymous with Asia; rather it is a central part of it. Although Eastern societies are extremely geographically, politically and economically spread, they largely share similar cultural values and philosophies and there are clear differences between Eastern and Western institutions, philosophies and cultural values. So although the issue is complex, it can be useful to consider cultural orientations as *cultural spaces*. Such cultural spaces include how people perceive and behave in the world they live in: both individually and collectively. Taking a collective approach to considering cultural spaces, we begin by considering three different, and often interrelated, cultural patterns across Eastern and Western cultural spaces: Individualism vs. collectivism, high- vs. low-context communication and hierarchy vs. equality. Again, we acknowledge the general nature of this discussion and our omissions of the cultural nuances within and across these cultural spaces (so are mindful of the risk of stereotyping). Nevertheless, an understanding of some of the issues can contribute to the development of your own intercultural competence. Indeed, the development of cultural competence is the first step to developing cultural and intercultural capability.[8]

Individualism vs. Collectivism

Arguably, one of the keenest differences across the East-West dichotomy that influences many other cultural dimensions, is the Eastern emphasis on collectivism in contrast to the Western emphasis on individualism.[7, 9–10] Indeed, the influence from Eastern countries is thought to stem from Confucianism and the values of *reciprocity* and *proper social relationships*.[11] It is essentially a culture of ethics. Over thousands of years an East Asian political and cultural value system has been influenced by Confucianism, having such a profound effect that it was adopted by many of the Chinese dynasties, the Yi dynasty in Korea and the Tokugawa shogunate in Japan.[12] Confucianism is a philosophy of human nature. It considers human relationships and motivation to be the basis of society across a number of interrelated principles of correct conduct including (in Mandarin using traditional/simplified characters where they differ, Pinyin and English): 仁 (*rén*: humanism) and 義/义 (*yì*: faithfulness, loyalty or justice), which comprise the ethical system; along with 禮/礼 (*lǐ*: propriety, rite, respect for social etiquette), 恕 (*shu*: reciprocity or empathy) and 智 (*zhì*: wisdom/liberal education); see Box 11.4 for further description.[12]

Box 11.4 Information: some of the interrelated principles of Confucianism philosophy (Mandarin, Pinyin and English explanations)

仁, *Rén*: the fundamental principal, summing up the core of Confucianism, it essentially means warm human feelings among people. *Rén* is like the seed from which all the ideal qualities of a person grow and which all people should aspire to possess.

義/ 义, *Yì*: the part of our nature that enables us to look beyond the self and our immediate gains, and towards the benefit of the common good.

禮/ 礼, *Lǐ*: being deferent to others and reserved, so follows from *Rén*. *Lǐ* includes acting with propriety, following etiquette and tradition. *Lǐ* is the 'social glue'.

恕, *Shù*: the embodiment of *rén* is related to *shù* (reciprocity). It is closely linked with empathy (understanding others).

智, *Zhì*: moral wisdom; knowing what is 'right' and 'wrong'. It is a process comprising *hsüeh* (what is learned) and *ssu* (critical thinking/reflection). A balance of each is required for moral wisdom.

Box 11.5 'Why can't you call me *aiya*?'

'In the Asian context… we have this brotherly and sisterly way of communication… even at the professional level using *aiya* (elder brother) and *akka* (elder sister). But I feel it's too intimate… because I myself feel very uncomfortable calling another doctor *aiya* in a ward (soft laughter) in front of patients or other doctors. Even though they have been in the faculty with us I would call the same person *aiya* or *akka* if we meet in a private setting… but I feel very uncomfortable calling *aiya* because it feels too intimate for the occasion… I had a small incident recently, I went to a ward… and there also a senior colleague of mine… and greeted him as: "Good morning doctor". Then he asked me, "Good morning what… why are you calling me doctor?"… Then I realized that he must be from our (soft laughter) faculty… He said, "Why can't you call me *aiya*?" Then I told him, "Because as a professional I think you should be called a doctor"… I didn't commit anything wrong… he got angry with me because I didn't call him *aiya*….'

Vidula, female, year 7, medical student, Sri Lanka

Related to these principles is the concept of 關係 (*guān xi*). This refers to both personal and group connections engendering trust and that people draw upon to perform a favour or a service which is then reciprocated. In the Western world the nearest equivalents are the concepts of social capital, *Gemeinschaft* and social networks, although there is a qualitative difference in Eastern societies as the group is a more central societal unit. So, for example, in Sri Lanka, as with other Eastern cultures, there is a tradition of referring to non-family members as if they are close relatives. In Sri Lanka, middle-aged people are called aunty or uncle, older people are referred to as grandmother or grandfather (*achchi* or *seeya*) and younger people as elder sister or brother and younger sister or brother (*akka*, a*iya*, *nangi* and *malli*). This kind of practice is important in maintaining harmony and a sense of collectiveness amongst people. However, although addressing people as family members is accepted in social environments, in professional settings this can be problematic as the relative appropriateness of this can be highly personal and contextual. Take a look at Vidula's narrative in Box 11.5, which will help you further to contextualize the issues discussed here. Vidula is a Sri Lankan female medical student in her final year. Her narrative concerns a dilemma she experienced whilst interacting with a slightly more senior colleague from the same faculty in which she was working. This is an interesting example as it interplays with the dimension of *hierarchy* versus *equality* (discussed later) and both people are from the same culture and faculty – so further underpins our opening assertion regarding within-cultural differences and the complexities of the issues at hand.

Unlike Eastern values, which stem from ethics, Western values emphasize: 'the dignity, indeed the sacredness, of the individual. Anything that would violate our right to think for ourselves, judge for ourselves, make our own decision, live our lives as we see fit, is not only morally wrong, it is sacrilegious.'[13, p. 142] It is easy to see how the origins of individualism have a basis in law, with its associations with liberalism and freedom: from the state, from association with others, along with freedom of speech and the right to freely participate in political life.[14] Individualism is also associated with the notion of human rights 'freedom' which are individualistically justified.[15] Thus the difference between the basis of Eastern (ethics) and Western (law) philosophies gives us a deeper understanding of core issues underlying Chang-Chi's dilemma at the start of this chapter.

Associated with these broad-brush notions of Eastern social relations and Western individualism come differences in communication style.[16] We now consider the concept of high- and low-context communication: a much-researched concept that was first introduced by the anthropologist, Edward Hall, in the 1970s, but one that is still very relevant today when we consider issues around different approaches to communication.

High-context communication vs. low-context communication

Across collectivist and individualist cultures people also differ in the way they communicate. Hall[16] identified a means through which we can effectively understand similarities and differences in perception and communication across different collective cultural spaces: cultures can be placed along a high-context/low-context continuum, and this is dependent upon the degree to which meaning is inferred from the settings in which communication occurs (high-context: HC) or from the words themselves (low-context: LC). Context has been defined as, 'the information that surrounds an event; it is inextricably bound up with the meaning of the event'.[17, p. 6] So, HC communication is one in which much of the information resides in the person, with little being explicitly transmitted as part of the message. On the other hand, communication that is LC is one in which the majority of information is verbally expressed.[16]

HC cultures are those which, because of tradition and history, change very little over time (e.g. Japan, China and Korea). In such cultural spaces, individuals are homogeneous in terms of experiences and information networks due to the strong social relations inherent in the culture: consistent messages tend to produce consistent responses, with information being conveyed through gesture, the use of space, silence and status (including age, gender, level of education, family background, title and so on). Alternatively, LC cultures are those in which the population is less homogenous (e.g. USA, Scandinavia, Germany).[16] Such a lack of common experiences necessitates more detailed background information during verbal interaction as very little is already embedded contextually.[11]

When interacting interculturally, the indirect-implicit (as in high-context) and direct-explicit (as in low-context) ways of interaction can become problematic: LC communicators might feel uncomfortable with the vagueness and ambiguity of HC communicators, and LC communicators might appear too direct by asking 'inappropriate' clarifying questions. Equally, HC communicators might feel impatient and irritated by the high-volume of 'unnecessary' information from their LC interactants, whose reliance on verbal information can make them appear less credible.[11,17] Following on from the understanding of how information can be embedded within the context, and how status is part of that context, we now consider the dimension of *hierarchy* versus *equality* and how this plays out across different individual cultural spaces, as in Vidula's narrative (Box 11.5).

Hierarchy vs. equality

Also related to individualism and collectivism is the issue of hierarchy vs. equality (which has additional links with aspects of power distance and gender egalitarianism in Box 11.2 above). So the concept of hierarchy can be understood through the Confucian saying, 'King is king; subject is subject; father is father; and son is son', with people *expected* to behave according to their social status. Even in modern day Asia, interaction is influenced by age, educational, institutional and economical levels. This includes within the extended family structure where individuals are placed in terms of their kinship (where people have certain ways of relating to equals, along with generational

---

Box 11.6 Stop and do: reflecting on Vidula's and related narratives

Discuss aspects relating to Maleki and de Jong's[7] nine clusters of cultural dimensions (Box 11.2) in terms of Vidula's narrative (Box 11.5).

Thinking about your own experiences of interacting with doctors on the wards, how might these cultural dimensions have been played out within an intercultural context and across LC-HC cultural spaces?

Consider the values of self-interest, harmony and receptiveness: how are these portrayed within Vidula's narrative?

Think of an experience you have had already that was interculturally challenging: critically reflect on this experience in terms of HC-LC communication.

---

obligations and responsibilities). This is despite the Great Cultural Revolution in China (1966–1976) during which time traditional hierarchies were challenged.[18]

Conversely, the concept of individualism is entwined with the Western value of equality: equal rights, right to vote and equal social status (within families and within other relationships where people in power appear to act as less powerful than they actually are). Although this is a value, reality is more complex: it has been acknowledged that the legal basis for social equality within Western cultures is more established than 'actual' social equality in practice,[19] with the issue of the 'old boys network' still continuing to undermine equality in the West.[20] The issue of social equality has already been discussed in detail in Chapter 9 on student abuse (in particular Box 9.1).

It is important to understand how these cultural dimensions of hierarchy and equality also translate into communication differences around assertiveness, accord and harmony. Essentially, cultures based on law tend to value and encourage assertion, whereas cultures based on ethics tend to value the subordination of self-interest in the interest of harmony and receptiveness.[21,22] Before moving onto the next section we suggest you look at the questions in Box 11.6 to further explore communication across different individual cultural spaces.

How can we Develop Cultural and Intercultural Capability?

We have now considered a few of the key ways in which people across different collective cultural spaces might interact. Understanding these issues is one way of developing your own cultural *competency* (i.e. developing your knowledge around how and why people identify with certain behaviours, language practices, beliefs, and values and what that means in terms of acting and interacting). We now turn to consider how events involving people across different individual and/or collective cultural spaces might result in professionalism dilemmas (for one or more people present). Here, the issues of cultural and intercultural *capability* are key (i.e. knowing the level of competence that is required in any given situation and developing the ability to exercise it wisely, making moral judgements in response to complex situations). The overarching aim of this section is to understand how to recognize and use cultural differences as a *resource for learning* and to develop a deeper understanding of what *effective action* might be when encountering professionalism dilemmas within and across interculturally complex situations.[1,23]

In order to understand how to act effectively and professionally when encountering intercultural dilemmas, we begin by considering the range of reactions individuals have to the issue of cultural difference, which some researchers believe comprise different stages we pass through (or become stuck within) as we develop through life.[24] We then take these a step further by outlining Friedman and Berthoin Antal's concept of *negotiating reality*:[1] this process of negotiating reality will enable you to recognize and understand intercultural professionalism dilemmas as they happen, as well as to develop effective strategies for dealing with them in the moment.

Responses to Cultural Difference

When dealing with cultural difference we can adopt a number of stances.[24] Using Chang-Chi's opening narrative around the 'unconsented DNR', we can see Bennet's six stages of cultural awareness in Box 11.7. While denial, defensive and minimizing approaches to intercultural dilemmas are inappropriate within professional interactions, acceptance, adaptation and assimilation also have their problems. The underlying assumption is that culture is an unproblematic and reasonably unitary construct. In other words, that culture affects all members in the same way. This deterministic approach to culture ignores the complexity within our cultural repertoires and how we respond to specific interactional events. It also assumes that we have full insight into our own cultural repertoire and can easily shift into other ways of thinking and behaving.[1] Another problem is that without actively exploring one another's cultural repertoires, we might end up shifting our thinking inappropriately (e.g. based on incorrect and/or stereotypical assumptions).

Box 11.7 Information: Bennett's (1998) stages of cultural awareness

Denial: Chang-Chi could have ignored (or denied) the cultural difference between himself and the patient's family concerning consent, continuing to behave as normal.

Defensive: involves organizing the world into *us* and *them*, drawing on negative stereotypes (for them) and positive stereotypes (for us): Chang-Chi was respectful when narrating his story, although he did assert the superiority of his cultural position, with the family's position being seen as inferior (ethnocentricity).

Minimizing: being unaware of his own particular culture, Chang-Chi might have interpreted the failure of other clinicians to use his style (consenting the patient for the DNR, rather than the patient's family) as a lack of professionalism, rather than as a fundamental cultural difference.

Acceptance: Chang-Chi could have accepted his own cultural viewpoint as just one of many, equally complex, worldviews, instead of asserting his way was right.

Adaptation: Chang-Chi could have adapted his worldview to incorporate facets of the family's cultural perspective, demonstrating his ability to shift his frame of reference across cultures.

Assimilation: Chang-Chi could have responded by fundamentally modifying his own cultural identity by integrating the cultural perspectives of the patient's family.

Negotiating 'Reality'

Friedman and Berthoin Antal[1] suggest a useful way for us to understand, recognize and use our cultural differences as a resource for learning within culturally complex situations, such as intercultural professionalism dilemmas, where there is no single correct solution. In doing so we can develop an intercultural capability to enable us to create new responses and to expand our own cultural repertoire for future interactions.[1] As healthcare students and professionals it is important that we learn from all of our experiences in order to develop our capability when dealing with other healthcare professionals and patients. So by actively, and without prejudice, developing an understanding of our own, and others' cultural icebergs, and how these affect our behaviours in a given context, we can generate much-needed cultural knowledge in the moment (although assimilation usually takes time). This can help facilitate and enact the appropriate next steps (rather than reacting automatically according to our hidden cultural assumptions). So this is a process of exploration and assumption-testing and a foundation, 'for learning new ways of seeing and doing something effectively with other people'.[1, p. 77]

Negotiating reality essentially entails knowing when (and how) to halt our automatic functioning and to engage in open enquiry about the reasons behind others' and our own actions.[25] In doing so, we are engaging in an exploration and visiblization of our own and others' cultural repertoires: attempting to remove the veils of culture and to critically consider different realities and move towards a *negotiated reality*. This is particularly important when dealing with intercultural professionalism dilemmas as it assumes no prior authority of one cultural interpretation over another. To achieve such an end point, an action strategy that combines high advocacy and enquiry is needed. This means jointly, and explicitly, exploring the logic of other ways of thinking whilst simultaneously being open to the inconsistencies or gaps in our own ways of thinking (see Box 11.8). Advocacy entails clearly expressing and advocating our own desired outcomes. Enquiry entails exploration and questioning around motivations for action. The combination of the two,

---

Box 11.8 Information: Friedman and Berthoin Antal's[1] advocacy-enquiry quadrant

High advocacy-high enquiry
- Clearly expressing and advocating your reasoning and intentions
- Striving to understand reasoning of others and self, encouraging all parties to question their own logic and gaps
- Internal commitment, facilitates intercultural learning

High advocacy-low enquiry
- Imposing your perspectives and reasoning on the situation
- Ignoring others' logic, intentions, perceptions and gaps
- Unlikely to result in commitment or intercultural learning

Low advocacy-high enquiry
- Suspending, denying, deferring, holding back your own reasoning, intentions and perspectives
- Exploring others' logic, intentions, perceptions and gaps
- Generates information, possible insights, but no intercultural learning

Low advocacy-low enquiry
- Hiding your own reasoning/intentions by deflecting questions ('don't you think we could...')
- 'Diplomatic' approach to pursuing your own agenda ('I quite understand your apprehension but ...')
- Feels manipulative to others, rarely generates intercultural learning

within a *high-advocacy/high-enquiry* conversational frame, facilitates learning as all parties explore these together until an equal and committed course of action is agreed upon.

So far in this chapter we have examined what culture is and where it is acquired, considered some of the different cultural dimensions underpinning values and practices (in particular, across Eastern and Western cultures), outlined some of the ways we might react in the face of intercultural professionalism dilemmas and proposed a strategy for negotiating outcomes to intercultural professionalism dilemmas. Drawing on our research conducted with healthcare students across the UK, Australia, Taiwan and Sri Lanka, we now turn to consider the different types of dilemmas they reported experiencing both 'at home' and whilst overseas during their healthcare electives.

What are the Professionalism Dilemmas Across Different Cultural Spaces?

Thinking about professionalism across different cultural spaces (Chapter 2), there are three distinct points to consider: how the same dilemma in one cultural setting might have different meanings in another cultural setting (culturally-interpreted dilemmas), how possible reactions to and actions within the same dilemma differ across cultural spaces (culturally-constrained dilemmas) and how some dilemmas seem to occur only in certain cultural spaces (culturally-specific dilemmas). We also need to consider the problem of attributing all apparent differences we see as being purely down to cultural differences, when sometimes social and economic factors are at play.[26] So bringing together our understanding of culture and of developing cultural competences and capabilities we will now consider some of the dilemmas we have found in our research across Eastern and Western cultural spaces. We will begin by identifying some of the dilemmas that can be considered to be the same types of dilemmas cross-culturally, we will then go on to look at more culturally-specific and socio-cultural dilemmas we have identified within Eastern cultural spaces, before looking specifically at intercultural dilemmas and how the model of negotiating reality can be used to develop intercultural capability in these settings.

Culturally-interpreted and Constrained Dilemmas: Same *Event*, Different *Dilemma*

Many of the professionalism dilemmas students talked about across both Eastern and Western cultural spaces appeared on the surface to be very similar in terms of the *type* of events that were discussed. Commonalities included situations concerning misrepresenting students' identities, witnessing and participating in breaches of patient safety and dignity, consent, student abuse and social media dilemmas; all of which we have previously discussed in depth across Chapters 5–10. But within these categories there were subtle differences that can only be fully understood in terms of differences across cultural spaces (as in culturally-interpreted and culturally-constrained dilemmas).

An example of culturally-interpreted dilemmas includes those attributed to hierarchy (e.g. between students and doctors, between different professional groups and between patients and doctors). We know that these are markedly different between Eastern and Western societies, with hierarchy being more accepted within Eastern cultures.[9] An example of this hierarchy between, for example, students and patients is neatly exemplified in Box 11.9 (narrative 1). Chih-Hung, a fifth-year medical student from Taiwan, tells

Box 11.9 Taiwanese and Sri Lankan and UK students' culture-related dilemma narratives

Narrative 1: 'I just sort of cry'

'I challenged my professor once just one month after I came back from [USA medical school], I challenged my professor and eventually I cry out (soft laughter). I just can't sustain my emotions there because my professor just blamed me for not respecting the tradition (soft laughter). One year ago, that made me a lot of frustration, because there was a lot of dispute between my professor and I about the history taking. My professor said that to take a history you need to be straight forward, and you need to be short like two minute to three minute. But I like to sit on the bedside and then talk to the patient and also the family. So when I start a conversation I would just say: "Oh how is everything going?" And the professor behind me just said, "Why are you saying that, that is not useful?" so they blamed me in front of the patient, so after a lot of blames I just sort of cry. Yeah that was a terrible situation.'

Chih-Hung, male, year 5, medical student, Taiwan

Narrative 2: 'within a few minutes the patient died'

'There was patient who was admitted with cardiac failure… she was deteriorating and [the consultant] asked us to connect her to a cardiac monitor and give CPR… the patient was intubated, but the ET [endotracheal] tube had inserted into the stomach. Registrar and the HO [House Officer] picked it up. But they were scared of taking it out and put it again because the consultant was so tough. And they were very scared to do it, because patient was also deteriorating. So they were keeping on giving oxygen but it was useless because tube is in the stomach. But they didn't do anything, ultimately within few minutes patient died. We were there at the incident but at that time they were trying to cover it up without telling it to the consultant.'

Sathi, female, year 7, medical student, Sri Lanka

Narrative 3: 'the patient really suffered'

'Well when I was working at pulmonary medicine, they had a patient with lung cancer and distant metastasis, and he suffered because of the swelling liver. But the family asked us not to tell him about the disease. It did make some difficulty because we could not treat him properly, we could only give him symptomatic treatment instead of surgery or chemotherapy because we have to get informed consent before we start chemotherapy… the patient really suffered when I was on duty, I could do nothing but observe. I believe they [family] were seeking some alternative treatment privately but the patient himself could not make a decision because he doesn't know about his status.'

Ren-Huei, male, year 7, medical student, Taiwan

Narrative 4: 'why you called me "Miss"?'

'In a clinic, one of the lady SHOs [Senior House Officers] wearing a skirt and a T-shirt, was consulting a very old lady. The lady has been calling the doctor "Miss" [term used by patients to call nurses]. Then the doctor scolded the patient, "Why you called me 'Miss'? I'm a doctor", very aggressively… The patient was very embarrassed and she almost cried… [A fellow doctor] said to that lady doctor, "If you wear a sari [traditional smart dress] everyone call you madam. If you do not wear a sari then these things can happen."

Hiruni, female, year 7, medical student, Sri Lanka

Narrative 5: 'just cross off these options'

'We learn a lot of medical ethics, or a general ethics, or professionalism… but in reality… different experts will provide different suggestions and the drug of choices, but then the doctors or the resident will say "the family seems to be more conservative and not economically capable"… then we don't tell them about the treatment. They just cross off these options. So they could maybe provide the patient with like less effective way of treatment for the sake of their economy. And although they're doing that for the patient's good, because they're afraid if the patient know about the better treatment, but he couldn't have it because of the economical issues, maybe more frustrated… but the medical ethics tell us to provide every options available for the patients to decide… it's kind of dilemma for me… I know [they're] thinking in the good ways of the patients, but it's contradicting with what we learn in ethics class.'

Guan-yu, male, year 6, medical student, Taiwan

---

us of a time when he had just returned from learning medicine in an American medical school and begins to use the knowledge and skills he learnt there to take a history from a patient. In essence, Chih-Hung explains that his clinical teacher unfairly criticizes him (so, same event – student abuse – as those outlined in Chapter 9) but the gist of his dilemma is different to those typically seen in Western cultural spaces. Here, Chih-Hung appears to be criticized by his clinical teacher for adopting a patient-centred approach (typified by a Westernized egalitarian student-patient relationship rather than a hierarchical one), which Chih-Hung seems to suggest his clinical teacher thinks culturally inappropriate.

An example of a culturally-constrained dilemma includes when a healthcare worker makes a mistake. In such situations, healthcare professionals attempt to cover up their mistakes by ignoring them, blaming students and colleagues, or asking students to cover them up. However, in our research there are qualitative differences between Western students narrating such incidents and Eastern students – in both the tone of the narratives and the ways in which students and others present are reported to react to dilemmas. For example, consider Sathi's narrative (Box 11.9, narrative 2). She tells us how she witnessed a registrar and house officer cover up their mistake (they had intubated into the patient's stomach rather than lungs) because they were scared of the female consultant. This was despite the patient being in a critical condition at the time. We can contrast this with Esme's narrative in Chapter 12 (Box 12.6, narrative 1). Esme is a female UK medical student who witnessed a clinician making a mistake then blaming the nurse. He accused the nurse of sabotaging the patient's care. When he then tried to get Esme to back him up, she spoke out and challenged him. Thinking about the differences culturally, this again links with the different cultural dimensions around power distance (Box 11.2). Eastern cultures value deference towards an ascribed authority, which contrasts with the Western value of self-assertion and an earned-authority. By speaking up, Esme believes she will earn the respect of others. Conversely, Sathi earns her respect by staying silent.

Culturally-specific Dilemmas

Although there are many dilemmas common across different cultures, there are also some that are culturally-specific. We have already seen an everyday example of consent issues around family versus patient consent (Chang-Chi's narrative). Other common situations include dilemmas where patients take Chinese medicine in addition to, or in place of, Western medicine (note, this dilemma is one that could occur in Western settings also). Examples of dilemmas that students experience in relation to this issue includes patients telling students about their use of Chinese medicine because of their student status, and telling them not to tell the doctor about this.

Often patients' failures to disclose their use of Chinese medicine (or reporting their use at a lower level than it actually is) stems from mistrust between patient and doctor, from their scepticism around Western medicine and their strong belief in the therapeutic effects of traditional remedies. Such scepticism might be related to differences in the cultural dimension of control (Box 11.2): the external (mastery) of Western medicine and the 'modern notions' of anatomy and pathology vs. internal (harmony) of Chinese medicine, which includes cosmological notions such as harmony between yin-yang. The dilemma itself for medical students appears to be whether to tell the patients' clinicians (which they invariably do not), and whether to try to dissuade the patient from using traditional Chinese medicine (which they invariably thought was futile). Furthermore, many of these dilemmas are extremely multifaceted and overlap across different themes (see Box 11.9, narrative 3 in which Ren-Huei illustrates how issues around consent and Chinese medicine intertwine). These complex dilemmas, where the patient's family act as *gatekeepers*, can result in healthcare providers withholding information and treatment from the patient, as illustrated earlier also in Chang-Chi's dilemma.

Other dilemmas occurring within Eastern contexts but not found in our Western data include healthcare professionals compromising patient care by giving preferential treatment to some patients due to personal or familial connections (關係 *guān xi*), again as a result of a strong collectivist culture. Examples include allowing patients to be seen in the clinic before other patients who had waited for longer. Within our narratives from a Sri Lankan context we also identified dilemmas that students encountered around identity, gender, hierarchy and dress code (linking with the cultural dimension of gender egalitarianism). Indeed, Hiruni, a female student (Box 11.9, narrative 4), told us how she witnessed a female senior house officer who was wearing a skirt and T-shirt (instead of a sari) admonish an older patient for calling her 'miss' (a term used by patients for nurses) instead of 'doctor' because she was not wearing her traditional Sri Lankan dress.

Socio-economic Dilemmas

In addition to professionalism dilemmas that can be mainly attributed to culture, there are dilemmas where it is apparent that socio-economic factors are at play.[26] Powerful examples of this come from both the Taiwanese and Sri Lankan cultures and include situations around health systems issues. In Taiwanese settings, while initial healthcare is covered by healthcare insurance, there are economic concerns around the cost of any treatment, with patients having to pay for drug therapies. In Sri Lanka, the cost of healthcare is available free of charge at the point of delivery, with this state-sponsored system being used by the vast majority of the population. However, even basic facilities are not available to all patients at all times due to limited financial capacity in the government sector. Therefore, patients, at times, are compelled to use private sector facilities, thereby bearing the health costs personally, which is often unaffordable for them. Within both of these contexts, students narrated situations in which doctors sometimes withheld information about expensive treatments because they felt that patients could not afford them (see Guan-yu's story in Box 11.9, narrative 5), or patients faced going without much-needed drug therapy. The dilemma for the student includes confusion (or frustration) when 'actual practice' goes against the formal ethics teaching they have received (as discussed earlier in Chapter 3 in terms of the hidden curriculum), and sometimes experiencing feelings of guilt or duty, which may lead them to go beyond professional boundaries for the sake of patient care. For example, consistent with Sri Lankan collectivist values, a Sri Lankan medical student reported purchasing antibiotics for a patient who could not afford his treatment.

How are Situations Culturally Interpreted? Intercultural Dilemmas on Medical Electives by Western Students

Although the majority of the dilemmas discussed so far have an intercultural dimension, in this final section, we consider intercultural dilemmas reported by Western medical students during their medical *elective* period. The elective offers healthcare students a unique opportunity to experience healthcare in an unfamiliar environment. Electives typically occur overseas, sometimes within countries whose scientific and economic standards and resources differ significantly. Within our research with medical students, they recounted a range of dilemma scenarios encountered in non-Western cultures, many of them being similar to those found in Western settings including: issues around how students' learning sometimes took priority over patient care; situations in which they were asked to act beyond their level of competence without supervision (or undertook to do so through their own volition); informed consent dilemmas; and dilemmas around healthcare professionals' actions, such as patient safety and dignity breaches. What differs between dilemmas experienced in non-Western cultures to those experienced at home, are the ways in which students subsequently acted and the types of explanations they gave for their actions that can be understood in terms of cultural differences and students' identities. Students' explanations for acting suggest a subtle shift in their goals from *learning how* to cure the sick to *attempting to* cure the sick: sometimes leading them to act beyond their levels of competency.

Narrative 1 in Box 11.10 demonstrates clearly how Neil's shifting identities of himself, and of others' perceptions of him, began with him complying to 'small' requests (to take blood) during an overseas elective before becoming a medical student. This quickly escalated over time, resulting in him complying with more and more requests to perform procedures requiring greater levels of experience and competence than he actually possessed, clearly placing patient safety at risk. Note how Neil constructs his situation as being one of his own making: in his narrative he does not suggest that he has made any attempt to highlight the extreme limits of his own competences to those who are making the requests for him to act. Contrast this with James, a cautious fifth year student nearing the end of his course, who declines to go beyond his competence level in a resource-poor county (Box 11.10, narrative 2). Perhaps he is over cautious, so is mindful not to take the child's history and run blood tests (something he is likely to be competent at doing) being aware that those are his limits: anything else takes him beyond his abilities, and also into the realms of having started something he cannot finish.

The final dilemma type, frequently encountered during overseas electives, are situations in which students' values and practices fundamentally differ from those of their host country. Such dilemmas include issues around (lack of) patient consent, dignity breaches and occasionally, religious practices. Consider Chris' narrative (Box 11.10, narrative 3) where he tells us of a situation he encountered whilst assisting with the circumcision of a six-year-old during his elective in Senegal. The local anaesthetic was not working and the

---

Box 11.10 Western students' electives dilemma narratives

Narrative 1: 'a kind of self reinforcing thing'

'First day I was working in this hospital in South Africa somebody handed me a tray with a load of blood tubes and forms and said, "Right those six need [bloods taking]"… and he disappeared, and I was left there holding the kit to take blood from six people and fortunately my cousin was around and I said, "Look [name] I've been asked to do this can you show me how to do this?" And he said, "Yes …" and I do remember thinking, "Okay I've just been shown this in a matter of seconds, do I? am I? do I feel confident enough to be able to do this? 'cause, once you start do this, you'll be expected to carry on with it." And, as part of perhaps of who I am, I went, "Yeah, okay…" and it worked… none of the patients complained too bitterly. But that was repeated… the second day it was putting in cannulas and running IV bags… the third day it was putting in catheters. Looking back it was kind of self-reinforcing thing… by the second week… we had a lot of trauma coming in, the surgeon said to me, "I need to have another pair of hands in theatre can you come in?" And I was there scrubbed in… I went in with literally an out of date first aid certificate, and within two weeks was assisting with major surgery… when I look back on it, it's absolutely terrifying. Not just for me but for poor bloody patients.'

Neil, male, year 1 medical student, UK

Narrative 2: 'I can't do it'

'I was in Pakistan, and it's quite, resources are quite limited… I was in the staff room. Basically, I get a knock on the door and it's a nurse saying, "Oh, there's like parents of the child who's developed a rash and we need you to, you know, deal with the matter". What that meant was, basically seeing the patient, diagnosing what's going on and prescribing, or doing any investigations that I needed to, because there was no other doctors around. And I felt, "Oh my god what am I supposed to do in this situation?" So then I just felt that, I just had to like decline… let the nurse know that basically I can't do it… her response was a bit negative… she was putting a lot of pressure on me because she was saying, "You know, they're in a very critical situation… and you're the only person who's got some sort of medical knowledge who could actually help." So that was a bit of a dilemma for me… when I thought it through, I just stood my stance… the parents were outside the room and that was extra pressure.'

James, male, year 5 medical student, UK

Narrative 3: 'I can't put up with it anymore'

'When I was in Senegal… we were doing circumcision… they kind of realized part way that the local hadn't fully worked, and it was horrible, and then they were saying to the kid like, "No just be brave… put up with it" and they were getting quite mean, and I just sat there thinking, "Maybe it's a cultural thing", and in the end I was like… "Don't talk to him like that it's just not right", and they were like, "What do you mean?" I was like, "He's in pain he's six years old", like, "That's just not funny", and they were kind of laughing… I think it's the language barrier as well. I think at first they thought I was joking. They really laughed, that was horrible… at first I thought, "Oh I'll put it down to cultural differences…" it took ages, and after about twenty minutes, I was like, "This can't go on any more, this just can't go on any more, I've got to say something because I can't put up with it anymore.'

Chris, male, year 3 medical student, UK

child was in pain. Instead of giving him further pain relief, the doctors laughed and told the child to be brave. The dilemma Chris experienced was knowing when – or if – to make a stand and speak out for the boy. After all, he did not wish to interfere in matters of local culture and practices. The result was that Chris became angry and frustrated, leading him to speak out (with the rest of the day being spent avoiding the doctors).

Thinking about Chris' narrative in terms of our earlier discussion of developing an intercultural capability through negotiation, we wonder how this scenario might have played out had Chris used a high advocacy-high enquiry approach. Rather than internally deliberating whether the disturbing scene he saw unfolding before him was 'a cultural thing', Chris might have engaged in an open enquiry with the doctors about their behaviours, and explained his own perspective. While, ultimately, such an approach might not have spared the young boy pain, it might have resulted in a better understanding between Chris and the doctors, enabling them to continue to work together after the event with less animosity.

Chapter Summary

This chapter has provided an overview of what culture is and its different dimensions, examples of different cultural orientations between Eastern and Western cultural spaces, suggestions about how healthcare students can develop their cultural and intercultural capabilities, the similarities and differences in terms of professionalism dilemmas experienced by healthcare students in Western and Eastern cultural spaces, and those experienced by Western students on their overseas electives (often in different cultural spaces). The key take-home messages for healthcare students and professionals from this chapter are summarized in Box 11.11. Suggestions for small group discussions around the topic of professionalism dilemmas across different cultural contexts can be found in Box 11.12 with reflective exercises in Box 11.13. Finally, Box 11.14 provides further recommended reading.

Box 11.11 Chapter summary points

- Healthcare students and professionals should apply what they know about culture and its different dimensions to understand cultural and intercultural professionalism dilemmas better
- Healthcare students and professionals should develop their own cultural and intercultural capabilities through developing awareness about their own and others' cultures
- Healthcare students and professionals need to understand how their professionalism dilemma experiences may vary depending on where they are in the world (e.g. home country vs. overseas)

Box 11.12 Small group discussion points

- What issues (if any) does this chapter raise for you in terms of Eastern healthcare students learning Western healthcare?
- What are the challenges for you of developing cultural and intercultural capabilities?
- What universal healthcare professionalism values do you think there are or do you think they are all culture-specific and why?

Box 11.13 Chapter learning activities

- Think about a recent or most-memorable cultural or intercultural professionalism dilemma of your own.
- Write down the details of the dilemma: what was the gist of your dilemma? Where and when did it take place? Who was there? What happened? What did you do and why? How did you feel?
- How can you understand your experience better by applying what you now know about culture from this chapter?
- Using what you now know about developing cultural and intercultural capabilities, how could you cope better with this dilemma if it happened again? What could you do differently next time?
- What advice would you give to one of your peers if they had this same experience?

Box 11.14 Chapter recommended reading

Ho M, Gosselin K, Chandratilake M, Monrouxe LV, Rees CE. Taiwanese medical students' narratives of intercultural professionalism dilemmas: exploring tensions between Western medicine and Taiwanese culture. *Advances in Health Science Education.* [Epub ahead of print] 10.1007/s10459-016-9738-x

Hofstede G, Hofstede G, Minkov, M. *Cultures and Organizations: Software of the Mind,* 3rd Edition. New York, NY: Mcgraw-Hill, 2010.

Monrouxe LV, Chandratilake M, Gosselin K, Rees CE Ho M. Taiwanese and Sri Lankan students' dimensions and discourses of professionalism. *Medical Education.* In press.

Maleki A, de Jong M. A proposal for clustering the dimensions of national culture. *Cross-Cultural Research* 2014;48:107–143.

Jha V, Mclean M, Gibbs TJ, Sandars J. Medical professionalism across cultures: a challenge for medicine and medical education. *Medical Teacher* 2014;37:74–80.

References

1 Friedman VJ, Berthoin Antal A. Negotiating reality: a theory of action approach to intercultural competence. *Management Learning* 2005;36:69–86.

2 Clemens E, Cook J. Politics and institutionalism: explaining durability and change. *Annual Review of Sociology* 1999;25:244–266.

3 Trandis H. *Individualism and Collectivism.* Boulder, CO: Westview Press, 1995.

4 Berthoin Antal A. What is culture? Discussion note. In A Berthoin Antal (Ed.) *Course Reader on Intercultural Management.* Berlin: WZB and Technical University Berlin, 2002.

5 Hong Y, Morris M, Chiu C, Bennet-Martinez V. Multicultural minds: a dynamic constructivist approach to culture and cognition. *American Psychologist* 2000;55:709–720.

6 Swidler A. Culture in action: symbols and strategies. *American Sociological Review* 1986;51:273–286.

7 Maleki A, de Jong M. A proposal for clustering the dimensions of national culture. *Cross-Cultural Research* 2014;48:107–143.

8 Fraser SW, Greenhalgh T. Coping with complexity: educating for capability. *British Medical Journal* 2001;323:799.

9 Hofstede G, Hofstede G, Minkov M. *Cultures and Organizations: Software of the Mind*, 3rd Edition. New York, NY: McGraw-Hill, 2010.

10 Schwartz SH. Mapping and interpreting cultural differences around the world. In H Vinken, J Soeters, P Ester (Eds) *Comparing Cultures, Dimensions of Culture in a Comparative Perspective*. Leiden, Netherlands: Brill, 2004: pp. 43–73.

11 Qingxue L. Understanding different cultural patterns or orientations between East and West. *Investigationes Linguisticae* 2003;9:21–30.

12 Yum JO. The impact of Confucianism on interpersonal relationships and communication patterns in east Asia. *Communication Monographs* 1988;55:374–388.

13 Bellah R, Madsen R, Sullivan W, Swidler A, Tipton S. *Habits of the Heart: Individualism and Commitment in American Life*. Berkeley: University of California Press, 1985.

14 Triandis H. Issues in individualism and collectivism research. In R Sorrentino, D Cohen, J Olson, M Zanna (Eds) *Cultural and Social Behavior: the Ontarion Symposium*. Mahwah, NJ: Lawrence Erlbaum Associates, 2005: pp. 207–215.

15 Depaigne V. Human rights and cultural identity in a constitutional framework. *Government and Opposition* 2002;37:450.

16 Hall E. *Beyond Culture*. New York: Doubleday, 1976.

17 Hall E, Hall M. *Understanding Cultural Differences: German, French and Americans*. Yarmouth: ME Intercultural Press, 1990.

18 Chu G, Ju Y. *The Great Wall in Ruins: Communication and Culture Change in China*. Albany, NY: State University of New York Press, 1993.

19 Scollon R, Scollon S. *Intercultural Communication: a Discourse Approach*. Beijing: Foreign Language Teaching and Research Press/Blackwell Publishers Ltd, 2000.

20 Blackwell M. Old boys' networks, family connections and the English legal profession. *Public Law* 2013;3:426–444.

21 Choi Y. *East and West: Understanding the Rise of China*. Bloomington, Indiana: iUniverse, 2010.

22 Moeran B. Individual, Group and Seishin: Japan's internal cultural debate. *Man* 1984;19:252–266.

23 Barnlund D. Communication in a global village. In M Bennett (Ed.) *Basic Concepts of Intercultural Communication Selected Reading*. Yarmouth, ME: Intercultural Press, 1998: pp. 31–51.

24 Bennett M. Intercultural communication: a current perspective. In M Bennett (Ed.) *Basic Concepts of Intercultural Communication Selected Readings*. Yarmouth, ME: Intercultural Press, 1998: pp. 1–34.

25 Argyris C, Schon D. *Theories in Practice: Increasing Professional Effectiveness*. San Francisco: Jossey-Bass, 1974.

26 Betancourt JR, Green AR, Carrillo JE. *Cultural Competence in Health Care: Emerging Frameworks and Practical Approaches*. Commonwealth Fund, Quality of Care for Underserved Populations, 2002.

12

Professionalism Dilemmas Across Professional Cultures

[I experienced] a nurse complaining and humiliating me in front of staff and patients. [I was in a] teenage cancer unit. Nurses and patients [were] present. The nurse said I hadn't used hand gel when I had. She also complained that I had my coat with me despite us not being provided with anywhere to put it, then completely bypassing it when another nurse failed to gel her hands and a social worker brought numerous personal belongings onto the ward. [I] apologized for not using alcohol gel. I knew she was just doing it for a power trip as most nurses hate medical students... I'm sick of being shot down and treated like rubbish by nurses just for studying medicine.

Catriona, female, year 5, medical student, UK

LEARNING OUTCOMES

- To compare the key roles of dentists, doctors, nurses, pharmacists and physiotherapists
- To compare healthcare learners in terms of the professionalism dilemmas they experience
- To discover the range of interprofessional dilemmas experienced by healthcare learners and how they arise
- To explore learners' reactions and actions in the face of interprofessional dilemmas
- To reflect on ways that interprofessional conflict can be managed

---

KEY TERMS

Professional roles
Professional identities
Interprofessional identities
Interprofessional dilemmas
Interprofessional hierarchies
Interprofessional conflicts

Healthcare Professionalism: Improving Practice through Reflections on Workplace Dilemmas, First Edition.
Lynn V. Monrouxe and Charlotte E. Rees.

Introduction

The healthcare workplace is typically interprofessional (see Box 12.1 for definitions), with many different healthcare professionals working (and learning) together for the good of the patient. Although roles are becoming increasing flexible in modern-day healthcare, variations exist across healthcare students' and professionals' roles and, therefore, the education and training they receive. We know from our own and others' research that healthcare students experience various interprofessional dilemmas involving hierarchies, roles and conflicts throughout their workplace learning.[1,2] This is illustrated by the above narrative from a medical student (Catriona), in which she narrates receiving unfair criticism from a nurse on a teenage cancer clinic; criticism which, Catriona implies, arises from the nurse's hatred of medical students. In this chapter, we discuss the similarities and differences in roles and education across the healthcare professions. We also compare healthcare students in terms of the professionalism dilemmas they face, drawing out highlights from Chapters 5 to 9. We then focus on the different types of interprofessional dilemmas experienced by healthcare students from our programme of research and how they react to them. Finally, we discuss key management strategies for tackling interprofessional conflict. This chapter should enable healthcare students to better understand their own and other healthcare students' and professionals' roles, in order to better manage any interprofessional conflicts. Ultimately, we hope this chapter will help healthcare students work towards a better awareness of their developing multiple identities – both their professional identity (as dentist, doctor, nurse, pharmacist or physiotherapist) and their interprofessional identity (as interprofessional healthcare team member) and managing how these multiple identities interrelate over the course of their healthcare education.

Box 12.1 Information: defining the terms interprofessional, patient, role and identity

Interprofessional: Interactions between individuals from two or more different professions (e.g. doctors and nurses). Interprofessional education has been defined as: 'occasions when two or more professions learn with, from and about each other to improve collaboration and the quality of care.'[3,4]

Patient: Although we use the term 'patient' in this chapter, we recognize that not all individuals seeking health and social care are comfortable being referred to as 'patients', instead preferring other terms such as 'clients'.[5]

Role: Outward indicators that you have a certain role (e.g. wearing a badge that says 'pharmacist'), consisting of a set of expectations from others about how you should act (as in *relational identity*). Wearing this badge and being recognized by others as a 'pharmacist', however, does not necessarily mean that you will feel like a pharmacist (*as in personal identity*), such as in the case of a newly qualified pharmacist who does not yet feel like a 'pharmacist'.[6,7]

Identity: Inward self-perception that you embody a certain identity (e.g. feeling like a 'doctor', as in *personal identity*). Feeling like a doctor, however, does not always mean that others recognize you as a doctor (as in *relational identity*) such as in the case of a person who has retired from medical practice and therefore no longer has a doctor role.[6,7]

What are the Roles of Different Healthcare Professionals?

There are innumerable similarities across the healthcare professions, with all focusing on the effective and safe delivery of healthcare, serving as 'patient' advocates morally bound by their duties and united by an 'ideology of caring'.[1,8] However, traditional understandings of the roles of different healthcare professionals, and their occupational boundaries, differ. In this chapter, although we talk about roles *and* identities, we focus mostly on *roles*, in contrast to other chapters (such as Chapter 5). While some identity scholars equate roles with relational identity,[9] others in healthcare education have tried to distinguish between roles and identity (see Box 12.1).

When thinking about professional roles, it is first helpful to revisit the healthcare hierarchies discussed earlier in Chapter 9 (see Box 9.6). Traditional roles of healthcare professionals (see Table 12.1 for a comparison from the UK NHS health careers website) are linked to typical healthcare hierarchies, where norms exist in terms of division of labour between the *things* doctors do, as opposed to what nurses do, and so on.[10] For example, some consider the doctor role to comprise things like ownership of the patient, decision-making responsibility, authority over medical knowledge and leadership.[11–17] Whereas doctors often perceive themselves as leaders and decision makers, other healthcare professionals such as nurses, therapists and pharmacists typically see themselves as 'team members' adopting holistic approaches to care.[18] For example, traditional understandings of the role of the nurse include patient advocacy, caring and promoting and optimizing health and quality of life, whereas the role of the physiotherapist includes focusing on patient mobility and physical stability.[12–17,19,20] Interestingly, researchers have outlined lines of occupation demarcation (or boundaries) in the healthcare professions; for example curing versus caring, skilled versus unskilled and diagnostic versus technical work.[1] Work through Box 12.2 to reflect on where you see these boundaries across different healthcare professionals. While ignoring the roles of nurse specialist and advanced nurse practitioner, see the shared role perceptions and expectations of doctors and nurses about their own and one another's roles in Box 12.3.

Table 12.1 **Information: comparison of roles in healthcare** (from http://www.healthcareers.nhs.uk).

Roles	Expectations
Dentist	'work with patients and the general public to prevent and treat dental and oral disease, correcting dental irregularities… and treating dental and facial injuries'
Doctor (example here relates to general internal medicine)	'diagnose, treat and manage the care of in-patients and outpatients with acute and chronic medical problems'
Nurse (example here relates to mental health nurse)	'promoting and supporting a person's recovery and enabling them to have more involvement and control over their condition'
Pharmacist	'experts in medicines and their use'
Physiotherapist	'work with people to help with a range of problems which affect movement, using exercise, massage and other techniques'

Box 12.2 Stop and do: reflect on and discuss boundaries across healthcare professions (Apesoa-Varano)[1]

Write the following healthcare roles on separate slips of paper or post-it notes. Here, we list them in alphabetical order: *dentist, dental hygienist, dental nurse, dietician, general practitioner, mental health nurse, occupational therapist, pharmacist, physician, physiotherapist, psychiatrist, registered nurse, specialist nurse practitioner, speech therapist, surgeon.*

- Now, on a sheet of paper or whiteboard, draw a line at the top along the horizontal plane. Write the word 'curing' at the end of the line on the left-hand side and 'caring' at the opposite end on the right.
- Working on your own or with your peers, arrange the slips of paper across the continuum in a manner that you think best represents boundaries between the healthcare professions in terms of curing and caring.
- Reflect on why you have put them in that order.
- What (if any) disagreements did you have with your peers about the order and why?
- Repeat the above steps for the skilled/unskilled and diagnostic/technical boundaries.

However, there is now considerable knowledge emphasizing the fluidity and flexibility of roles.[1] Indeed, professional boundaries are in a constant state of flux as professional roles change over time and new types of healthcare workers come into being.[6] Things like role ambiguity, blurring, erosion and extension are now commonplace in modern healthcare.[16] Burford *et al.*,[10] for example, talk about 'pragmatic hierarchies', which can contravene typical healthcare hierarchies in that the primary driver is getting the job done, such as when junior doctors defer to the greater experience and expertise of senior nurses.[1,10,21] Exploring the complexity of interprofessional collaborative practice on a distributed transplant team, Lingard *et al.*[22] found that professional roles were changeable depending on the circumstances, and that the team's expertise was about being cognisant and responsive to such changes in roles.

Linked with different roles across the healthcare professions are key differences in healthcare students' educational experiences. For example, although length of education varies across countries and depends on degree (e.g. Bachelor, Master) and whether students have prior degrees, there are marked differences across the healthcare professions in terms of duration of training (e.g. ranging from three years of undergraduate

---

Box 12.3 Information: shared role expectations of doctors and nurses[23]

Roles in patient management: doctors to manage the patient, prescribe medication, explain diagnoses and management to patients; nurses to follow up patients during hospital stay, provide psychological support, execute medical orders

Roles in clinical reasoning and diagnosis: doctors to perform reasoning and decision making through medical knowledge; nurses to bring doctors' decisions into action through nursing knowledge

Roles in the team: doctors and nurses to work as team, communicating and sharing information; nurses as link between patient and doctor

study for UK nursing and physiotherapy students to five years of undergraduate study for UK medical students plus many more years of postgraduate training; see: http://www.healthcareers.nhs.uk). While all healthcare students have workplace learning experiences, there is also considerable variation in the amount of time healthcare students spend learning in the healthcare workplace, and what students engage in during that learning. For example, pharmacy students in our study spent little time doing clinical placements during their degrees compared with other healthcare students, and medical students in our study spent little time during their placements doing 'hands-on' practical work in contrast to nursing, physiotherapy and dental students.

How do Professionalism Dilemmas Compare Across Healthcare Students?

There are more similarities than differences in professionalism dilemmas across the five healthcare student groups in our research programme. For example, as illustrated across Chapters 5–10, all healthcare students experience identity, patient safety, patient dignity, student abuse and e-professionalism dilemmas, and all except pharmacy students experience patient consent dilemmas.[24] Furthermore, healthcare students are often similarly distressed by the dilemmas and all healthcare student groups become more morally distressed (a pattern we call disturbance) with increased frequency of dilemmas that cannot be justified for student learning.[25] Furthermore, healthcare students from all groups can go along with lapses in professionalism because of the complexities of healthcare hierarchies. However, we have noticed some interesting differences over the years across the five healthcare student groups.[24–26] For reasons of brevity, in this section, we provide an illustrative example for each healthcare student group only, examples that serve to emphasize the uniqueness of each profession in terms of their different roles and/or educational experiences.

Medical Students and Patient Consent

As discussed in Chapter 6, the consent dilemmas captured across our programme of research came disproportionately from medical students, reflecting their different student roles in the healthcare environment (e.g. observer, learner) compared with dental, nursing and physiotherapy students, who often act as care providers to patients with and without supervision depending on their competency. Indeed, at the core of these dilemmas for the medical student was that much of their hands-on interactions with patients (through examinations or procedures) was done to benefit themselves rather than the patient (see narrative 1, Box 12.4). Furthermore, medical students were the only healthcare group that became habituated (i.e. less morally distressed) to dilemmas occurring frequently that were thought to be justifiable for their learning, such as consent dilemmas.[25]

Nursing Students and Physical Dignity (Patient and Self)

As discussed in Chapter 8, the patient dignity dilemmas disproportionately came from nursing and medical students. Interestingly, nursing students cited more physical patient dignity-related professionalism dilemmas, as well as physical student abuse

---

Box 12.4 Unique aspects of professionalism dilemmas across student groups

Narrative 1. Medical students and patient consent

'A fellow student performed an unconsented rectal examination on an anaesthetized patient… I politely reminded the student before he performed [the procedure] the university guidelines to gain consent. The surgeon said I was out of order and did not believe consent was necessary and that I would not progress as a surgeon if I thought like that. The student performed the examination. I considered reporting it further but thought that my superiors would be on the surgeon's side so did not. No one else in the operating room seemed to think there was a problem with this behaviour. I avoid that particular student and am extra careful myself to consent patients beforehand.'

Kathryn, female, year 5, medical student, UK

Narrative 2. Nursing students and physical dignity

'Nurse Z insisted on moving a client to the bathroom on a trolley covered only by a small towel. [The] client had cerebral palsy and was on a mixed dorm. I asked on more than one occasion why it was necessary to undress the client in the bedroom and then transfer to the bathroom. The bathroom was more than big enough to cope with the procedure… due to the nature of cerebral palsy [the patient] exposed themselves to other students in the corridor. [I] covered the client up immediately… [I] reported the nurse to my mentor.'

Sara, female, year 3, nursing student, UK

Narrative 3. Dental students and patient safety

'[I was] asked to extract a premolar in a patient unsupervised. [Present was] just myself, patient and patient's father in the surgery. [I] extracted the tooth in question as competent to do, however adjacent tooth was attached by soft tissue and was also extracted. [I] advised patient I required a superior's opinion and attempted to find senior clinician. [I] did not wish to worry the patient and had not previously been told about what to do in this eventuality. The tooth was re-inserted and was firm, patient was advised regarding the situation and I was cleared of blame, however I was stressed at the time and still worry that I could have acted faster to reinsert the tooth, increasing its prognosis if I had been advised on management of complications.'

Lotta, female, year, 4, dental student, UK

Narrative 4. Pharmacy students and identities

'The pharmacy that I work at part-time… pharmacist is silent except for when telling me to check a prescription, when I ask a question sometimes I am ignored or answered in a mumble. Pharmacist has also not applied for my counter assistant training and so I have missed the deadline. [I did] nothing – pharmacist is the manager… but will just wait until the old manager returns.'

Meg, female, year 2, pharmacy student, UK

> **Narrative 5. Physiotherapy students and (lack of) emotion talk**
>
> 'On one of my... placements... we were on the wards and they didn't... really draw curtains around for treatment of patient and the patient I think had dementia but she was... wearing hospital gown but it was quite loose... and her sheet wasn't really covering her so she was quite exposed... and... they didn't do anything to try and sort of preserve her dignity very much, I think it was like exposing the breast or something... they didn't sort of cover her back up but I think... I ended up doing it at the end of the session... I think they were listening to her chest, I think the way they did it, it could have preserved the dignity a bit more.'
>
> Poppy, female, year 3, physiotherapy student, UK

dilemmas perpetrated by patients, often around personal care activities.[26] Again, these differential experiences probably reflect nursing students' different roles in the workplace, with their being involved in the hands-on delivery of patient care, including intimate care activities such as feeding, bathing, toileting and lifting (see narrative 2, Box 12.4).

Dental Students and Patient Safety

As illustrated in Chapter 7, the most striking patient safety dilemmas that involved students' actions (rather than witnessed by students) were from dental students, largely because of their relatively hands-on provision of dental care, including invasive procedures with relatively dangerous equipment. For example, we collected numerous examples of dental students working beyond the limits of their competence inside patients' mouths, sometimes using powerful and sharp instruments and conducting irreversible procedures without sufficient supervision (see narrative 3, Box 12.4). Within this context, participants narrated numerous stories of students (self and peers) making mistakes and then covering them up (e.g. going through the roof of a patient's mouth and trying to hide it).[24]

Pharmacy Students and Identities

Pharmacy students' workplace professionalism dilemmas were sometimes situated in the context of their working in community pharmacies as counter assistants as part of paid work, creating interesting identity dilemmas not discussed by other healthcare students (see how Meg criticizes the pharmacist in the pharmacy she works at for not applying for her counter assistant training: see narrative 4, Box 12.4). Indeed, pharmacy students struggled with their dual identities as counter staff and pharmacy student,[24] alongside the lapses of other non-professional staff within pharmacies: 'A lot of them [counter staff] are essentially retail staff... so in a way you can't really expect them to have the same... [code of ethics]' (Cassie, female, year 4, pharmacy student, UK). That many of our pharmacy students' dilemmas related to their roles as counter staff, probably reflects the shorter time they spent in clinical placements as part of their undergraduate degree compared with other healthcare students.

Physiotherapy Students and Emotion

The most notable difference found between physiotherapy and other healthcare students in our programme of research was that physiotherapy students typically recounted their oral professionalism dilemmas with less emotion talk (e.g. less negative emotional talk in abuse narratives and less anger talk in patient safety and dignity dilemmas: see narrative 5, Box 12.4).[24] By exploring the content of physiotherapy students' oral narratives, it was clear that their professionalism dilemmas seemed less serious, traumatic and life-threatening compared with those recounted by other healthcare students, possibly reflecting their narrower scope of practice as allied health students compared with, say, the medical profession and their more close supervision compared with, for example, nursing students.[24]

Interprofessional Dilemmas: Hierarchies, Roles and Conflict

Just over ten per cent of the professionalism dilemmas across our programme of research were interprofessional.[2] As already illustrated in Chapters 5–9, healthcare students experienced interprofessional dilemmas around student identities (e.g. Box 5.2), patient consent (e.g. Box 6.9), patient safety (e.g. Box 7.7), patient dignity (e.g. Box 8.12), and student abuse (e.g. Boxes 9.12). From the perspective of interprofessional working, many of these dilemmas had at their core various intersecting issues of hierarchies, roles, and conflict,[2] as illustrated in Catriona's narrative at the start of this chapter. Before we discuss these issues in more detail, complete the activity in Box 12.5.

Interprofessional Hierarchies

As we discussed in Chapter 9, multiple hierarchies exist in the healthcare workplace, including levels of seniority and specialties within healthcare professions, and across the different healthcare professions themselves, with medical practitioners often considered to be at the top and other professionals like nurses lower down.[17,27,28] Imbued with power asymmetries, such hierarchies mean that students observe healthcare professionals engaging in power play, and enacting and resisting the power of one another, with students sometimes getting caught in the middle. Students in our research programme observed innumerable communication violations between healthcare practitioners from different professions, including aggressive orders, challenges, criticisms, disagreements, reprimands and insults, along with back-biting. In narrative 1 (Box 12.6), a medical student illustrates a doctor abusing interprofessional hierarchies by blaming a nurse for one of his own mistakes.

Box 12.5 Stop and do: reflect on your own interprofessional dilemma experiences

- Have you ever experienced any interprofessional dilemmas?
- If so, write down your most memorable experience: What was the gist of your dilemma? Where were you? Who was present? What happened? What did you do? Why? How did you feel?
- What interprofessional issues were involved in this dilemma? Hierarchies? Roles? Conflict? Boundary issues? Something else?
- How has this experience (if at all) influenced your thoughts about interprofessional working?

Box 12.6 Illustrative examples of narratives involving interprofessional hierarchies

Narrative 1. 'A doctor made a mistake and blamed it on a nurse'

'A doctor made a mistake and blamed it on a nurse, he then tried to get me to join in. [I was] in an anaesthetic room, with a doctor and a nurse. The doctor pulled out a cannula by accident then accused the nurse of doing it and trying to sabotage the patient's care. I did nothing until he asked me to join in, then I told him that I saw it was his fault. He was trying to bully her, and he expected me to join in just because I was his junior. I am glad I challenged him, and I would do it again, doctors have greater respect for students who stand up for themselves.'

Esme, female, year 5, medical student, UK

Narrative 2. 'The nurse came back once the doctor left and kicked us off the ward'

'[I was] on a GI ward with about six other students, a patient and a doctor. A nurse came into the bay where a group of students and doctor were with a patient and said: "These students cannot be here, they have to leave now," and threw the patient's folder onto his bed where he was sitting. The doctor explained this was the only time that we had ward teaching timeta-bled and that the patient was agreeable to talk with us so the nurse left and the doctor moved on to talk with another group of students whilst we took a history. The nurse came back once the doctor left and kicked us off the ward. [We] apologized to the patient, left the ward and returned to the teaching room to await the doctor and explain what had happened...'

Phillipa, female, year 2, medical student, UK

In another example of students getting caught in the middle of interprofessional hierarchies, Phillipa, a medical student, describes a ward nurse challenging her supervising doctor by telling him that medical students (including Phillipa) needed to leave the ward (see narrative 2, Box 12.6). Although the doctor refuses her directive and the medical students continue to interview the patient, the nurse returns once the doctor has gone and tells the students to leave again. So, while this nurse defers to the superordinate status of the doctor, she simultaneously resists this typical hierarchy by enacting power over the medical students who are subordinate to her in terms of clinical expertise and experience.

Interprofessional Roles

Interestingly, at the heart of these interprofessional dilemmas were issues concerning role boundaries, described as socially constructed sites of 'practice and power play'.[6,11] Several studies have now explored interprofessional boundary work and found various critical incidents involving different boundary dilemmas.[1,29] As illustrated in Box 12.7, these include: (1) professionals acting outside the boundaries of their training; (2) professionals performing others' non-medical tasks such as bathing and feeding patients; (3) professionals doubting their counterpart's expertise; (4) professionals criticizing other professionals' work to the patient; (5) professionals dismissing others' recommendations or requests; (6) professionals disagreeing over patient management; and (7) lack of communication between professionals.[1,29]

Box 12.7 Illustrative examples of interprofessional dilemmas involving role boundary dilemmas

1. Professionals acting outside the boundaries of their training

JAMIE: I've had this one particular nurse in the dental school… overstepping her professional role as a nurse… the roles set in the profession are quite strictly defined, what procedures they can do and what their role is expected to be and at the end of the day the dentist is the head of the team and the others should… fulfil their role in accordance with the dentist's wishes and this nurse really oversteps her role… she moved my drill without saying… we had done a treatment and she was suggesting doing more treatment and I didn't want to do that treatment… I found it quite hard to be polite with her but I did quite frankly go and say to her, 'No… I don't think that's appropriate today'…

MARY: It's the whole student status again, if we are in practice and you were the qualified dentist you would not hesitate to put her in her place but she is a qualified nurse… but even though technically we are in charge.'

Jamie, and Mary, male and female, year 4, dental students, UK

2. Professionals performing others' tasks

'I was on neurosurgery [placement] again and this patient… we were doing tracheal care on him and chest physio and he opened his bowel and I said, "Oh, I'll get some wipes and clean him," and she [physiotherapy supervisor] said, "No, that's not what the physio job is, the nurse will take care of that," and I said, "Yes, but the nurse might be ten, fifteen minutes, I can just do it quickly"… You don't have to be a nurse to give nursing care do you?'

Juliette, female, year 3, physiotherapy student, UK

3. Professionals doubting their counterpart's expertise

'I witnessed [a] clinician talking badly about nurses, calling them "stupid". [I was in the] doctors' mess, [present were the] consultant, registrar and me. The consultant was making generalizations about all nurses being stupid and not knowing anything. I kept a very straight face making no agreement (because I didn't agree) and no disagreement (because I didn't want to offend him)… I was quite offended by this as my boyfriend's mother is a nurse who I know well and respect. I've also met many nurses who I look up to and respect immensely for their intelligence.'

Louisa, year 3, female, medical student, UK

4. Professionals criticizing their counterpart's work to the patient

'[I was] in [an] outpatient clinic with [a] nurse specialist. [He] was giving incorrect information to patient. Whilst trying to describe postural hypotension called it BPPV (Benign paroxysmal positional vertigo) repeatedly. [The] patient said they understood. [I] corrected the nurse and told [the] patient, "What he has just told you is incorrect." [I did this because the] mother seem[ed] very anxious about their child. [I felt it was the] correct step. Nurses tend to put medical students down… [It is] really disheartening. Some of the reasons why many doctors may well leave the NHS.'

Fred, male, year 5, medical student, UK

5. Professionals dismissing others

'[I] thought a patient had a DVT (Deep vein thrombosis), [so I] referred it to a doctor who seemed to dismiss my concerns. [I was] at X [with] my clinical educator. My clinical educator carried out the subjective assessment (which was positive) and helped me refer the situation to the doctor. [We] wrote-up the medical notes and spoke to the nursing staff, told them to keep an eye on [the] patient. [I] felt concerned, it was an abnormal situation for the patient in the two weeks that I had got to know the patient. As it turns out the patient didn't have a DVT but I felt like the doctor ignored me.'

Trisha, female, year 3, physiotherapy student, UK

6. Professionals disagreeing over patient management

'I witnessed [a] patient denied medication. [I was] placed on a unit for challenging behaviour and complex needs [and the] doctor prescribed compound analgesics for an infected wound [but the] nurse prescriber decided these should not be administered. [The] named nurse questioned the decision and requested a "best interest meeting". [I] checked BNF for medication benefits and side effects, look at PRN ["where necessary"] protocol policy to collate evidence to support the use of the medication. I feel it is cruel to knowingly make anyone live in pain. [The] best interest meeting overturned the decision [to withhold the analgesics].'

Sally, female, year 3, nursing student, UK

7. Lack of communication between professionals

'... The patient was nil by mouth as he was aspirating. There was no sign at his bedside to say this... the HCA [healthcare assistant] was with the patient on the opposite side of the room. The patient started to drink the water when SALT [speech and language therapist] walked into the room and confronted the HCA. The HCA explained that the doctor had consented to giving the patient some water, which the doctor immediately denied. I stayed out of the situation and said nothing... The HCA was stuck between the doctor who denied giving consent in front of his colleagues and the SALT who was angry that the HCA was putting the patient's health at risk.'

Mavis, female, year 2, physiotherapy student, UK

Interprofessional Conflict

By examining how narrators describe their interprofessional dilemmas presented in this chapter, we can see clearly the conflicts between different healthcare professional groups. The metaphoric talk of two medical students (see Catriona's narrative at the start of the chapter and narrative 2, Box 12.6) illustrates this conflict, such as 'shot down', 'kicked off the ward', 'kicked us off the ward', which implies the conceptual metaphor of doctor-nurse relationship as war.[2,30,31] The metaphoric entailments of war here indicate that doctors and nurses are enemies within a battle, with relationships marked by hostility and violence.[2] Other students similarly illustrated the conflict between nurses and other healthcare professionals (e.g. dentists and doctors respectively), using terms like 'put her [dental nurse] in her place' and 'nurses tend to put medical students down' (see narratives 1 and 4, Box 12.7), which implies the conceptual metaphor of interprofessional relationships as hierarchy.[30,31] The hierarchy metaphor also has entailments, including healthcare professionals being at opposite ends of a hierarchy (up or down), with relationships marked by power asymmetries, and students typically being at the bottom of the pile.[30,31]

How do Dilemmas Around Role Boundaries Come About?

Previous research has suggested a number of factors influencing role boundaries in the interprofessional workplace, operating at a number of levels: structural influences include physical space, workloads, staff turnover, hierarchy and team composition; interpersonal influences include professionals' understandings of one another's roles, trust and leadership; and individual influences include a healthcare practitioner's approach to care, perspectives about other healthcare professionals and willingness to engage in collaborative practice.[32] Examples of factors contributing to dilemmas around role boundaries from our research can be seen in Box 12.8.

Box 12.8 Illustrations of different contributory factors to role boundaries

Individual factors

Nurse's communication skills: 'The nurse who approached me was a Polish lady whose English communication was not brilliant and she seemed to think I was a doctor… approaching me for things beyond the scope of my abilities/responsibilities.'

Peta, female, year 5, medical student, UK

Doctor's perspectives about nurses: 'Doctor X stated that I was an embarrassment to my medical school and that I should be ashamed of my performance… he proceeded to say that my performance was, quote, "worse than a lay person, no, worse than a nurse", which is derogatory of nurses.'

Stella, female, year 5, medical student, UK

Interpersonal factors

Phlebotomist's lack of trust in student competence: 'When taking blood supervised by an F2 (PGY2 doctor), a phlebotomist shouted across the corridor I was doing it wrong in front of all staff and patients.'

Mel, female, year 5, medical student, UK

Surgeon's lack of trust in nurse competence: 'The nurse did not have a piece of equipment so he (consultant surgeon) had to ask for it, the surgeon flipped and started shouting that she should know what he needs and when and have it ready instantly.'

Tess, female, year 4, medical student, UK

Structural factors

Cultural norms: 'Poor hand washing practice is something I've observed on a number of placements, with doctors being the most negligent. Although sometimes hand washing facilities aren't always [there], alcohol gel typically is and should be used.'

Steph, female, year 3, physiotherapy student, UK

Hierarchy: 'I was in neurosurgery and one patient had a final diagnosis [cancer] and he wasn't aware of it… Three or four or five days we were actually treating him without actually telling him [he had a couple of months to live at most]… So it was a dilemma, how can you be an advocate for your patient when your patient doesn't even know… you just have to wait for the consultant to turn up and have a chat with your patient… its back to hierarchy in a way.'

Grace, female, year 3, physiotherapy student, UK

What are Students' Reactions and Actions in the Face of Interprofessional Dilemmas?

As with professionalism dilemmas occurring *within* the professions (outlined in Chapters 5–10), interprofessional dilemmas (i.e. ones involving interactions between multiple different healthcare professionals) were often recounted with negative emotional talk such as 'sick', 'hard', 'annoyed', 'offended', 'concerned', 'cruel' and 'badly', illustrating how emotionally difficult it could be for healthcare students to be caught up in interprofessional conflict. Not only did students narrate finding interprofessional conflicts challenging, but they also reported discontent around their own lack of action in the face of interprofessional dilemmas. In several of the narratives presented in this chapter, healthcare students did not directly challenge perpetrators (see Catriona's narrative at the start of the chapter, plus narrative 2, Box 12.6 and narratives 3 and 7, Box 12.7), giving numerous reasons for their inaction: (1) opinions that students would not be believed against the word of qualified healthcare professionals; (2) reluctance to offend the perpetrators; (3) avoidance of receiving bad grades from perpetrators; and (4) general lack of confidence to challenge. However, by failing to challenge, interprofessional conflicts tended to be unresolved, leaving students confused about the perspectives and decisions of other healthcare professionals. This also led students to label other healthcare professionals as 'unprofessional', resulting in them avoiding other healthcare professionals and places (such as wards) where interprofessional conflicts took place. Finally, students sometimes developed the belief that doctors and nurses inherently dislike each other.

However, other students (e.g. narrative 1, Box 12.6, and narratives 1 and 2, Box 12.7) did narrate challenging perpetrators of interprofessional lapses. While they sometimes narrated how 'hard' it was to challenge (narrative 1, Box 12.7), they often spoke positively about doing so, feeling 'glad' (narrative 1, Box 12.6), and they liked that they had done the 'correct' thing (narrative 4, Box 12.7). Interestingly, students who challenged sometimes did so because they did not want to appear complicit in the lapses of their own professional group, because they thought that healthcare professionals had more respect for students who did challenge, that students needed to challenge because of their vital role in service improvement and because students needed to do the right thing by patients. In the following narrative, Tina, a physiotherapy student explains how she disagreed with the medical team's management plan to discharge an elderly, frail patient, with positive outcomes (see Box 12.9).

Box 12.9 'From a physio point of view I didn't feel they were ready to be discharged'

I was on a placement and… and I read in the medical notes that the nurse and the medical staff wanted to discharge this patient but… from a physio point of view I didn't feel they were ready to be discharged and I think I ended up treating the patient just after the ward round one day or just before a ward round and then they, the doctors came round and he was sort of the consultant and registrar and all his minions behind him… and… he was just sort of asking me about the patient and how she's doing and you know sort of said, "Oh, you know, she's ready to be discharged", and I thought… "Do I just go along with it because I am just a student and (sighs) my opinion may not be valued as much and they

> may just go ahead and discharge them anyway or do I sort of say something' and I ended up, you know, saying, "Oh, in my opinion she's not ready to be discharged, I think we should keep her a few more days until you know she's ready" and… he was, "Oh no that's fine, she can stay as long as she wants"… it was really positive…'
>
> Tina, female, year 3, physiotherapy student, UK

How can Interprofessional Conflict be Managed?

We know that interprofessional conflict can be associated with poor educational experiences, personal stress for learners, and more significant medical errors and adverse patient outcomes (see Chapter 7).[20,33] For example, the 187 residents reporting conflict with two or more professionals on a national survey reported serious medical error rates of 51% and 16% for adverse patient outcomes.[33] We have seen such interplays between interprofessional conflict and patient safety dilemmas earlier in this book (see Box 7.7). Therefore, the management of interprofessional conflict is crucial for maintaining safe and effective healthcare, for patients and staff alike.

Preventing Interprofessional Conflict?

Preventing conflict is not always possible or desirable. Indeed, interprofessional conflict within the healthcare workplace is 'normal' and not always negative, as conflict can be productive: it can help surface problems, ensure better decision-making, facilitate change, improve quality, and so on.[20,34] However, in terms of preventing destructive conflict, a potential strategy is thought to be learners developing their 'dual' identities, that is, their professional *and* interprofessional identities (see Box 12.10).[35,36] We see this development as students improving their awareness of their complex multiple identities (e.g. as professional *and* interprofessional healthcare team member) and how these multiple identities interrelate over the course of their undergraduate and postgraduate education.[37,38]

While stage theories can oversimplify complex social processes involved in human development,[39] Khalili *et al.*[35] suggests that the development of dual professional *and* interprofessional identities occurs through a three-stage process after learners have developed their professional identities. In the first stage, it is important to break down any barriers between professions, such as challenging students' pre-existing views and stereotypes about other professions through interprofessional interactions, including debate and discussion. In the second stage, interprofessional role learning and collaboration is important in order for students to better understand one another's roles, knowledge, skills and values. In the final stage, students are thought to develop dual identities involving both a sense of belonging to their own profession and to interprofessional healthcare teams.[35] Some identity theories, for example, suggest that an individual's professional identity (e.g. 'physiotherapist'), may be completely embedded in other identities (e.g. 'allied healthcare professional', 'healthcare professional', 'interprofessional team member'), with one identity gaining dominance over another depending on the context.[37] For example, in a professional supervisory encounter, a physiotherapy teacher may foreground their dominant 'physiotherapist' identity, whereas in a multidisciplinary team meeting, he or she might foreground a dominant 'interprofessional healthcare team member' identity.

Box 12.10 Information: professional and interprofessional identities

Several authors talk about healthcare professionals needing to possess 'dual' professional identities, that is, professional *and* interprofessional identities.[35,36,40]

- **Professional identity:** identification with your own professional group (e.g. doctor), leading individuals to view their own profession (e.g. medicine) as different to or special in comparison with other professions (e.g. nursing).[35]
- **Interprofessional identity:** identification with the wider interprofessional group (e.g. healthcare professionals) with whom you work as part of an interprofessional team, leading individuals to view the broader interprofessional healthcare team as belonging to the same group (in-group).[35]

Box 12.11 Stop and do: reflect on and discuss conflict management styles within the narratives

- Re-read the seven narratives about role boundary dilemmas in Box 12.7.
- What conflict management styles (if any) do you think are articulated within these narratives?
- Which ones do you think are effective and why? Which are ineffective and why?
- Which conflict management styles might have been more appropriate within the context of each narrative and why? How might that style have been achieved?
- Discuss your thoughts with your peers.

Managing Interprofessional Conflict

In Chapter 9, in summarizing bullying prevention and management strategies at the individual, relationship and organizational levels, we touched on conflict management training at the interpersonal level (see Box 9.13). Different conflict management styles may be required for different conflicts, although there is little evidence identifying which styles are appropriate for which conflicts.[41] Conflict management styles, according to the Thomas-Kilmann Conflict Mode Instrument (TKI), can include competing (trying to satisfy one's own concerns over another's expense), accommodating (satisfying the other's concerns at the expense of oneself), avoiding (side-stepping the conflict), collaborating (finding a solution that satisfies everyone's concerns fully) and/or compromising (finding a solution that partly satisfies everyone's concerns).[42] We can see some of these styles at work within the narratives already presented in this chapter (see Box 12.7). Work through Box 12.11 to identify any conflict management styles exhibited in students' narratives.

As part of their conflict resolution training with healthcare professionals in Canada, Zweibel *et al.*[34] reported on features of their workshop that were perceived to be positive by their workshop participants: (1) reframing conflict as potentially positive; (2) taking a systematic and thoughtful approach to analysing conflict; (3) using 'interest analysis' to better understand others' perspectives, needs and concerns; (4) understanding better own conflict management styles; and (5) better communication through active listening and avoiding negative trigger words like 'but', 'never', 'always'. Finally, as suggested by the Canadian National Interprofessional Competency Framework,[43] we also recommend that students think about how patients can be involved in helping to resolve interprofessional conflicts. For example, thinking about the narrative presented in Box 12.9 about discharge planning, think about how a simple act of asking the patient whether she felt ready to be discharged could have resolved any interprofessional conflict.

Before we summarize this chapter, it is worth saying that we have many examples in our data of students receiving support, mentorship and supervision from other healthcare professionals, as has been illustrated in other studies.[10,21,44] While several students talked about hateful nurse-doctor relationships (see Catriona's narrative at the start of this chapter), healthcare professionals from different professions to students often helped students manage conflict. For example, we had multiple examples from medical students of being aided by nurses, with nurses sometimes helping students to carry out their clinical tasks, and other times helping students who were abused by patients or senior medical colleagues: 'He stood there and shouted at me in front of everyone until a nurse came and rescued me' (Prudence, female, year 4, medical student, UK). Furthermore, we had numerous examples of medical students being simultaneously horrified by the behaviour of their senior medical colleagues towards patients and impressed by the good work of nurses to protect and comfort patients: 'The nurses were very good at checking the patient was okay' (Debra, female, year 5, medical student, UK). It is therefore prudent for healthcare students to invest time and energy in getting to know other healthcare professionals, not only to help them manage their professional and interprofessional identities, but also to help them manage conflicts both intra- and interprofessionally.

Chapter Summary

This chapter has provided an overview of the different roles and education of diverse healthcare professionals. It provides a comparison of the professionalism dilemmas experienced by different healthcare students, including key variations based on roles and education. We have learnt that healthcare students experience interprofessional dilemmas involving hierarchies, roles and conflicts and we have discussed how those dilemmas come about. We have also talked about how learners react to interprofessional dilemmas and how interprofessional conflict can be managed. The key take-home messages for this chapter are summarized in Box 12.12, with suggestions for small group discussions in Box 12.13 and reflective exercises in Box 12.14. Finally, Box 12.15 outlines some recommended reading.

Box 12.12 Chapter summary points

- Different healthcare professionals have different roles and education but roles are increasingly flexible
- Similarities but also some differences exist across healthcare learners in terms of the professionalism dilemmas they experience
- Healthcare students experience a range of interprofessional dilemmas involving hierarchies, roles and conflict
- Healthcare students and trainees need to develop their own ways for managing interprofessional conflict

---

Box 12.13 Chapter discussion points

- Think about your workplace learning experiences with other healthcare professionals. How have those interactions facilitated or hindered your learning?
- Think of positive interprofessional experiences you have directly experienced or witnessed in the healthcare workplace. Share your experiences with your colleagues and explain what it was about those experiences that made them positive.
- To what extent are you aware of your developing multiple professional identities as both a professional (e.g. dentist, doctor, nurse, pharmacist, physiotherapist), as well as your interprofessional identity (e.g. as interprofessional healthcare team member)?

Box 12.14 Chapter learning activity

- Many of the interprofessional dilemmas in our research involve healthcare assistants (e.g. see narrative 7, Box 12.7). Sometimes healthcare students recounted dilemmas from a time where they were themselves HCAs.
- Read the paper by Lloyd *et al.*[45] about healthcare assistant roles/identities.
- Thinking about the issues raised in this paper, put yourself into the shoes of the HCA in the narrative on 'lack of communication' (narrative 7, Box 12.7).
- Given HCAs' constant engagement with direct patient care, how might healthcare professionals better interact with HCAs for the good of the patient?

Box 12.15 Chapter recommended reading

Burford B, Morrow G, Morrison J, Baldauf B, Spencer J, Johnson N. Newly qualified doctors' perceptions of informal learning from nurses: implications for interprofessional education and practice. *Journal of Interprofessional Care* 2013; 25(5):394–400.

Khalili H, Orchard C, Laschinger HK, Farah R. An interprofessional socialization framework for developing an interprofessional identity among health professions students. *Journal of Interprofessional Care* 2013;27(6):448–453.

Lloyd JV, Schneider J, Scales K, Bailey S, Jones R. Ingroup identity as an obstacle to effective multiprofessional and interprofessional teamwork: findings from an ethnographic study of healthcare assistants in dementia care. *Journal of Interprofessional Care* 2011;25:345–351.

References

1 Apesoa-Varano EC. Interprofessional conflict and repair: a study of boundary work in the hospital. *Sociological Perspectives* 2013;56(3):327–349.

2 Rees CE, Monrouxe LV, Ajjawi R. Professionalism in workplace learning: understanding interprofessional dilemmas through healthcare student narratives. In D Jindal-Snape, EFS Hannah (Eds) *Exploring the Dynamics of Personal, Professional and Interprofessional Ethics*. Bristol: Policy Press, 2013: pp. 295–310.

3 Centre for Advancement of Interprofessional Education (CAIPE). *Definition of Interprofessional Education* (revised), 2002, http://caipe.org.uk. (Accessed 2 December 2016).

4 Barr H. *Interprofessional Education – a Definition*. London: CAIPE Bulletin No. 13,1997.

5 Rees CE, Knight LV, Wilkinson CE. 'User involvement is a sine qua non, almost, in medical education': learning with rather than just about health and social care service users. *Advances in Health Sciences Education* 2007;12(3):359–390.

6 Sims D. Reconstructing professional identity for professional and interprofessional practice: a mixed methods study of joint training programmes in learning disability nursing and social work. *Journal of Interprofessional Care* 2011;25:265–271.

7 Michalec B, Hafferty FW. Role theory and the practice of interprofessional education: a critical appraisal and a call to sociologists. *Social Theory & Health* 2015;13(2):180–201.

8 Kopelman LM. What is unique about the doctor and patient medical encounter? A moral and economic perspective. *The American Journal of Bioethics* 2006;6(2):85–88.

9 Schwartz SJ, Luyckx K, Vignoles VL. *Handbook of Identity Theory and Research*. New York, USA: Springer, 2011.

10 Burford B, Morrow G, Morrison J, Baldauf B, Spencer J, Johnson N, *et al*. Newly qualified doctors' perceptions of informal learning from nurses: implications for interprofessional education and practice. *Journal of Interprofessional Care* 2013;25(5):394–400.

11 Whitehead C. The doctor dilemma in interprofessional education and care: how and why will physicians collaborate? *Medical Education* 2007;41:1010–1016.

12 Lingard L, Vanstone M, Durrant M, Fleming-Carroll B, Lowe M, Rashotte J, *et al*. Conflicting messages: examining the dynamics of leadership on interprofessional teams. *Academic Medicine* 2012;87(12):1762–1767.

13 Nugus P, Greenfield D, Travaglia J, Westbrook J, Braithewaite J. How and where clinicians exercise power: interprofessional relations in health care. *Social Science & Medicine* 2010;71:898–909.

14 Brown J, Lewis L, Ellis K, Stewart M, Freeman TR, Kasperski MJ. Conflict on interprofessional primary health care teams – can it be resolved? *Journal of Interprofessional Care* 2011;25:4–10.

15 Wright A, Hawkes G, Baker B, Lindqvist SM. Reflections and umprompted observations by healthcare students of an interprofessional shadowing visit. *Journal of Interprofessional Care* 2012;26:305–311.

16 King N, Ross A. Professional identities and interprofessional relations: evaluation of collaborative community schemes. *Social Work in Health Care* 2003;38(2):51–72.

17 Thistlethwaite J. Hidden amongst us: the language of inter- and outer-professional identity and collaboration. In FW Hafferty, JF O'Donnell (Eds) *The Hidden Curriculum in Health*

Professional Education. Dartmouth, USA: University Press of New England, 2014: pp.158–168.

18 Baker L, Egan-Lee E, Martimianakis MA, Reeves S. Relationships of power: implications for interprofessional education. *Journal of Interprofessional Care* 2011;25:98–104.

19 Robinson SG. The unique work of nursing. *Nursing* 2013;March:42–43.

20 Brinkert R. A literature review of conflict communication causes, costs, benefits and interventions in nursing. *Journal of Nursing Management* 2010;18:145–156.

21 Tamuz M, Giardina TD, Thomas EJ, Menon S, Singh H. Rethinking resident supervision to improve safety: from hierarchical to interprofessional models. *Journal of Hospital Medicine* 2011;6(8):448–456.

22 Lingard L, McDougall A, Levstik M, Chandok N, Spafford MM, Schryer C. Representing complexity well: a story about teamwork, with implications for how we teach collaboration. *Medical Education* 2012;46:869–877.

23 Muller-Juge V, Cullati S, Blondon KS, Hudelson P, Maitre F, Vu NV, *et al*. Interprofessional collaboration on an internal medicine ward: role perceptions and expectations among nurses and residents. *PLOS One* 2013;8(2):e57570. doi:10.1371/journal.pone.0057570.

24 Monrouxe LV, Rees CE, Endacott R, Ternan E. 'Even now it makes me angry': healthcare students' professionalism dilemma narratives. *Medical Education* 2014;48:502–517.

25 Monrouxe LV, Rees CE, Dennis A, Wells S. Professionalism dilemmas, moral distress and the healthcare student: insights from two online UK-wide questionnaire studies. *British Medical Journal Open* 2015;5:e007518. doi:10.1136/bmjopen-2014-007518.

26 Rees CE, Monrouxe LV, McDonald LA. My mentor kicked a dying woman's bed: analysing UK nursing students' most memorable professionalism dilemmas. *Journal of Advanced Nursing* 2015;71(1):169–180.

27 Norredam M, Album D. Prestige and its significance for medical specialties and diseases. *Scandinavian Journal of Public Health* 2007;35:655–661.

28 Eisler R, Potter T. Breaking down the hierarchies. *Nursing Management* 2014;21(5):12. doi:10.7748.nm.21.5.12.s13.

29 DeJesse LD, Zelman DC. Promoting optimal collaboration between mental health providers and nutritionists in the treatment of eating disorders. *Eating Disorders* 2013;21:185–205.

30 Rees CE, Knight LV, Wilkinson CE. 'Doctors being up there and we being down here': a metaphorical analysis of talk about student/doctor-patient relationships. *Social Science & Medicine* 2007;65(4):725–737.

31 Rees CE, Knight LV, Cleland JA. Medical educators' metaphoric talk about their assessment relationship with students: 'You don't want to sort of be the one who sticks the knife in them'. *Assessment & Evaluation in Higher Education* 2009;34(4):455–467.

32 MacNaughton K, Chreim S, Bourgeault IL. Role construction and boundaries in interprofessional primary health care teams: a qualitative study. *BioMed Central Health Services Research* 2013;13:486; https://bmchealthservres.biomedcentral.com/articles/10.1186/1472-6963-13-486 (Accessed 2 December 2016).

33 Baldwin DC, Daugherty SR. Interprofessional conflict and medical errors: results of a national multi-specialty survey of hospital residents in the US. *Journal of Interprofessional Care* 2008;22(6):573–586.

34 Zweibel EB, Goldstein R, Manwaring JA, Marks MB. What sticks: how medical residents and academic care faculty transfer conflict resolution training from the workshop to the workplace. *Conflict Resolution Quarterly* 2008;25(3):321–350.

35 Khalili H, Orchard C, Laschinger HK, Farah R. An interprofessional socialization framework for developing an interprofessional identity among health professions students. *Journal of Interprofessional Care* 2013;27(6):448–453.

36 Thistlethwaite JE, Kumar K, Roberts C. Becoming interprofessional: professional identity formation in the health professions. In RL Cruess, SR Cruess, Y Steinert (Eds) *Teaching Medical Professionalism*, 2nd Edition. Cambridge, USA: Cambridge University Press, 2016: pp.140–154.

37 Roccas S, Brewer MB. Social identity complexity. *Personality and Social Psychology Review* 2002;6(2):88–106.

38 Walsh CL, Gordon MF, Marshall M, Wilson F, Hunt T. Interprofessional capability: a developing framework for interprofessional education. *Nurse Education in Practice* 2005;5:230–237.

39 Rees CE. Proto-professionalism and the three questions about development. *Medical Education* 2005;39:7–11.

40 Clouder DL, Davies B, Sams M, McFarland L. 'Understanding where you're coming from': discovering an [inter]professional identity through becoming a peer facilitator. *Journal of Interprofessional Care* 2012;26:459–464.

41 Leskell J, Gardulf A, Nilsson J, Lepp M. Self-reported conflict management competence among nursing students on the point of graduating and registered nurses with professional experience. *Journal of Nursing Education & Practice* 2015;5(8):82–89.

42 Kilmann TK. *Thomas-Kilmann Conflict Mode Instrument*. Mountain View, CA: CPP Inc, 2007.

43 Canadian Interprofessional Health Collaborative. *A National Interprofessional Competency Framework*. University of British Columbia, Vancouver: Canadian Interprofessional Health Collaborative, 2010, http://www.cihc.ca/files/CIHC_IPCompetencies_Feb1210.pdf (Accessed 2 December 2016).

44 Mattick K, Kelly N, Rees CE. A window into the lives of junior doctors: narrative interviews exploring antimicrobial prescribing experiences. *Journal of Antimicrobial Chemotherapy* 2014;69(8):2274–2283.

45 Lloyd JV, Schneider J, Scales K, Bailey S, Jones R. Ingroup identity as an obstacle to effective multiprofessional and interprofessional teamwork: findings from an ethnographic study of healthcare assistants in dementia care. *Journal of Interprofessional Care* 2011;25:345–251.

13

Conclusions

When we set out on this book-writing journey, we wanted to provide healthcare students, trainees and educators with a unique type of 'core textbook' on healthcare professionalism: A book that focuses on students' and trainees' experiences, that links theory with practice, that draws on our own personal and professional lives in order to offer solutions – rather than mere descriptions – to have a real impact on the professional practice of healthcare students and professionals. So, by drawing on thousands of professionalism dilemma narratives across our decade-long research programme, alongside current evidence in the field, we hoped to unpack wider issues facing today's healthcare learners as they become tomorrow's healthcare practitioners. In this concluding chapter, we discuss in more detail two crosscutting themes that permeate our book: the first comprises interrelated constructs of power, hierarchy, conformity and resistance; the second comprises those of negative emotions, empathy and moral distress. We then take a forward-focused look at the implications of our research on future education, training and practice, and further research on professionalism education. Finally, we end this concluding chapter with our own personal reflections on the processes of undertaking this research; specifically considering how we shaped the research, and in turn, how it shaped us.

Power, Hierarchy, Conformity and Resistance

'As a relationship amongst two or more persons, power relies upon a subordinate's participation and response.'[1 p. 1333]

The first of our crosscutting themes focuses on power and related issues of hierarchy, conformity and resistance. The French philosopher, Michel Foucault, asserts that 'power is everywhere'.[2] By this he means that power is the interactional force that we attempt to exert towards each other as we negotiate our way through life. Power is therefore intertwined with the hierarchical nature of healthcare environments (see Chapters 9 and 12 for further details). Furthermore, where there is power, there is also compliance or resistance to those enacting power. Such compliance and resistance in turn further impacts upon this repetitive and everyday use of power. So power is inevitable, and rather than being possessed by individuals, it is relational, moving between

Healthcare Professionalism: Improving Practice through Reflections on Workplace Dilemmas, First Edition.
Lynn V. Monrouxe and Charlotte E. Rees.
© 2017 John Wiley & Sons Ltd. Published 2017 by John Wiley & Sons Ltd.

people as they get on with their daily business. Power also operates in hidden (latent) ways through institutions, architecture and symbols (see Chapter 3). As such, in many ways power is frequently *routinized*, often accepted as an inevitable force that works upon us, rather than within us.[1]

As we have seen across Chapters 2–12 of this book, the issue of power in all its forms permeates through the defining, teaching and assessing of professionalism (Chapters 2–4) and across each and every dilemma narrative as students and trainees navigate their ways through workplace learning (Chapters 5–12). So, professionalism is defined as contextual and hierarchical (Chapter 2). Professionalism is frequently taught and assessed via powerful others within an environment that inculcates the acceptance and reinforcement of traditional professional and interprofessional hierarchies whereby individuals are positioned at various levels within their chosen profession and across professions (Chapters 3, 4, 9 and 12). Power is discussed openly by healthcare learners in the context of student abuse, whereby the *power games* played by those in superordinate positions can lead to discrimination and harassment in the workplace (Chapter 9). Furthermore, the strong hierarchical culture has been identified as acting as a *latent* factor contributing to patient consent, patient safety and patient dignity-related professionalism dilemmas (Chapters 6–8). Here, power relations between students and patients, healthcare practitioners and patients, and students and healthcare practitioners can lead to the instigation and maintenance of consent, safety and dignity violations.

Due to the relational nature of power, with it moving between people and not residing at any one level, across our chapters we have seen numerous examples of situations in which students and trainees highlight their resistance to professionalism lapses, including direct and indirect verbal and bodily challenges and reporting perpetrators. In this way, rather than thinking of power as an inevitable and hierarchical force, power is used *productively*.[2,3] Moreover, it is through these narrated acts of resistance[4] that healthcare students and trainees can establish their professional identities within a strong moral framework (Chapters 2 and 5).

However, throughout this book we have also seen numerous examples of healthcare learners in a position of powerlessness, going along with the hierarchical status quo and conforming to a healthcare culture accepting of professionalism lapses. But these *conformity narratives* not only reveal a stark recognition of existing power relations, they also reveal how learners' understandings of and reactions to such forces of power are far from straightforward. Rather than being fully socialized into accepting existing power relations,[1] we often witness students' personal *desires* to act professionally, resulting in emotional distress when they do not. As such, the judgement of whether to resist or comply is an emotionally charged one, in which the empathy felt for the recipient of the professionalism lapses (often the patient) is balanced by the perceived consequences of resisting or complying.[5]

Negative Emotions, Empathy and Moral Distress

The narratives presented in the chapters of this book are littered with negative emotional talk. Students commonly reported being negatively affected by others' professionalism lapses, sometimes even weeping (see the opening narrative to this book in

Chapter 1), or narrating their emotional trauma due to the harsh treatment patients received at the hands of uncaring healthcare students and professionals (e.g. Chapters 6–8), thereby revealing narrators' empathic connection with patients.[6–8] Sometimes emotions comprised reasonably low levels of distress, for example 'uncomfortable' and 'awkward' feelings were common for learners as they witnessed or breached patient consent (Chapter 6). At other times, more powerful emotions were narrated, including feelings of 'anger', 'fear', 'distress', 'shock', 'disgust', 'stress', 'irritation', 'sadness' and 'shame': words frequently appearing in narratives about patient safety and patient-dignity related professionalism dilemmas (Chapters 7–8). Further, learners occasionally reported the need to vent their emotions, sometimes online, leading to e-professionalism dilemmas (Chapter 10).

Although we are mindful that sharing difficult experiences encountered during students' workplace learning were often deeply upsetting for our research participants, we found this heartening, as well as a cause for concern (due to their well-being). Contrary to previous reports, from the perspective of students' narratives, alongside their self-reported moral distress, we saw no evidence in our data that healthcare students lost their empathy over time.[8] The thousands of students taking part in our studies typically remained empathically connected to the patients they met as part of their healthcare education. What is absent across the narratives presented in this book, however, is a consideration of the emotional state of their senior clinical teachers, who were often the instigators or perpetrators of the professionalism dilemmas and lapses narrated. So we have reports of clinical educators and educational supervisors shouting and swearing–thus displays of emotional states–and we note a distinct lack of empathic positioning of the narrators towards their senior clinical teachers. Rather, we see a *them and us* form of narrative in which learners position themselves positively as they draw on various character tropes including *patient-advocate, hero* and *victim*. By contrast, their clinical teachers are often positioned more negatively, drawing on the character tropes of *neglectful caregiver, bully, villain* and so on.[9]

Looking Forward: Education, Training and Practice

From these two crosscutting themes, we now consider where to go from here. In this section we now turn to four key areas for education, training and practice that have the potential to impact on the development towards a more caring and compassionate healthcare workplace environment for the benefit of patients, learners and healthcare professionals alike: resistance, emotional regulation, interprofessional education and leadership. Taken together these aspects should help to facilitate a shared perception of personal, interpersonal and organizational ethical practice by taking both bottom-up and top-down approaches towards the development of a strong ethical climate for healthcare learning and practice.[10]

Resistance
Relating to both crosscutting themes above is the *dilemma*: that is, the difficult judgement narrated by most of our study participants around whether to go along with or resist professionalism lapses. While healthcare learners in our study were subject to formal professionalism curricula in their various institutions, to our knowledge, none

received any significant formal education on how to resist in the face of professionalism dilemmas. Yet learners seemed to develop their own ways of dealing with these issues through their employment of various direct and indirect acts of resistance including: direct verbal acts (e.g. verbally challenging perpetrators), directly raising concerns about perpetrators, indirect verbal acts (e.g. soft correction), indirect bodily acts (e.g. openly washing hands when others fail to adhere to hygiene regulations), withdrawing verbally or emotionally, direct bodily acts (e.g. removing oneself from the situation) and debriefing from professionalism dilemmas (e.g. with peers for social support).[11] Rather than leave these processes to chance, we believe that students and trainees should be taught explicitly a range of low-risk resistance strategies through active teaching methods – such as rehearsing resistance via role-play simulations. We belief that such learning activities should facilitate learners' personal confidence and empowerment, thereby enabling them to feel more in control of their actions. Indeed, throughout this book we see examples of narrators reporting a sense of achievement and pride when they do resist professionalism lapses, alongside a stronger sense of commitment to their professional identity.

Emotional regulation

Related to the second crosscutting theme above, we believe that educating healthcare learners and practitioners to regulate their emotions is another way of moving things forward positively in terms of healthcare professionalism. Indeed, negative emotion left unchecked can lead to substantial ill-health and even suicide.[12] However, the use of certain emotion regulation strategies has been shown to be detrimental for personal health and interpersonal rapport building (e.g. suppression results in increased sympathetic nervous system arousal, coronary heart disease, along with reduced rapport and inhibited relationship formation).[13,14] Emotion regulation can be seen as a subset of resilience training.[15] Given that many healthcare learners report experiencing a range of negative emotional reactions during their workplace learning,[16] and that some report such emotions lasting many months and even years,[7,8] an understanding of how best to regulate one's emotions will be greatly beneficial. Furthermore, we believe that failure to regulate emotions – such as venting anger, anxiety or frustrations during stressful events – potentially leads to instances of workplace abuse (Chapter 9). Thus we can understand some of the reported actions by senior healthcare professionals as situations in which they failed to successfully regulate their emotions. Indeed, workplace abuse is not only a dignity at work issue but also a patient-safety issue, and we believe that incorporating emotion regulation training within continuing professional development to be an important way forward for improved workplace dignity, clinician well-being and patient care.

Interprofessional education

We think another crucial way forward is through interprofessional education (IPE) in which a range of healthcare learner groups learn with, from and about one another (see Chapter 12).[17,18] We think there is no better place for IPE to occur than within professionalism education as we know how many professionalism dilemmas crosscut healthcare professional boundaries. Furthermore, having an opportunity to learn more about one's own and others' roles will facilitate students' abilities to take on one another's perspectives. Such perspective-taking has been shown to be highly efficacious in removing stereotyped thinking,[19] and as such learners' active engagement within

IPE should help resolve common role boundary-related interprofessional dilemmas. Although IPE can be relatively expensive to arrange, educators can build on opportunities within educational institutions that already have multiple healthcare professional education courses running alongside one another. Furthermore, we suggest IPE learning takes place in small group settings to facilitate teamwork and effective communication between healthcare student groups. In such settings, students should be able to feel relatively safe to share their authentic personal experiences around professionalism dilemmas they have experienced. We hope that this book will facilitate students' frank and open sharing within interprofessional small groups so that everyone can bear witness to, and dwell in, each other's viewpoints and experiences. Indeed, research has demonstrated that when successful, IPE not only enables students' understanding of other healthcare professional's roles but also of their own professional identity and how each fits within the healthcare team, ultimately leading to improvements in patient care.[20,21]

Leadership

As evidenced by the narratives across this book, the healthcare workplace all too often displays evidence of a weak ethical climate in which there is low member agreement about appropriate ethical practice and how ethical issues should be managed.[10,22] Thus, we have seen time and again in this book how the mere existence of regulatory policy and laws of the state are insufficient in preventing professionalism dilemmas and lapses: ethical leaders who are committed towards preserving others' dignity and human rights are required to develop and shape organizational values, to communicate those values through their role-modelling practices, as well as facilitating the good practices of others in authority. Leaders should also provide opportunities for learners and healthcare professionals to safely raise their concerns about dubious workplace practices without fear of admonishment or retribution. Together with the bottom-up approach of developing healthcare learners' abilities to manage professionalism dilemmas ethically and with emotional sensitivity, this top-down ethical leadership should facilitate the development of a strong ethical workplace climate in which there is high-consensus regarding the *right thing* to do.[10]

Looking Forward: Research

Having discussed *what next* for education, training and practice, we now turn our attention to consider *what next* for research. We have reported copious narratives by healthcare learners regarding professionalism dilemmas encountered by them during workplace learning, originating from our ten-year research programme. However, as we have seen, important viewpoints are missing. So, although the original idea of investigating these highly emotional situations came from our study of patient involvement in medical education,[23–25] so far patients' voices are mainly represented through students' voices in this body of research. Likewise, we also fail to give voice to those who are commonly placed in the role of the perpetrator. The healthcare educators and practitioners have all too often been cast in the roles of *villains, bullies, neglectful caregivers* and *dictators*. We therefore acknowledge these omissions and call for further research to examine professionalism dilemmas from the much-needed perspectives of these important stakeholders. Indeed, as we already highlight at the beginning of this chapter, most healthcare professionals are hard-working patient-centred professionals who are just as appalled by the events narrated in this book as we are. Many are also constrained by the high-pressured and poorly-staffed workplace cultures, making it hard for them to raise concerns about their colleagues behaviours, so can be seen as victims themselves.

In addition to calling for further research from healthcare professionals and patients, we also believe that further research across different healthcare and cultural groups would be advantageous. So far our investigation of professionalism dilemmas has been limited to five healthcare professional student groups (dentistry, medicine, nursing, pharmacy and physiotherapy) and four countries (Australia, Taiwan, Sri-Lanka and the UK, which itself comprises the four countries of England, Scotland, Wales and Northern Ireland). As such there is a great deal of scope to study a wider range of healthcare professional groups across a greater number of countries. An understanding of a greater breadth of healthcare professional groups and countries would be useful to learners and educators within cultural settings different to those focused on in this book. For example, individuals with different cultures express emotions differently and respond to power hierarchies differently.[26] Such information would also be of interest to healthcare educators and employers who work cross-culturally, such as situations where trainees move to different countries to complete their training or students learn overseas as part of their electives.[27,28]

Finally, in terms of further research, we turn to consider the question of *who* should instigate and carry out this work. Across the ten years of our research programme specifically investigating professionalism dilemmas, along with other interrelated research projects in which these issues have serendipitously arisen, we have been fortunate to work with a wide range of research colleagues: nursing, medical, pharmacy, dental and physiotherapy educators alongside medical and dental students (see our acknowledgements earlier in this book). Our work is therefore truly interdisciplinary. We urge future ventures to continue in this vein, building research teams across a range of healthcare professional groups and including students as collaborative partners. Furthermore, we urge students themselves to take the lead. To develop and conduct a range of inquiries to fit within their courses, including audits, evaluations and research projects related to topics covered in this book. As today's healthcare students are tomorrow's practitioners and leaders, student engagement with such activities is the first step towards building ethical leadership for tomorrow and a strong personal commitment to changing the system. Indeed, we have had numerous reports from our student research colleagues who, by virtue of working with us on this data, have felt empowered to take a strong moral stand in the face of their own professionalism dilemmas going forward, something they felt would not have happened had they not collaborated with us. In essence, their engagement with this programme of research has helped to facilitate the development of their identities as patient-centred professionals.

Looking Back: Researcher Reflexivity

We now come to the end of this book. Having spent time discussing our hopes for the future, we now take a moment to look back and reflect. How have we, as women and as social scientists working in healthcare-related contexts, shaped this research? And how, in turn, have we been shaped *by* this research?

In terms of how we have shaped this research, from the outset we aimed to bring a strong theoretical basis to this work. We made a conscious decision to focus on narratives of lived experiences, rather than merely exploring people's attitudes. By working with these personal, and sometimes quite harrowing stories, we have been able to draw on our knowledge of social science theory to ask a range of questions around both *what* is narrated and *how*. So we have sometimes examined relatively *off piste* questions such as how participants have used laughter to cope with the act of narrating difficult events, as well as to cope with the difficult event itself; how participants distance themselves from their professionalism lapses through their explanations; how they construct their moral identities through narrative acts; and how they construct themselves and others by drawing on numerous story plots and character tropes often found in wider societal discourses.[7,9,22,29] In addition to our identities as social science researchers, we also believe that our identities as women have shaped the course of our research. For example, the questions we have explored around student abuse[30,31] – including sexual harassment and gender discrimination – have been driven by our personal experiences, along with commitments to equality and diversity. Furthermore, questions related to intimate examinations being conducted without valid consent were also partly influenced by our own gendered identities and experiences of intimate examinations as patients.[22]

It is fair to say that over the past ten years, our engagement with this international and interdisciplinary programme of work has impacted on us personally in a multitude of ways. Narrative interviewing demands that we listen, we witness, we engage with the narrator and later, we report. At the beginning of our research programme, narrative after narrative brought forth a range of emotions within us: disbelief, shock, anger, sadness and sometimes even excitement as we realized that we could report these stories to the educational community and people would have to listen. But as time went on we seemed to become socialized into the dilemmas – a *normalizing* process had begun: another student being abused, another coerced examination, another patient's dignity violated, another ... mirroring students who experience these instances time and again, we became *unshockable*. Or so we thought. Moving our research across country and healthcare student group boundaries brought back the shock-factor, and once again our emotions flowed. As time went on we began to learn more about issues such as equality and diversity, the shifting nature of workplace culture and the importance of leadership. As time went on we began to move into leadership positions ourselves. These moves have enabled us to practise lessons learned from engaging with this research area; like our student research colleagues we have become more emboldened to speak out.

Coda

In this chapter we have considered the crosscutting themes of power and emotion alongside the *what next* for education and research. We have also taken a moment to reflect on how we have affected the research and been affected by it. We started our book by giving voice to Fiona, who shared a harrowing colonoscopy narrative with us that made us both cry. Here, we end our book giving voice to Stuart, another Australian medical student, whose intimate examination narrative has given us hope for the future of healthcare professionalism. Stuart tells us about a time when a 17-year-old patient was coerced into allowing him to witness her intimate examination. As Stuart narrates this event to us, he clearly articulates his own ethical reasoning processes, demonstrating his commitment to putting the patient above his own learning needs to preserve her dignity, as well as upholding the positive self-image of the doctor. In short, Stuart demonstrates his professional and ethical leadership practices: practices, we hope, this book has inspired you to emulate.

> 'I can remember being in a GU [genitourinary] clinic... they'll say, "Oh you don't mind if there's a medical student present do you?"... Of course the doctor says, "Oh you don't mind if there's a medical student here while... I examine you", and this woman, sort of part spreadeagled on the bed, and the nurse is pulling down her jeans at the same time, and it was all very complicated, and you could see her, she was about 17... and she's sort of, "Um er er er er", and I thought, "This is a really awkward situation so I'm going to take the decision out of the patient's and the doctor's hand", and I just turned around and said, "Actually, I think I'll go for a cup of coffee", and I left the room. And I thought it was best in that situation where she was clearly uncomfortable, and the doctor obviously wasn't going to take "no" for an answer, so I thought, "No, I'd take the decision myself", and I left the room and went and had a cup of coffee and then came back in afterwards.'
>
> Stuart, male, year 3, medical student, Australia

References

1 Ewick P, Silbey S. Narrating social structure: stories of resistance to legal authority. *American Journal of Sociology* 2003;108:1328–1372.
2 Foucault M. *The History of Sexuality*. New York: Pantheon Books, 1979.
3 Foucault M. *The Birth of the Clinic*. London: Tavistock, 1973.
4 Rees C, Monrouxe LV. Contesting medical hierarchies: nursing students' narratives as acts of resistance. *Medical Education* 2010;44:433–435.
5 Prinz JJ. Can moral obligations be empirically discovered? *Midwest Studies In Philosophy* 2007;31:271–291.
6 Monrouxe LV, Rees CE. 'It's just a clash of cultures': emotional talk within medical students' narratives of professionalism dilemmas. *Advances in Health Sciences Education* 2012;17:671–701.
7 Monrouxe LV, Rees CE, Endacott R, Ternan E. 'Even now it makes me angry': health care students' professionalism dilemma narratives. *Medical Education* 2014;48:502–517.
8 Monrouxe LV, Rees CE, Dennis I, Wells SE. Professionalism dilemmas, moral distress and the healthcare student: insights from two online UK-wide questionnaire studies. *British Medical Journal Open* 2015;5. e007518 doi:10.1136/bmjopen-2014-007518.
9 Monrouxe LV, Rees CE. Hero, voyer, judge: understanding medical students' moral identities through professionalism dilemma narratives. In KI Mavor, M Platow, B Buzumic (Eds) *The Self, Social Identity and Education*. Abingdon, UK: Psychology Press, 2017: pp. 297–319.
10 Victor B, Cullen J. A theory and measure of ethical climate in organization. *Research in Corporate Social Performance and Policy* 1987;9:51–71.

11 Monrouxe LV, Rees CE, Rees-Davies L, Sweeney K. "*Oh I'd better wash my hands because you're there*": effects of medical students' acts of resistance during medical workplace learning encounters. *Association for the Study of Medical Education Annual Scientific Meeting*, Edinburgh, 15th–17th July 2009.

12 Beyondblue. National Mental Health Survey of Doctors and Medical Students. http://www.beyondblue.org.au (Accessed 1 September 2016).

13 Aldao A, Nolen-Hoeksema S. Specificity of cognitive emotion regulation strategies: a transdiagnostic examination. *Behaviour Research and Therapy* 2010;48:974–983.

14 Gross JJ. Emotion regulation: affective, cognitive, and social consequences. *Psychophysiology* 2002;39:281–291.

15 Troy A, Mauss I. Resilience in the face of stress: emotion regulation as a protective factor. In S Southwick, B Litz, D Charney, M Friedman (Eds) *Resilience and Mental Health: Challenges Across the Lifespan*. Cambridge: Cambridge University Press, 2011: pp. 30–44.

16 Monrouxe LV, Bullock A, Rees CE, Mattick K, Webb L, Lall K, Lundin R. Foundation doctors, transitions and emotions: final report to the General Medical Council. http://www.gmc-uk.org/about/research/28224.asp (Accessed 2 December 2016).

17 Barr H. *Interprofessional Education – a Definition*. London: CAIPE Bulletin, 1997.

18 Centre for Advancement of Interprofessional Education (CAIPE). https://www.caipe.org/ (Accessed 2 December 2016).

19 Galinsky A, Moskowitz G. Perspective-taking: decreasing stereotype expression, stereotype accessibility, and in-group favoritism. *Journal of Personality and Social Psychology* 2000;78:708–724.

20 Bridges DR, Davidson RA, Odegard PS, Maki IV, Tomkowiak J. Interprofessional collaboration: three best practice models of interprofessional education. *Medical Education Online* 2011;16:10.3402/meo.v3416i3400.6035.

21 Campion-Smith C, Austin H, Criswick S, Dowling B, Francis G. Can sharing stories change practice? A qualitative study of an interprofessional narrative-based palliative care course. *Journal of Interprofessional Care.* 2011;25:105–111.

22 Rees CE, Monrouxe LV. Medical students learning intimate examinations without valid consent: a multicentre study. *Medical Education* 2011;45:261–272.

23 Knight LV, Rees CE. 'Enough is enough, I don't want any audience': exploring medical students' explanations of consent-related behaviours. *Advances in Health Sciences Education* 2008;13:407–426.

24 Rees CE, Knight LV, Wilkinson C. 'User involvement is a sine qua non, almost, in medical education': learning with rather than just about health and social care service users. *Advances in Health Sciences Education* 2007;12:359–390.

25 Rees CE, Knight LV, Wilkinson C. Doctors being up there and we being down here: a metaphorical analysis of talk about student/doctor-patient relationships. *Social Science & Medicine* 2007;65:725–737.

26 Maleki A, de Jong M. A Proposal for clustering the dimensions of national culture. *Cross-Cultural Research* 2014;48:107–143.

27 Dowell J, Merrylees N. Electives: isn't it time for a change? *Medical Education* 2009;43:121–126.

28 Rees-Davies LN, Knight LV, Rees CE. 'It doesn't matter if you kill the patients ha ha': medical students' explanations of behaviour of professional dilemma situations during overseas electives. Presented at: 'Quality Counts: Developing Theory and Practice in Medical Education Research', Cardiff, UK, 2008.

29 Rees CE, Monrouxe LV. 'Oh my God uh uh uh': laughter for coping in medical students' personal incident narratives of professionalism dilemmas. In C Figley, P Huggard, C Rees (Eds) *First Do No Self-Harm: Understanding and Promoting Physician Stress Resilience*. Oxford: Oxford University Press, 2013: pp. 67–87.

30 Rees CE, Monrouxe LV. 'A morning since eight of just pure grill': a multi-centre qualitative study of student abuse. *Academic Medicine* 2011;86:1374–1382.

31 Rees CE, Monrouxe LV, Ternan E, Endacott R. Workplace abuse narratives from dentistry, nursing, pharmacy and physiotherapy students: a multi-school qualitative study. *European Journal of Dental Education*, 2015;19:95–106. doi:10.1111/eje.12109.

Afterword

Healthcare Professionalism: Improving Practice through Reflections on Workplace Dilemmas

Textbooks on professionalism are sometimes rather dull. This one is anything but: I found it hard to stop reading the manuscript, even though I found it challenging, even harrowing at times. But (and this is the crucial thing) I also found it *recognizable*. The dilemmas that emerge are authentic and, in many cases, familiar to me from my long experience of working with healthcare trainees – and also from my own experience of being a patient.

As a consequence, I think the book has another unique attribute among professionalism texts. In addition to being readable, it is, I believe, *useful* in a direct practical sense. I think the healthcare trainee reading this book will be enlightened and empowered, both in terms of changing their own subsequent mental attitudes to professionalism challenges after due reflection, but also in being provided with a series of possible strategies to help them deal with the challenges at the time.

I believe that many accounts of medical and healthcare professionalism suffer from what I have called 'pious platitudes' about professionalism. When practitioners are asked to define professionalism, they may respond with what they think they *ought* to say, rather than by drawing on the challenging circumstances they have actually observed or experienced. Moreover, healthcare professionals are no more immune to the pressures of *belonging to a profession* than are other professionals such as lawyers and policemen. George Bernard Shaw's dictum that: 'All professions are conspiracies against the laity' (with, of course, medicine as the profession under discussion) may seem a little harsh. But consider Rueschemeyer's comment: 'Individually and... collectively, the professions "strike a bargain with society" in which they exchange competence and integrity against the trust of client and community, relative freedom from lay supervision and interference, protection against unqualified competition as well as substantial remuneration and higher social status.[1] Or Johnson's definition of professionalism as the process by which occupations seek to gain status and privilege in accord with their ideology,[2] and similarities begin to emerge.

Typically professions form *in-groups*, which define themselves against *out-groups*,[3] and the *out-groups* may be other health professionals or even patients. In my view, only by recognizing and coming to terms with these negative aspects of 'professionalism' can we ever hope to reduce lapses in professionalism: those behaviours – acts of commission or

Healthcare Professionalism: Improving Practice through Reflections on Workplace Dilemmas, First Edition.
Lynn V. Monrouxe and Charlotte E. Rees.
© 2017 John Wiley & Sons Ltd. Published 2017 by John Wiley & Sons Ltd.

omission – which harm patients, and which may arise either by a failure to act in the way conventionally described as professionalism, or by acting in accordance with negative social norms associated with Shaw's definition, acting perhaps through the hidden curriculum as discussed in this book.

One interesting example of this is in the book's treatment of cheating in medical exams – or rather, its lack of treatment, because it is rarely mentioned. The authors tell me that this is because cheating was less frequently narrated in their interviews compared to the key professionalism dilemmas covered in this book. This may be because it is rare, although this seems unlikely, or because, as Tonkin suggests, it is normalized:[4] it does not present trainees with a professionalism dilemma because it is regarded as a common occurrence, with perhaps a degree of complicity by medical schools and other organizations.

Another area which remains to be explored further is that of selection. It has been shown that not only negative behaviours in medical school predict the probability of later disciplinary action, but so, too, do low exam scores.[5,6] This is doubly surprising, in that disciplinary action is generally not about simple failures of knowledge, and we do not generally associate being good at exams with being a good person. I've hypothesised that the common factor may be the 'trait' of conscientiousness,[7] already known from work psychology to be the strongest single predictor of performance in the workplace generally. If this is true, and if conscientiousness in simple tasks in learners can be correlated with later failures of conscientiousness in clinical practice *and* if (note the string of conditionals) such a 'trait' can be detected before entry into healthcare professions, then selection for characteristics such as conscientiousness and resilience may be at least as important as teaching in ensuring good professional practice in later practice.

Of course, much of the power of this book comes in the main from its narrative approach – humans are story-telling animals (we grandly style ourselves *Homo sapiens*, but might better be described as *Homo fictogenesis*). But this is also a challenge. As the authors indicate, stories can align with common plotlines and narrative tropes, and can change over time and depending on who is listening and the purpose of the story. While the authors have done quantitative studies on professionalism dilemmas,[8] it is hoped that further quantitative work will confirm and extend the insights provided in this book.

Another area which will be interesting to explore subsequently will be the outcomes associated with cross-cultural medical schools, where Western medical schools open campuses in other countries with different cultural values, or conversely where medical schools are opened in one country but cater solely to foreign students.

But these comments are not intended as significant criticisms of this book. On the contrary, I think this is a uniquely valuable work, specifically because it looks unflinchingly at the realities of healthcare professionalism dilemmas. Since students and trainees will be better able to address failures of professionalism in themselves and in others as a result of studying, and reflection on, this book, I suspect that it will make a significant contribution, not only to healthcare education, but also, in the long run, to patient well-being.

School of Medicine, University of Central Lancashire   *John C. McLachlan*

References

1 Rueschemeyer D. Professional autonomy and the social control of expertise. In R Dingwall, P Lewis (Eds) *The Sociology of the Professions*. London: McMillan, 1983: pp. 35–58.

2 Johnson TJ. *Professions and Power*. London: Macmillan, 1972.

3 Burford B. Group processes in medical education: learning from social identity theory. *Medical Education* 2012;46(2):143–152.

4 Tonkin AL. 'Lifting the carpet' on cheating in medical school exams. *British Medical Journal* 2015; 351: doi: http://dx.doi.org/10.1136/bmj.h401.

5 Papadakis MA, Hodgson CS, Teherani A, Kohatsu ND. Unprofessional behavior in medical school is associated with subsequent disciplinary action by a state medical board. *Academic Medicine* 2004;79(3):244–249.

6 Papadakis MA, Teherani A, Banach MA, Knettler TR, Rattner SL, Stern DT, *et al.* Disciplinary action by medical boards and prior behavior in medical school. *New England Journal of Medicine* 2005;353(25):2673–2682.

7 McLachlan J. Measuring conscientiousness and professionalism in undergraduate medical students. *The Clinical Teacher* 2010;7(1):37–40.

8 Monrouxe LV, Rees CE, Dennis A, Wells S. Professionalism dilemmas, moral distress and the healthcare student: insights from two online UK-wide questionnaire studies. *BMJ Open* 2015;5:e007518. doi:10.1136/bmjopen-2014-007518.

Index

Healthcare Professionalism: Improving Practice through Reflections on Workplace Dilemmas, First Edition.
Lynn V. Monrouxe and Charlotte E. Rees.
© 2017 John Wiley & Sons Ltd. Published 2017 by John Wiley & Sons Ltd.

Printed and bound by CPI Group (UK) Ltd, Croydon, CR0 4YY

27/10/2024

14580197-0002

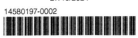